Praise for *Diagnosis and Tr*
Chronic Fatigue Syndrome and My

"Dr. Sarah Myhill does it again, shedding light on chronic illness and patterns of fatigue and extreme brain fog. I was first introduced to the idea that mitochondrial damage was the basis of all disease in the early '90s while battling my own health issues, and later, again, in naturopathic medical school in the mid '90s. One of my professors taught me that the first sign of mitochondrial damage was fatigue. In a world where we are chronically overfed and undernourished and riddled with 'holes in our bucket,' as Dr. Myhill points out, our mitochondria are in constant battle against dietary indiscretions, lifestyle imbalance, and toxicants, making it difficult to run our internal motors effectively and efficiently. Dr. Myhill explains how we got here and how we can turn it around, offering hope to thousands."

—Dr. Nasha Winters, coauthor of *The Metabolic Approach to Cancer*

"Conventional medicine has failed to bring relief to the many thousands of people suffering from Chronic Fatigue Syndrome or Myalgic Encephalitis, in part because these conditions have roots in mitochondrial damage that are not well understood. Explaining the role of diet, gut health, inflammation, and much more, Dr. Sarah Myhill offers detailed recommendations so that readers can take control of their own recovery."

—Tom Cowan, MD, author of *Human Heart, Cosmic Heart*

"This is a *must* read for anyone with Chronic Fatigue Syndrome or Myalgic Encephalitis! It's not only an excellent resource on these two common health conditions but also a clear example of the failings of the conventional medical establishment and the profit-over-patient paradigm that Big Pharma operates on.

"Right from the beginning of the book, it becomes immediately clear that conventional medicine is far too ill-equipped or ill-trained to deal with such complex disorders. With many possible causes that can lead to wide-ranging symptoms, CFS/ME is a prime example of the need for personalized healthcare and treating the whole *person*, not just symptoms. However, with the limitations intrinsic to conventional 'cookie-cutter' healthcare, it's almost always symptoms management.

"In the age of easy access to information, and with this amazing book being so readily accessible, democratizing their own healthcare is now a reality for CFS/ME patients. With clear guidelines on what tests are useful and why, and various treatment options that can be adjusted for each individual situation, this book may just be the resource that rejuvenates tired bodies around the world."

—Dr. Lee Know, author of *Mitochondria and the Future of Medicine*

"Dr. Myhill has written an extraordinary book. She is the number one authority on CFS in the UK. Whereas many doctors dismiss the condition, she explains what it is, what has gone wrong in the body, using appropriate tests that are not done by mainstream medicine, and tells people what they can do about it. Whereas mainstream medicine only uses drugs to deal with a particular symptom, Dr. Myhill explains the reasons 'Why'. In my opinion, you will never cure anything unless you understand and deal with the why."

—Dr. P. J. Kingsley, MB BS, MRCS, LRCP, FAAEM, DA, DObst, RCOG

"If the first edition of this book became a key reference that was readable and upbeat, full of information explaining complex issues of cell biology together with practical tips, three years later, the second edition supersedes it with a wealth of added helpful points in the light of more recent developments in the world of 'functional' and environmental medicine. Many important tests are explained in detail together with their role in a person's recovery plan. The folly of the mainstream approach to ME is exposed and is truly shocking. The style is flowing; the evidence is poignant and the references are meticulously made, yet easy to follow. Dr. Myhill has opened the minds of thousands of ME sufferers, and their carers, as to how to seize control of their health in an era when evidence is mounting that the causes of many chronic conditions can be traced to our life-styles and environment."

—Dr. Apelles Econs, MRCS, LRCP, Allergist

"Brilliant! This book offers the most complete, logical, practical and optimistic guide for people trying to recover from CFS that I am aware of. If every doctor could also take its contents on board, the management of CFS would be revolutionised."

—Dr. Charles Forsyth, MB BS, FFHom

"Over the years, working as a General Practitioner, I have recommended Dr. Myhill's work to hundreds of patients. Her approach combines an in-depth understanding of human physiology with years of practical experience, and the use of cutting-edge laboratory testing, to diagnose and treat the root causes of complex chronic diseases. Written with humour and compassion, Dr. Myhill has put together a simple step-by-step guide for patients, to take back control of their own health and start their journey to recovery. I am delighted that I can now recommend this book to every patient."

—Dr. Jens Rohrbeck, MD, MPhil, GP, Functional Medicine Physician

"This book is a 'must have' for everyone suffering from CFS (and their doctors). It explains all the different aspects of this complex condition, and details ways that each patient can contribute to their own recovery. Dr. Myhill has tirelessly dedicated much of her career to improving the quality of life of CFS patients for whom conventional approaches (antidepressants, cognitive behavioural therapy and graded exercise) have not been enough. Her commitment, genius and sense of humour come across wonderfully in these pages, encouraging and supporting those with this terrible condition not to give up."

—Dr. Nicola Hembry, BSc, MB BS, MSB, PGDip

"The brilliant work of John McLaren-Howard, Sarah Myhill and Norman Booth reveals that CFS / ME is due to mitochondrial dysfunction. This discovery revolutionizes the world's understanding of CFS and how to investigate and treat the biochemical abnormalities. Dr. Myhill's book has never been more needed. In 2016 NHS data found that 26 per cent of young women aged 16 to 24 years had mental health problems and 9.1 per cent of young men. Most first use of antidepressants is in adolescent girls aged 15 to 19 years using non-oral progestin-only contraception. Progestins increase MAO activity upsetting brain and blood vessel functions. Four women have mitochondrial function tests for every one man. The epidemic of CFS, like breast cancer, has increased since contraceptive hormone and HRT use became widespread. Mitochondrial dysfunction has many causes, including toxic DNA adducts, but avoiding progestin and oestrogen use is vitally important for recovery from CFS."

—Dr. Ellen Grant, MB ChB, DObst, RCOG

"Dr. Myhill breaks new ground in her approach to chronic fatigue syndrome and demonstrates clearly, with compelling scientific evidence, that this condition is not psychological but has treatable physical causes. She gives detailed guidance on practical ecological measures that need to be followed to effect recovery. This is a book which should cause many doctors and health professionals to radically revise their understanding of CFS and gives sufferers real encouragement and hope for their future health."

—Dr. John Meldrum, MB ChB, MRCGP, DA, DCH, DObst, RCOG, HTD

"What really struck me about this book is the degree to which it allows people with CFS to be in charge of their own recovery, and to have the confidence, through the authority of the author, to know what to ask for from health professionals. It explains with real clarity the complex biochemical processes underlying chronic disease and CFS, and the link with allergies, diet, micro-organisms and aspects of the Western lifestyle. There is a detailed and clear discussion of the tests available, how to interpret them, and what to do to get better. All this without ignoring the importance of good lifestyle habits, psychological health and the right kind of exercise. A fantastic book for all health professionals too."

—Dr. Dee Marshall, MB BS, MFHom, WellnessMedical, London, UK

"Dr. Myhill's wonderful book presents the clearest and most helpful information I have ever read on what chronic fatigue syndrome actually is and what the many possible causes of it are. This is the only book that I've found that presents a comprehensive approach for assessing the underlying causes of CFS and treating them that may be tailored for the individual patient. Understanding how mitochondrial failure can arise, why mitochondrial function problems are often a major factor in CFS and the approaches for restoring good mitochondrial function should form part of all medical training. Dr. Myhill's book should be a standard text in all medical schools as well as being essential reading for all CFS patients and their doctors. It is easy to read, laden with information and shows practical ways of actually assessing and treating CFS. Loved it!"

—Paul Robinson, BSc (Hons),
author of *Recovering with T3 and The Ct3m Handbook*

"Drawing on decades of clinical experience, and unparalleled success in restoring health, hope and energy to thousands of CFS patients, Dr. Myhill brings solid scientific evidence together with biological common sense to explain how to recover from this ghastly and increasingly common illness. She describes the underlying cellular mechanisms in a way that everyone can understand, demonstrating simply the physiological basis of low energy production in CFS. This is an aspect that is largely ignored by most current approaches to CFS, but Dr. Myhill shows clearly that CFS is in your mitochondria, not in your mind! This book is an invaluable step-by-step guide to recovery, for patient and physician alike. I would not be without a copy in my clinic!"

—Dr. Jenny Goodman, MA, MB ChB

Diagnosis and Treatment of
Chronic Fatigue Syndrome and Myalgic Encephalitis

Diagnosis and Treatment of Chronic Fatigue Syndrome and Myalgic Encephalitis

It's Mitochondria, Not Hypochondria

DR. SARAH MYHILL, MB, BS

Edited by, and with a chapter by,
CRAIG ROBINSON

Chelsea Green Publishing
White River Junction, Vermont

Original edition published in 2017 by Hammersmith Books, London, United Kingdom, under exclusive license for all formats, languages and territories.

This edition published by Chelsea Green Publishing, 2018. This edition is authorized for sale only in North America.

Printed in Canada.
First printing February, 2018.
10 9 8 7 6 5 4 3 2   19 20 21 22

Our Commitment to Green Publishing

Chelsea Green sees publishing as a tool for cultural change and ecological stewardship. We strive to align our book manufacturing practices with our editorial mission and to reduce the impact of our business enterprise in the environment. We print our books and catalogs on chlorine-free recycled paper, using vegetable-based inks whenever possible. This book may cost slightly more because it was printed on paper that contains recycled fiber, and we hope you'll agree that it's worth it. *Diagnosis and Treatment Chronic Fatigue Syndrome and Myalgic Encephalitis* was printed on paper supplied by Marquis is made of recycled materials and other controlles sources.

Library of Congress Cataloging-in-Publication Data
Names: Myhill, Sarah, author.
Title: Diagnosis and treatment of chronic fatigue syndrome and myalgic encephalitis : it's mitochondria, not hypochondria / Dr. Sarah Myhill, MB, BS ; edited by, and with a chapter by, Craig Robinson.
Other titles: Diagnosing and treating chronic fatigue syndrome
Description: Second edition. | White River Junction, Vermont : Chelsea Green Publishing, 2018. | Revised edition of: Diagnosing and treating chronic fatigue syndrome : it's mitochondria, not hypochondria. London : Hammersmith Health Books, 2014. | Includes bibliographical references and index.
Identifiers: LCCN 2017050651 | ISBN 9781603587877 (pbk.) | ISBN 9781603587884 (ebook)
Subjects: LCSH: Chronic fatigue syndrome--Diagnosis--Popular works. | Chronic fatigue syndrome--Treatment--Popular works. | BISAC: HEALTH & FITNESS / Diseases / Chronic Fatigue Syndrome. | MEDICAL / Diseases. | MEDICAL / Holistic Medicine. | MEDICAL / Nutrition. | MEDICAL / Healing.
Classification: LCC RB150.F37 M98 2018 | DDC 616/.0478--dc23
LC record available at https://lccn.loc.gov/2017050651

Chelsea Green Publishing
85 North Main Street, Suite 120
White River Junction, VT 05001
(802) 295-6300
www.chelseagreen.com

This book is dedicated to:

Dr John McLaren-Howard of Acumen Laboratory

His brilliance lies in taking cutting-edge, biochemical research techniques and applying them to clinical conditions. Without his logical thinking and intellectual generosity the underlying pathophysiological mechanisms that result in CFS/ME could not have been elucidated.

Dr Norman Booth of Mansfield College Oxford

Who applied his analytical skills and academic prowess to prove that the Acumen tests are effective in identifying the biochemical lesions that underpin CFS/ME and that the treatments applied result in clinical benefit.

And also to my long-suffering patients. They have all known the right questions to ask. It has taken me far too long to find out some of the answers and in the interim patients have suffered. Thank you all for your faith, perseverance and tolerance during our steep, and indeed ongoing, learning curve.

DR SARAH MYHILL

Once again it has been an absolute pleasure and privilege to work with Sarah. Whilst it is not conventional for an editor to dedicate his editing, this book was not borne from conventional thinking. So, with that in mind, I dedicate this book to my two children, Gina and Conor. They have never known me without CFS/ME; I hope that one day they will. In any case, one thing is for sure; I have learnt more from them than they have from me. They are my pride and joy and I have been inspired by them more than they will ever know.

CRAIG ROBINSON, Editor

Gina Robinson

'Always be a little kinder than necessary'
J M BARRIE (9 May 1860 – 19 June 1937)

Conor Robinson

'At the end of the game, the king and the pawn
are placed in the same box'
OLD ITALIAN PROVERB

CONTENTS

PART III

Practical

The foundation stones of recovery – what everyone must do

PART IV

Appendices

ACKNOWLEDGEMENT

Quite simply, without Craig as editor, this book would not have happened. Like all journeys, it is easy to forget, or take for granted, the early stages. It is tempting to concentrate on the recent, fashionable and cutting edge. Craig has constantly pulled me back to reality and reminded me of our roots. Where I gloss over, he explores in detail. When I rush to the recent, he pulls me back to what is possible. When I am light on detail, he insists. This means this manual of treatment fully empowers the CFS/ME sufferer to cure themselves with practical interventions that are within the grasp of all.

HOW TO USE THIS BOOK

The idea of this book is to supply all of the information, together with access to all the relevant tests (I'm working on this), to allow you to fashion your own recovery.

The first section of the book is the theory. The problem is that many people with CFS have foggy brains and will not be able to read, let alone absorb, this. In this event, skip straight to Part III (page 175) – the practical steps you must take in order to start to recover. Take a leap of faith and just do it! As your energy improves and your brain fog clears, then you can go back to the beginning and learn how you started to recover.

Through understanding the symptoms and mechanisms of those symptoms, you will be able to further fine-tune your recovery. Indeed, the interventions I recommend are also a blueprint for good health for life. You may have lost years of your life through this wretched, miserable illness, but stick to your guns, never give up fighting and those years will be stuck on to the end of your life.

PART I

Introduction

CHAPTER 1

Why is CFS/ME the worst treated condition in Western medicine?

Because of the Name, the Blame and the Shame

The Name – when the name masquerades as a diagnosis

The practice of medicine used to be an honourable occupation undertaken by doctors who listened to patients, catalogued their symptoms and tried to make sense of why they were suffering such. Having established the cause, there were clear implications for treatment. This is called diagnosis – with the cause established, the treatment followed naturally and logically.

In the treatment of chronic conditions, doctors no longer diagnose. They may be good at recognising and giving names to clinical pictures, but this now masquerades as a diagnosis. Patients feel comforted and reassured that their illness has been recognised because it has been named. What I shall call 'CFS/ME' throughout this book (see page 18) has been called 'the disease of a thousand names'. Its clinical picture is variously recognised under the names of yuppie 'flu, myalgic encephalitis, post-viral syndrome, Royal Free syndrome, systemic exertion intolerance disease (SEID), chronic fatigue immune dysfunction syndrome (CFIDS) and many others, some of which include:

Poliomyelitis names:
atypical poliomyelitis
abortive poliomyelitis
encephalitis stimulating poliomyelitis
encephalitis resembling poliomyelitis
post-polio syndrome
posterior poliomyelitis
sensory poliomyelitis

Location-based names:
Akureyi disease
Coventry disease
English disease
Iceland disease
Lake Tahoe mystery disease
Lyndonville chronic mononucleosis
Otago mystery disease
Tapanui 'flu

Neuromyasthenia-related names:
acute infective encephalomyelitis
benign encephalomyelitis
benign myalgic encephalomyelitis
benign subacute encephalomyelitis
epidemic diencephalomyelitis
epidemic encephalomyelopathy
epidemic myalgic encephalomyelitis
lymphoreticular encephalomyelopathy

Myalgia-type names:
Damadian's ache
epidemic malaise
epidemic myositis
fibromyalgia syndrome
fibromyositis
fibrositis
lymphocytic meningo encephalitis with myalgia and rash
muscular rheumatism
myofascial syndrome
persistent myalgia following sore throat
syndrome polyalgique idiopathique diffus (SPID)

Personal names:
Beard's disease
Da Costa's syndrome

Symptom-based names:
effort syndrome
English sweats
la spasmophilie
lazy man disease
Raggedy Ann syndrome
tetanie chronique idiopathique

Combined virus/symptom names:
persistent viral fatigue syndrome
post-viral fatigue syndrome (PVFS)

Immune-based names:
allergic fatigue syndrome
antibody negative lupus
antibody negative Lyme disease
chronic activated immune dysfunction syndrome (CAIDS)
chronic immune activation syndrome (CIAS)
chronic immune dysfunction syndrome (CIDS)
ecological disease
low natural killer cell syndrome
multiple chemical sensitivity syndrome
naxalone-reversible monocyte dysfunction syndrome (NRMDS)

Epstein-Barr virus-based names:
chronic active Epstein-Barr virus syndrome (CEBV)
chronic Epstein-Barr virus infection (CAEBV)
chronic infectious mononucleosis
chronic mononucleosis
chronic mononucleosis-like syndrome
familial chronic mononucleosis

Hypothalamic names:
epidemic vegetative neuritis
habitual chronic hyperventilation syndrome
neurocirculatory asthenia
vasomotor instability
vasomotor neurosis
vasoregulatory asthenia

The 'atypical' names:
atypical migraine
atypical multiple sclerosis

Miscellaneous names:
epidemic vasculitis syndrome
soldier's heart

Quite naturally and understandably, patients assume, once their illness has been named, that appropriate treatment, addressing the causes, will follow. But this is where it all starts to go horribly wrong.

Conventional medicine offers a package of treatment that bears no resemblance to causation. In fact, the treatments make things much worse, be they antidepressants or graded exercise therapy. Many patients are told that they are depressed, but so often the CFS intolerance of medication means that the drugs prescribed make them much worse. Meanwhile, it is an intellectual disgrace that graded exercise therapy is offered in a condition which, by definition, is exacerbated by exercise.

We have arrived at this intellectually risible situation because Western medicine is now run for profit and driven by Big Pharma. Big Pharma established its reputation early with the discovery of antibiotics. These miracle drugs have saved millions of lives, have been and continue to be a massive medical asset. The problem with antibiotics is that, whilst they save lives, they do not make big money for Big Pharma because people are cured.

Pharmaceutical companies quickly worked out that the way to register big profits is to get patients and doctors dependent on symptom-suppressing drugs which they have to take for life. Having been dazzled by the antibiotic miracle, doctors are now wooed by Big Pharma so that they no longer act as free-thinking, intelligent, responsive and responsible individuals. They have been sucked into a mechanistic tick-box set of algorithms which masquerade under the names of diagnosis and treatment.

Nowhere is this worse than in the treatment of CFS/ME where fatigue is called 'depression' – this really makes CFS/ME sufferers angry. 'No,' they cry, 'not depressed, but seriously frustrated because I do not have the energy to get on with life.' In the eyes of the doctor, the tears of frustration further confirm the diagnosis of depression. The essential doctor–patient trust is then lost.

To counterbalance this state of affairs, this book has been organised as follows. It starts with the symptoms, describes the mechanisms that underpin the causes of those symptoms, and finally explains the 'tools of the trade' that we need to effect a cure. Diagnosis should be about identifying the underlying causes of symptoms and tackling those – I go into this in much more detail in my book *Sustainable Medicine*. This Sherlock Holmes-detective approach results in a package of treatments which is unique and tailored to individual patients and their clinical setting.

The Blame – when compensation should be due

There are many triggers for CFS/ME and a common cause is acute infection. Almost invariably there will have been a package of stress (and life is full of such), which has led up to the trigger. However, we now recognise increasingly that many people are switched into CFS/ME by other factors about which the patient has no knowledge, no say and no control. In my 35 years of seeing, I estimate, over 6,000 patients with CFS/ME, I have seen many other triggers, viz:

Sheep dip 'flu (poisoning by organophosphate pesticides)
Aero-toxic syndrome (poisoning by engine fumes, including organophosphates)
Dental amalgam fillings (mercury leaks out of fillings from the moment they are inserted)
9/11 syndrome (poisoning by burnt plastics and fire retardant chemicals)
Gulf War syndrome (multiple triggers including vaccination, organophosphates, chemical warfare and depleted uranium)
Sick building syndrome (poisoning by volatile organic compounds used in carpets, paints, glues and solvents)
Vaccination (this is pro-inflammatory with the potential to switch on the immune system – vaccinations are immuno-toxic)
Silicone poisoning from breast and other implants (silicone migrates out of implants from the day they are inserted; it migrates through the body and switches on inflammation – it is immuno-toxic)
Carbon monoxide poisoning
Prescription drugs (the Pill, HRT and fertility drugs are a major risk factor and trigger for CFS. Statins are a particular hate of mine)
Outdoor air pollution (from pesticide drift, polluting industry)
Poisoning by formaldehyde (farmers in chicken-rearing sheds)
'Recreational' drugs (alcohol, cannabis, amphetamines, etc)

What is common to many of the above conditions is that there have been huge patient-driven campaigns to recognise these syndromes so that appropriate litigation and compensation can follow. I have often been involved. The outcome is predictable – the Establishment ignores, denies and buries the problem to ensure a cheap conclusion. Where compensation has resulted in individual cases, a gagging clause has been applied so that no others can follow that route.

To achieve the above, successive governments have colluded with doctors to bury the proper diagnosis of CFS/ME and continue to run with clinical pictures that pander to the different Establishment pressure groups. Millions of pounds of government and industry money have been spent to establish CFS/ME as a psychiatric disorder, culminating in what is known as the PACE trial,[1] which was published in *The Lancet* in 2011 and cost in the region of £5million.[2] Those wishing to investigate the true nature of CFS/ME can only dream of receiving such sums of money; in fact, these researchers have been left out in the cold.

The PACE study

Much has been written about the PACE study and an almighty battle has been going on to get its authors, through the relevant institutions, to be open about their work and release their original data. Its authors repeatedly refused to let their trial data be open to such scrutiny. Numerous Freedom of Information Act requests were made to Queen Mary University of London (QMUL) and also to King's College London (KCL) for such data to be released. In October 2015, the Information Commissioner's Office (ICO) ruled that such disclosure should be made;[3] this was appealed by QMUL but on 11 August 2016 (promulgated 12 August) the First-Tier Tribunal (General Regulatory Chamber) decided 'by a majority, to uphold the decision notice dated 27 October 2015, and dismiss the appeal.[4] (While waiting for this decision, even the online publisher PLoS ONE [which published a PACE-related open-access paper online[5]] had been approached because of its policy of open access to data and yet there had been more refusals). In response to the Tribunal's decision, the authors have at last released their detailed findings (of which more below) so we can start to answer the question 'Why have these institutions (QMUL and KCL) been so determined not to release the data?'

But even before the release of the data we did know some things about PACE from the concerns that had been raised in an open letter to the editor of *The Lancet*, Dr Richard Horton, by the eminent scientists Ronald W Davis (Professor of Biochemistry and Genetics, Stanford University), Jonathan C W Edwards (Emeritus Professor of Medicine, University College London), Leonard A Jason (Professor of Psychology, DePaul University), Bruce Levin

(Professor of Biostatistics, Columbia University), Vincent R Racaniello (Professor of Microbiology and Immunology) and Albert L Reingold (Professor of Epidemiology, University of California, Berkeley). They were particularly concerned about the reporting of the PACE study because, as they said, it had such 'widespread international influence' on 'government policy, public health practice, clinical care, and decisions about disability insurance and other social benefits' as well as 'public attitudes'. The need for the study to be indisputably scientifically sound was therefore paramount, yet it suffered from serious flaws in method that raised issues of 'validity, reliability and integrity of the findings'. Davis et al pointed out in their open letter that because the study was 'unblinded' – the researchers and patients knew what treatments each patient in the study was receiving and therefore could be influenced by expectations and consequently subject to bias – 'strict vigilance' was needed, yet on the contrary, the following failings were clear but had never been addressed or explained by the study's authors:

The Lancet paper included an analysis in which the outcome thresholds for being 'within the normal range' on the two primary measures of fatigue and physical function demonstrated worse health than the criteria for entry, which already indicated serious disability. In fact, 13 per cent of the study participants were already 'within the normal range' on one or both outcome measures at baseline, but the investigators did not disclose this salient fact in *The Lancet* paper. In an accompanying *Lancet* commentary, colleagues of the PACE team defined participants who met these expansive 'normal ranges' as having achieved a 'strict criterion for recovery'. The PACE authors reviewed this commentary before publication.

During the trial, the authors published a newsletter for participants that included positive testimonials from earlier participants about the benefits of the 'therapy' and 'treatment'. The same newsletter included an article that cited the two rehabilitative interventions pioneered by the researchers and being tested in the PACE trial as having been recommended by a UK clinical guidelines committee 'based on the best available evidence'. The newsletter did not mention that a key PACE investigator also served on the clinical guidelines committee. At the time of the newsletter, two hundred or more participants – about a third of the total sample – were still undergoing assessments.

Mid-trial, the PACE investigators changed their protocol methods of assessing their primary outcome measures of fatigue and physical function. This is of particular concern in an unblinded trial like PACE, in which outcome trends are often apparent long before outcome data are seen. The investigators provided no sensitivity analyses to assess the impact of the changes and have refused requests to provide the results per the methods outlined in their protocol.

The PACE investigators based their claims of treatment success solely on their subjective outcomes. In *The Lancet* paper, the results of a six-minute walking test – described in the protocol as 'an objective measure of physical capacity' – did not support such claims, notwithstanding the minimal gains in one arm. In subsequent comments in another journal, the investigators dismissed the walking-test results as irrelevant, non-objective and fraught with limitations. All the other objective measures in PACE, presented in other journals, also failed. The results of one objective measure, the fitness step-test, were provided in a 2015 paper in *The Lancet Psychiatry*, but only in the form of a tiny graph. A request for the step-test data used to create the graph was rejected as 'vexatious'.

The investigators violated their promise in the PACE protocol to adhere to the Declaration of Helsinki, which mandates that prospective participants be 'adequately informed' about researchers' 'possible conflicts of interest'. The main investigators have had financial and consulting relationships with disability insurance companies, advising them that rehabilitative therapies like those tested in PACE could help CFS/ME claimants get off benefits and back to work. They disclosed these insurance industry links in *The Lancet* but did not inform trial participants, contrary to their protocol commitment. This serious ethical breach raises concerns about whether the consent obtained from the 641 trial participants is legitimate.

Such flaws have no place in published research.

The authors of the letter urged *The Lancet* 'to seek an independent re-analysis of the individual-level PACE trial data, with appropriate sensitivity analyses, from highly respected reviewers with extensive expertise in statistics and study design. The reviewers, they said, should be from outside the UK and outside the domains of psychiatry and psychological medicine. They should also be completely independent of, and have no conflicts of interests involving, the PACE investigators and the funders of the trial.' Considering the flaws identified, this would seem the only way to lay the matter to rest but would of course require access to the data sets that were being so closely guarded.

For those readers who are interested, Dr Tuller (currently Academic Coordinator of the concurrent Master's degree programme in Public Health and Journalism at the University of California, Berkeley) has written about further problems with PACE in exquisite detail in his *Trial by Error* blogs[6] which can be found at www.virology.ws/2015/10/21/trial-by-error-i and follow on sequentially. Yet more criticisms of PACE by Professor Malcolm Hooper and the Countess of Mar can be found at www.meactionuk.org.uk/Update-on-the-PACE-Trial-110712.htm and specifically in the paper *Magical Medicine: how to make a disease disappear*.[7]

Finally, Rebecca Goldin had the criticism below to offer.[8] She is Professor of Mathematical Sciences at George Mason University, Virginia, USA, and Director of STATS.org. She received her undergraduate degree from Harvard University and her PhD from the Massachusetts Institute of Technology. She taught at the University of Maryland as a National Science Foundation post-doctoral fellow before joining George Mason in 2001. Her academic research is in symplectic geometry, group actions and related combinatorics. In 2007, she received the Ruth I Michler Memorial Prize, presented by the Association for Women in Mathematics. It is fair to say she knows about statistics! This is what she says about PACE:

> *The PACE design changed so significantly as to leave many wondering whether there is value in the study itself. How can we judge whether the improvements seen in primary and secondary outcomes associated with CBT and GET are "real" if "recovery" does not always require clinically meaningful improvement, and if the meaning of "normal" is distorted to include averages for people in their 80s? How can we judge whether improvements are real when they are only self-assessed? APT is described as "based on the theory that one must stay within the limits of a finite amount of 'energy'," while CBT includes, "collaborative challenging of unhelpful beliefs about symptoms and activity". Will these different philosophies result in different patient self-rated overall well-being and relative improvement over the year in the study?*
>
> - *How can we generalize to the patients with ME/CFS who are too sick to travel to the hospital, if all PACE participants are able to attend hospital visits?*
> - *How do we contextualize major changes in protocol impacting results, and the unwillingness of the PACE authors to provide outcomes based on the initial planned data analysis? Do these changes impact patients in particular branches more than in others, biasing the study's outcomes?*
> - *It seems that the best we can glean from PACE is that study design is essential to good science, and the flaws in this design were enough to doom its results from the start.*[8]

With the release of the PACE data in August it has been possible for an independent group of scientists and mathematicians to re-work the analysis and their preliminary conclusions were published on 21 September 2016 in *Virology Blog* with this summary:

> *This re-analysis demonstrates that the previously reported recovery rates were inflated by an average of four-fold. Furthermore, in contrast with the published paper by the trial investigators, the recovery rates in the cognitive behavioural therapy and graded exercise therapy groups are not significantly higher than with specialist medical care alone.*[9]

With this finding, along with my extensive clinical experience, it seems not only were significant amounts of public money wasted but also many thousands of CFS/ME sufferers have been severely harmed by the application of highly inappropriate treatment regimes. The evidence of harm of CBT and GET to CFS sufferers has long been documented and I simply reference one paper, collated by Tom Kindlon.[10]

The words of the PACE study have sent a clear and simple message to doctors and politicians that these patients are idle hypochondriacs. The persecution of CFS patients is complete: they receive treatments (CBT and GET) which make them worse, they are often denied their justified State Benefits because it is somehow 'their fault' that they remain ill and the final insult is that real research and treatment of their complex and extremely debilitating illness are denied to them.

We should all do well to remember just how ill CFS patients are. As Dr Nancy Klimas, AIDS and CFS researcher and clinician, University of Miami, said:

> *I split my clinical time between the two illnesses, and I can tell you if I had to choose between the two illnesses (in 2009) I would rather have H.I.V. But C.F.S., which impacts a million people in the United States alone, has had a small fraction of the research dollars directed towards it.*[11]

The Shame – when good doctors are hounded out

Doctors who practise outside the narrow confines of conventional medicine soon feel the chill wind of Establishment opprobrium. I spent 20 years in unblemished NHS practice. Within a few months of full-time private work specialising in the treatment of CFS/ME I received the first of many broadsides from the Establishment. These continued for the next 11 years. A Freedom of

Information Act search conducted by me in December 2015 of the General Medical Council (GMC) has revealed that I am the most investigated doctor since the GMC started keeping records in 2006. Since 2001 I have been subject to 30 separate investigations by it involving seven separate GMC Court Hearings. All these 30 complaints had come either from other doctors or from the GMC itself – not a single patient had complained about my practice (bless them all). No patient had been harmed, indeed no patient had been put at risk. The accusations ranged from recommending nutritional supplements and vitamin B12 injections to the use of thyroid hormones in patients with chronic fatigue syndrome and the development of mitochondrial function tests. All investigations were eventually dropped, the most recent five in January 2015, with no case to answer. The only accusation of which I was really proud was the accusation that I had brought the reputation of the medical profession into disrepute!

I made very extensive Data Protection Act searches of my GMC records and still the most astonishing comment I have ever seen was this:

> *My main concerns with all the Myhill files are that all of the patients appear to be improving and none of them are likely to give WS [witness statements] or have complained about their treatment.*
>
> INTERNAL GMC MEMO dated 10 February 2006

It appears to be of 'concern' to the GMC that my patients are 'improving'!

Sadly, I am not alone in this harassment. Many other doctors have been subject to General Medical Council investigations for the very same reasons I was – their use of treatments outside of conventional guidelines. They too were trying to diagnose properly, establish underlying mechanisms and treat patients with natural therapies. Those doctors included:

- Dr Len McEwen (who developed Enzyme Potentiated Desensitisation)
- Dr Gordon Skinner (who pioneered thyroid treatments for CFS/ME patients)
- Dr Brian McDonagh (ditto)
- Dr Barry Durrant Peatfield (who recognised and developed adrenal support therapies for CFS/ME)
- Dr Andy Wright (one of the first doctors to treat patients for Lyme disease)
- Dr Peter Mansfield (who flagged up the many disease problems caused by vaccination)

Dr Jane Donogan (ditto)
Dr Andrew Wakefield (ditto)
Dr Patrick Kingsley (who successfully treated thousands of patients with multiple sclerosis using natural remedies)
Dr Jean Munro (who used chelation therapy to reduce heavy metal burdens)
Dr Nigel Speight (who worked with children with CFS/MS)
Dr Peter Behan (for his outspokenness)
. . . and many others.

I went into private medicine simply because I did not have the intellectual freedom to be an effective doctor within the NHS. This was a bad move financially – doctors within the NHS are paid regardless of success or ability. So long as they practise tick-box medicine they will be assured a regular salary, sick pay, holiday pay and early retirement. Many of my contemporaries are seeking early retirement with comfortable wealth and are happy to say good-bye to the intellectual voids and constraints of modern medical practice. No wonder NHS morale is at an all-time low.

I have spent 35 years trying to re-educate the medical profession. I have failed miserably. I now realise that in asking them to diagnose and treat CFS/ME correctly I am asking them to rethink the whole of their medical practice. This is not just an intellectual revolution for these doctors but also potentially a complete financial disaster for them personally. This must instead be a grass-roots revolution. The idea of this book is to wrest power away from the professional doctors and teach the 'amateur' patients to do it themselves. This book provides them with the Rules of the Game and the Tools of the Trade to allow each and all to take control of their disease and walk their own path to recovery.

Remember, the Titanic was built by professionals but amateurs built the Ark. Yes – I know it's a myth but it leads to a good joke:

The animals came in two by two including the zebras. Zebra one was looking happy, indeed smug, while zebra two was surly and fed up.

'What on earth is wrong with you?' asked Noah. 'You are one of the lucky ones.'

Zebra two replied, 'It's not fair . . . I have both the tapeworms.'

CHAPTER 1 SUMMARY

Why is CFS/ME the worst treated condition in Western medicine?

- CFS/ME is the worst treated illness in the Western World because of:
    - **The Name:** Doctors have confused both themselves and patients with a multitude of names for CFS/ME – the 'disease of a thousand names'.
    - **The Blame:** The real physical causes of CFS/ME have been buried and psychiatrists have published flawed studies purporting to show the efficacy of such dangerous treatments as CBT and GET, of which the PACE study has been the most destructive and is also the most disputed because of flaws in the scientific methodology that have now been clearly demonstrated.
    - **The Shame:** Those doctors who have stood up against these spurious, constructed arguments and looked for alternative causes and treatments have faced persecution from the Medical Establishment.
- Efforts to educate doctors in general about the true physical nature of CFS/ME have largely failed. (Of course, there are honourable exceptions.)
- So now it is time for patients to take control of their illness and walk their own path to health.

CHAPTER 2

The roadmap to recovery

Health is like wealth –
you don't know you've got it until you've lost it.

Popular saying

Energy

Energy is a vital part of life but is medically neglected. The commonest complaint in general medical practice is fatigue – it even has its own acronym, 'TATT' (tired all the time) – but it is the worst treated symptom in modern Western medicine as Chapter 1 explains.

We would all like to have more energy. Energy is like money – it is great fun spending it, but very hard work earning it. Think of energy as money in the bank, but our energy bank is one which we cannot go overdrawn on – we cannot borrow energy. If our bank runs out of energy, then we die. Energy is the difference between life and death. This is why fatigue is such an important symptom – it protects us from death. Henry Worsley, who tried to walk across Antarctica unsupported, died in January 2016 of 'complete organ failure'. He had poured all his energy into physical exertion and had nothing left to run his body on. He simply ran out of energy. Similarly, Napoleon was only interested in soldiers who ran themselves into the ground:

The first virtue in a soldier is endurance of fatigue;
courage is only the second virtue.

Napoleon Bonaparte (15 August 1769 – 5 May 1821)

This book is all about increasing the energy we need to live life to its full. Whilst its main application is for people with debilitating fatigue, the same principles apply also to athletes for peak performance and to healthy people who simply wish to live to their full potential. We all live on the same energy spectrum – athletes are at the top and some of my patients with CFS/ME are near the lower end. However, we can all move up that spectrum by putting in place the interventions in this book. It is a case of definition – one of my patient's definition of CFS was that he could only run his marathons in 2 hours 30 minutes. By dint of eating a ketogenic diet, taking supplements to support mitochondria and correcting his thyroid function, he subsequently won the Potteries marathon in a personal best time. I may not get most of my CFS/ME patients back to medal-winning performance but the majority can substantially improve their lot.

The same principles apply to all those who wish to live life to the full – fatigue is an inevitable part of the ageing process. Indeed, many of my CFS/ME patients tell me that they have the energy and abilities of a 90-year-old. Anyone, and that includes me, who wishes to live a long and energetic life can maximise their potential to achieve such by attention to the details in this book.

To achieve this level of energy is not an easy or a comfortable path to follow. It requires determination and discipline. To succeed in this, people need to be empowered by knowledge and understanding. As I say to my patients, 'I can point you in the right direction and shout words of encouragement, but you have to walk the path to recovery yourself.'

What follows is based on my experience of treating CFS/ME for over 35 years of both NHS practice and private practice since I qualified in medicine in 1981. Proper help will not come from the medical profession in its current state simply because it is not asking the question 'Why?'. (Much more about this question can be found in my second book, *Sustainable Medicine*.) This new edition of my first book gives CFS/ME sufferers the knowledge and the 'Tools of the Trade' to fashion their own recovery.

I hope what follows will satisfy scientific curiosity as well as provide a simple road map to recovery for the serious CFS/ME sufferer who initially may not have the brain power to get to grips with many of the difficult ideas I present. Not all my ideas may be 'correct', but they are at least biologically plausible and have stood the test of clinical application over 35 years of medical practice and, crucially, they abide by the 'First, do no harm' principle as first laid down in the Hippocratic Corpus.

The road map

There are some powerful analogies which help us to understand why we suffer the symptom of fatigue and where we are on the recovery path.

Fatigue is the symptom we experience when energy demand exceeds energy delivery:

> *Annual income twenty pounds, annual expenditure nineteen pounds nineteen and six, result happiness. Annual income twenty pounds, annual expenditure twenty pounds nought and six, result misery.*
>
> MR MICAWBER in *David Copperfield* (Charles Dickens)

. . . and so it is with energy.

This gives us the overall strategy: look at how energy is being delivered in the body and at how it is being spent. It is attention to both sides of the equation that gets the result.

Energy delivery in the body

THINK OF THE BODY AS A CAR:

Engine	mitochondria
Fuel	diet and gut function
Oxygen	lungs
Fuel and oxygen delivery	heart and circulation
Accelerator pedal	thyroid gland
Gear box	adrenal glands
Service and repair	sleep
Tool kit	methylation cycle
Cleaning – oil	antioxidants
Catalytic converter	detoxification
A driver	the brain in a fit state!

Energy expenditure in the body

Two thirds of all energy spent goes into staying alive – the so-called basic metabolic rate (BMR). This leaves one third of our energy to spend physically, mentally and on the essential evolutionary reason that we are alive – to reproduce.

To use yet another helpful metaphor, the two potential holes in what I call 'the energy bucket' are the emotional hole and the immunological hole. The latter is a major problem – many cases of CFS/ME have an infectious trigger. At the same time, be aware that the immunological hole embraces not just chronic infection but also allergy and autoimmunity. This helps us with the naming of the disease since names should reflect the underlying causes:

Chronic fatigue syndrome = poor energy delivery mechanisms
Myalgic encephalitis = CFS + inflammation (infection, allergy, autoimmunity)

Fatigue is an essential symptom to maintain life. Without the symptom of fatigue we would all be dead in 11 days. No-one has survived that long without sleep.

Fatigue is a powerful symptom – it prevents athletes winning gold medals.

Fatigue is the clinical picture that arises when, as I have said, energy demand exceeds energy delivery. Diagnosis is all about identifying the reasons for this because that gives clear indications for management. We have to ask the two questions:

- Is our energy pot, or 'bucket', too small?
- Are there wasteful holes in it?

We must maximise our 'Energy In' and keep our 'Energy Out' within reasonable bounds. At the very least, these must be in balance.

Finally, sometimes in my clinical work, I see 'step change' improvements in a patient's symptoms, or sometimes a 'flip' from a CFS state to a non-CFS state. My editor, Craig Robinson, who is a first-class mathematician, saw that these cases could be modelled by reference to 'Catastrophe Theory', whereby sudden shifts in behaviour, or states, arise from small changes in circumstances. This is discussed further by Craig in the final chapter of this book (see Chapter 24, page 271).

Dealing with these various issues around energy delivery and energy demand all at the same time is no easy task and requires much self-discipline and determination. One has to be defiant in the face of a seemingly unbeatable enemy.

CHAPTER 2 SUMMARY

The roadmap to recovery

- The key to recovery is to understand how your body delivers and uses energy.
- The goal is to *maximise* the delivery of energy and *minimise* the expenditure of energy, especially the wasteful expenditure of energy.
- We can maximise the delivery of energy by looking at factors such as:
    - mitochondria
    - diet and gut function
    - thyroid gland
    - adrenal gland
    - sleep
    - methylation cycle
    - antioxidants
    - detoxification
- We can minimise wasteful energy expenditure by looking at such factors as:
    - the 'emotional hole' – stress and worry
    - the 'immunological hole' – infection, allergy, autoimmunity, inflammation
- Chronic fatigue syndrome (CFS) occurs where there are poor energy delivery mechanisms.
- Myalgic encephalitis (ME) is CFS + inflammation – that is, CFS concurrent with infection, allergy or autoimmunity.

CHAPTER 3

The clinical picture of CFS/ME

Symptoms are important because they give us vital clues as to causation and treatment. Current symptoms give us an idea of whether the underlying cause has to do with poor energy delivery mechanisms or with inflammation. However, the history – that is to say, any symptoms prior to onset of the fatigue, together with any details of obvious triggers – is equally vital to establishing causation. It is a doctor's duty, through careful questioning, to elicit the necessary clues. But many doctors are bad at this. Indeed, one of my patients told me that when she went to visit her GP she was only allowed to report one symptom per consultation. More than one needed a second consultation, perhaps weeks later!

The medical history – past problems and current symptoms

The clinical pictures that I see evolve from:

A. Susceptible individuals with predisposing factors, so that their health and constitution start to erode.
B. These individuals are then further subjected to increasing levels of stress (physiological, immunological and emotional) and start using addictions to mask these symptoms (so they do not realise they are close to the edge of disaster) leading to a dangerous tipping point.
C. Then follows the *coup de grace* – a final trigger that kicks them over the edge (to mix my metaphors wildly).

Past problems

A. Susceptible individuals with predisposing factors

Predisposing factors may include one or more of the following:

Diet

Modern Western diets may be rich in calories (highly desirable from an evolutionary perspective) but they are deficient in micronutrients (vitamins, minerals, etc). This puts us at risk of infection, which is a major trigger for CFS/ME. High-sugar, high-carbohydrate diets cause metabolic syndrome and this, too, is a risk factor for CFS/ME. Metabolic syndrome is the clinical picture which arises when the body is fuelled with sugars and starches instead of fat and fibre. (Members of the medical profession do not diagnose this until it is well advanced, with high blood pressure, high blood sugars and central obesity.) It is a major risk factor for diabetes (and also heart disease, cancer and dementia).

Metabolic syndrome is a particular problem because CFS/ME sufferers do not have the energy to cook. They feed themselves on convenience foods which need minimal preparation, such as bread, cereals, biscuits, crisps, fruit, sweets, chocolate and dairy products. Worse still, these foods provide a very short-term, addictive buzz of energy. There is a particular vicious cycle here because these are the very foods which result in metabolic syndrome, fermenting gut, allergy and micronutrient deficiencies all of which deplete energy as you will see later. Worse still, even, the symptoms these foods create mean that those with CFS/ME turn to other addictions to relieve those symptoms – to caffeine, nicotine and possibly others. Much more detail can be found in my third book, *Prevent and Cure Diabetes*.

Chronic lack of sleep

It is a *sine qua non* that sufficient amounts of good quality sleep are essential for good health. All forms of life, even bacteria, need windows of time when the internal biochemistry can be shut down so that healing and repair can take place. The business of staying alive results in cell damage. Lack of sleep is a risk factor for CFS/ME. Recovery is hastened by quality sleep.

Typically, CFS/ME sufferers are owls. Our circadian rhythm (our internal 'body clock') is ultimately determined by light and the impact that light has on the hormones which pass its 'message' on to the rest of the body. These messenger hormones are melatonin and the thyroid and adrenal hormones; the CFS/ME owl needs all these 'messenger' hormones to be measured – see later (Appendix 1, page 291).

Sleep is often disturbed, not only because of pain or discomfort, but just because we wake up. A common cause of this is poor fuel delivery. We used to call this 'hypoglycaemia' – that is, a lack of sugar (glucose) in the bloodstream – but we cannot take such a simplistic view any more because there are at least three other fuels that the body can use. These are (1) short-chain fatty acids from the fermentation of fibre in the lower gut, (2) new glucose derived from protein, and, most importantly, (3) fuel from fat. It seems to be a feature of CFS/ME sufferers that they do not easily switch into burning fat as a fuel. This lack of energy delivery often manifests with vivid dreams or sweating or waking in the night.

Sleep may also be disturbed because of sleep apnoea; this may be central (the body forgets to breathe) or obstructive. Obstructive sleep apnoea occurs because the airways are narrowed; there are three common causes of this: Pickwickian syndrome (too fat), hypothyroidism (causing oedema, or swelling, of the larynx) or allergy (typically to dairy products, causing allergic swelling). I suspect, but do not know, that central sleep apnoea is also a mitochondrial symptom; I suggest this because many conditions known to be associated with central sleep apnoea are also associated with mitochondrial failure, such as heart failure, dementia and possibly cot death (see page 199).

Personality

The people in whom CFS often takes a hold are those driven, workaholic, goal driven, perfectionist,'never say die' characters. This is because these people ignore the normal cues that make us stop striving – they continue despite symptoms of fatigue and pain in order to achieve. The achievement is at the expense of their health. Furthermore, these personalities are more likely to turn to addictions to mask symptoms in order that they can keep going.

The Pill and HRT

Female sex hormones are immunosuppressive (and so women are more likely to get infections) and induce metabolic syndrome (again see my third book, *Prevent and Cure Diabetes*). In my practice, women with CFS/ME outnumber men by more than two to one and I suspect this is an effect of female sex hormones – endogenous (produced by the body) and exogenous (from outside the body, so the Pill for example).

Addiction

Addiction to any drug (including sugar – yes, I consider that to be a drug) is a risk factor. A past history of eating disorder (bulimia or anorexia) has its roots in addiction. Some people seem to be natural addicts and easily get hooked on something. Many go through their lives on the addiction ladder – that is, starting with sugar and chocolate in childhood and moving up through nicotine, alcohol and other such social highs. Even when coming down the addiction ladder they achieve this through swapping to 'safer' addictions. This is a good start – vaping is preferable to smoking – but eventually all addictions should be cut out if possible as they are so counterproductive.

Addiction too runs in families.

Allergy

Allergy is interesting because the allergen may be constant through life but its manifestation may change with time. Dairy allergy is common, typically presenting in babies with three-month colic, moving on to toddler diarrhoea, then catarrhal conditions, recurrent tonsillitis and glue ear. Eventually sufferers 'grow out' of those problems only for them to be replaced by migraine, irritable bowel syndrome and psychological problems (yes, allergy affects brain function). Later in life we see arthritis and fatigue resulting. Allergy is the great mimic and can produce almost any symptoms, but I always think 'allergy' if there is a shopping list of symptoms dating back many years.

Poor mitochondrial function

CFS/ME runs in families. I often see mother/son or mother/daughter combinations. One of the common causes of CFS is poor mitochondrial function. The genes for mitochondria come down the female line, so we inherit our mother's mitochondria. Poor mitochondrial function means our energy bucket is not as large as it should be. Sometimes this manifests with poor athletic performance – these people suffer at the school cross-country race when they simply do not have the stamina to compete. However, we know that mitochondrial function can be greatly improved by the regimes detailed in this book – simply because there is a genetic tendency does not mean that nothing can be done.

Poor thyroid function

Consultant endocrinologist Dr Kenneth Blanchard estimates that 20–40 per cent of Western women are hypothyroid. This alone is a cause of CFS, but it also makes us more susceptible to a major trigger – namely, infection.

Gut problems

We are seeing epidemics of people with gut symptoms. I used to think that allergy was the major cause of this, but I now think that fermentation in the upper gut (see Chapter 7, page 107) is the big problem. This has arisen because high-carbohydrate diets and snacking overwhelm our ability to digest so that foods are fermented instead. The commonest symptoms of this are wind and bloating, indigestion and reflux. The non-thinking doctor's favourite symptom-suppressing prescription is for acid-blocking drugs, such as proton pump inhibitors (Omeprazole, Lansoprazole, etc) and H2 blockers (Zantac). These wipe out stomach acid production, resulting in so-called hypochlorhydria. This is a disaster! Stomach acid is a frontline defence against infection. Why? Most microbes enter the body through the mouth – even inhaled microbes stick onto mucus and are coughed up and swallowed so that they can be killed in the stomach's acid bath. Acid blockers put the taker at risk of infection. Many cases of post-viral CFS are triggered by gut viruses, such as Epstein-Barr virus (glandular fever or 'mono'), cytomegalovirus and HHV6. Despite the Establishment's crushing* of Dr Judy Mikovits, my view is that her thesis that mouse viruses spread by vaccination are a major cause of CFS/ME has yet to be disproved. Furthermore, an acid stomach protects against upper fermenting gut. Acid

---

* **Historical Note:** Judy A Mikovits, PhD, is an CFS/ME researcher and was previously the research director at the Whittemore Peterson Institute (now the Nevada Center for Biomedical Research). Dr Mikovits led the team that published a paper suggesting a connection between the XMRV retrovirus and CFS/ME. As a result of this paper, Mikovits felt the full force of scientific prejudices regarding CFS/ME, and eventually she was fired from the WPI in 2011. After her sacking, there was a legal dispute with the WPI – Dr Mikovits was actually arrested at this time. All charges, including criminal charges of theft, brought by the WPI against Dr Mikovits, were eventually dropped. This book is not the place for a full recounting of the circumstances surrounding these events but, for example, at one time, Dr Mikovits was banned from even setting foot on the NCI (National Cancer Institute) campus, a prohibition which would be enforced by security. The full story is told in the excellent book, *Plague: One Scientist's Intrepid Search for the Truth about Human Retroviruses and Chronic Fatigue Syndrome (ME/CFS), Autism, and Other Diseases*, written by Kent Heckenlively (a former attorney) and Judy Mikovits.[12]

is required for the absorption of minerals and so hypochlorhydria renders us further deficient in essential raw materials, leading to a myriad of associated problems, including poor immune, mitochondrial, thyroid and adrenal function.

Toxic environment

We live in an increasingly polluted world and are inevitably exposed to toxic metals, pesticides and chemicals. They bio-accumulate in the body. Indeed, we are being internally pickled. How do I know that? Morticians tell me that bodies don't rot like they used to do! Whilst we are alive these chemicals mess up the system – imagine throwing a handful of sand into a finely tuned engine; it messes things up in unexpected ways, so, no surprise, they wear out faster. Mitochondria, the engines of our bodies, are directly inhibited, causing fatigue in the short term and accelerated ageing in the longer term. These toxic chemicals are directly carcinogenic, mutagenic (damaging to DNA and therefore cause cancer and birth defects), immunotoxic (disrupt the immune system, which may result in an inadequate response to infectious challenge or a worthless inflammation, such as allergy or autoimmunity), neurotoxic (result in autism, behavioural disorders, depression, dementia, Parkinson's disease, etc) and also hormone mimicking (which can be behind almost any symptom).

Ageing

Youth is wasted on the young.

OSCAR WILDE (1854–1900)

As you age you can stay just as fit and well but you have to work harder at it. This means taking care of your energy delivery systems (remember, doctors cannot be trusted to do this – you must work it out for yourself) and effectively avoiding or dealing with the emotional and immunological holes (wasters of energy) as and when they appear. However, the energy gap slowly narrows, and indeed this determines the ageing process. Eventually we do not have enough energy to power our organs; then we go into organ failure; that is why no one lives forever. However, the narrower the energy gap, the less energy we have to deal with stressful events, which leads us to the next issue . . .

B. Increasingly stressful events or lifestyle

The patient has had a period of intense stress. This may be mental, emotional, immunological, physical or financial. He/she tries to cope with this stress by spending more energy – working longer hours or perhaps exercising hard on the grounds that he/she can get fitter. This kicks a large hole in the energy bucket and the person becomes increasingly fatigued. Often the worry of the situation means sleep is disturbed or hours of sleep are lost – another risk factor for CFS/ME. Then the unexpected happens – a bereavement, job loss, virus or house move, perhaps. As demands increase and energy declines, then the quality of the diet declines as the person has neither the time nor the energy to cook and eat well. He or she turns to easy convenience foods ('junk food'), which yield a short-term energy spike but erode health longer term.

All the above is often compounded by addiction. Addiction masks the symptom of stress and affords short-term relief. It allows us to ignore the miserable symptom of fatigue and battle on – again this is short-term gain. We have addiction uppers like caffeine, and addiction downers like chocolate and nicotine. Alcohol is particularly pernicious because it is cheap, readily available and socially acceptable; it allows us to forget our worries and stop caring – but it is toxic and places great demands on the liver, further eroding our ability to deal with other toxins. Sugar and fruit sugar have both effects – a boost of energy together with a feeling of calm ('comfort eating'); sugar is also the cheapest addiction, so no wonder it is the commonest.

The stress hormones are poured out so that we can gear up to demands – truthfully, great things are achieved on adrenaline. We come to believe that we can function at this higher level long term. Indeed, it still astonishes me that people can carry on for as long as they do with high levels of unremitting stress, poor diet, poor sleep and, dare I say, toxic prescription drugs dished out to further suppress the symptoms and draw them towards the dangerous tipping point (see Catastrophe Theory, Chapter 24, page 271).

C. Triggers – the last straw that breaks the camel's back

There are many triggers which come on the back of the above and symptoms help determine causation. However, these can be confusing – symptoms of acute inflammation may arise from infection, allergy, autoimmunity or even chemical poisoning. So, for example, looking at a hay fever sufferer, without clinical details, one might diagnose a cold. Looking at an inflamed patch on the skin, without clinical details, I might not be sure if this was allergic eczema, sunburn, chemical burn, infected cellulitis or viral or autoimmune rash. The history, together with context and chronology, is vital.

Infectious triggers

Infectious triggers often present with **symptoms of acute inflammation**, such as:

Acute fatigue: This is an essential symptom to enforce rest so that the immune system has the energy available to fight. The fittest person may be rendered bed-bound for days with a nasty virus. This beautifully illustrates the power of the immune system to kick an immunological hole in the energy bucket.

Malaise and 'illness behaviour': Men seem much better at this than women (ho ho!).

Fever: Most microbes are killed by heat.

Swollen lymph nodes ('glands').

Mucus and catarrh: These physically wash out microbes.

Runny eyes: Ditto.

Cough and sneeze: These physically blast microbes out of the airways.

Airways narrowing, wheezing and asthma: These result in the air we breathe becoming more turbulent so microbes (and allergens or toxic particulates) are thrown against and stick to the mucus lining of the airways to be coughed up and swallowed and denatured by the acid bath of the stomach.

Vomiting: This is an essential defence against food poisoning and overloading of the gut.

Diarrhoea: Ditto.

Colic: Ditto.

Cystitis: Empty the bladder of urine and therefore of microbes.

Pain: This alerts us to the fact something is wrong, so we can rest. That is why aching joints are also an important symptom.

With acute infection, such as 'flu, it is potentially dangerous to use symptom-suppressing medications, which interfere with these natural defences. They have the potential to make problems much worse because the infecting microbe loves a cold body in which it can remain and an immune system lacking energy. (I would caution against prescribing symptom-modifying medication which interferes with the body's natural processes of eliminating microbes. Indeed, I suspect this is why we are currently seeing epidemics of post-infection fatigue syndromes. We should only be using interventions to reduce the infectious load and improve our immune defences. Central to this are rest, warmth, great food, love and super-nutrition [vitamin D, zinc, selenium and various herbals] – that is to say, good old-fashioned nursing care that every mother used to know about. As a child with pneumonia I can remember the glory of being able to spend the day in my parents' bed because they had a fire in their room – and, boy, did I love a fire! Still do.)

Infections may be:

Viral: Dr Martin Lerner estimated that in over 80 per cent of all post-viral CFS/ME patients, Epstein-Barr virus (glandular fever or 'mono') was causal (see Appendix 6, page 319).

Bacterial: Thankfully we have antibiotics which are highly effective in treating bacterial infections. However, and increasingly so, infections are missed and may become chronic. A common cause of CFS/ME used to be tuberculosis, happily now recognised and treated. The spirochete that is syphilis went through a similar evolution before treatment became available. Interestingly, another spirochete is coming to the fore as a major cause of fatigue – namely, *Borrelia burgdorferi* resulting in Lyme disease (see Chapter 12, page 161). Biological warfare in the Gulf War meant many veterans came away infected with 'mycoplasma incognita' – that is, a biologically plausible explanation for why many family members of Gulf War veterans, who had never visited the Gulf, came down with similar symptoms.

Fungal: I suspect these are most commonly seen as part of the fermenting gut issue (see Chapter 7, page 107). The problem is not so much infection as allergy to fungi. Although allergy and infection have different causations, the former being due to a worthless reaction to an allergen and the latter being due to the body's defence against a pathogen, they are both immune responses, and they both result in similar symptoms of acute and chronic inflammation. Allergy and infection present to the clinician as almost indistinguishable. In some cases, such as fungi, the pathogen (here a fungus) elicits an allergic response as much as it does a pathogenic response and so the causation mechanism also becomes blurred.

Parasitic.

The important point is that we now have good and reliable tests for these infections which have a high level of sensitivity and specificity. See later (Appendix 1, page 291).

Chemical triggers

A high level of suspicion is required to diagnose chemical involvement. The clinical pictures that I have actually seen in my practice (from long-term and short-term exposures) that result in CFS/ME, and may additionally switch on multiple-chemical sensitivity, can be seen in Appendix 4 (page 312).

PRESCRIPTION DRUGS

Many prescription drugs inhibit mitochondria directly – the best example would be **beta blockers**. Nearly all my CFS/ME patients are made worse by these. In addition, we have:

Statins are a particular hate of mine. They inhibit the body's own production of coenzyme Q10, the most important antioxidant (the 'oil of the engine') in mitochondria.

Antibiotics may inhibit mitochondrial function because, from an evolutionary perspective, mitochondria are bacteria. As with all drugs, they must be used with care.

General anaesthetics may trigger CFS/ME, and surrounding such are other stresses (worry about the hospital admission, etc) which obviously are contributory straws that may break the camel's back.

Major and minor tranquillisers, antidepressants and antipsychotics may all cause fatigue.

Bisphosphonates, such as alendonic acid to treat osteoporosis, inhibit mitochondria.

Many drugs are metabolised in the liver and this imposes extra strains on liver detox, so, for example, many CFS sufferers are made ill by normal doses of antidepressants.

CHEMICALS CREATED OR RELEASED FROM WITHIN THE BODY

These chemicals may arise from:

- **Gut fermentation:** In CFS/ME sufferers we often see a fermenting gut (see Chapter 7, page 107). This produces toxins such as alcohols (ethyl, propyl and butyl derivatives), 'right-handed' sugars (such as D-lactate), noxious gases (such as hydrogen sulphide) and bacterial endotoxin, all of which have to be detoxified in the liver. All the blood from the gut is carried in the portal vein directly to the liver. It does not immediately pass into the systemic circulation – if it did so we would rapidly fall unconscious and die because this portal-vein blood is so toxic. Indeed, this is what happens when people go into liver failure. Such sufferers are routinely prescribed antibiotics and antifungals to kill all the microbes in the gut, prevent fermentation and reduce the toxic load on the liver. The liver can be overwhelmed by several possible mechanisms:
  - Toxic overload from the gut, including sugar and products of fermentation

    - Toxic overload from the gut from foods such as aspartame, caffeine, alcohol and chemical residues in food
    - Toxic overload from the gut from prescription drugs
    - Toxic overload from the outside world – toxic metals, pesticides, etc
    - Insufficient raw materials to deal with toxic stress (vitamins, minerals, essential fatty acids, glutathione, etc)
    - Insufficient energy to power the necessary enzyme reactions.
- **Immune activity:** The way that the immune system kills microbes is by shooting free radicals at them. These free radicals have to be mopped up by a good antioxidant system, otherwise the body is damaged by 'friendly fire'. Free radicals damage mitochondria. Indeed, it is biologically plausible that this is the mechanism by which viruses switch on chronic fatigue syndrome. The fatigue results from an immunological energy hole combined with friendly fire damaging mitochondria.
- **Normal products of metabolism,** such as neurotransmitters and hormones: Many have to be detoxified in the liver.
- **Over-doing things** and switching from aerobic to anaerobic metabolism: Lactic acid is produced which must be recycled to pyruvate in what is called the Cori cycle (see page 187). This can only take place in the liver and is greatly demanding of energy.
- **Chemicals mobilised from fat:** In the short term, the body can 'hide' toxins by dumping them in fat. As we detox through weight loss, exercise, heating regimes or such, we mobilise these into the bloodstream and this can cause acute poisoning. Levels of toxins in fat are 100–1000 times higher than those in blood.

SILICONE

Silicone is in a league of its own. With silicone I am not just looking for the obvious breast implant or silicone injections – many other prostheses contain biologically active materials. Examples include testicular implants, lens implants, Norplant contraceptive devices (silicone rods), TMJ work, facial contouring, meshes for hernia repairs, etc. In the veterinary world reactions to suture materials are well documented.

Silicone itself is chemically inert but immunologically active. The trouble is that it 'out-gases' from implants, is picked up by the white cells and spreads into the rest of the body where, in susceptible people, it acts as an immune adjuvant, switching on the immune system, causing widespread inflammation wherever it ends up. Silicone is a large, tough molecule which cannot be broken down by any biological enzyme system. It cannot pass through cell membranes and cannot be excreted from the body, so there are no known detox techniques to get rid of it. I have seen over 250 women with fatigue syndromes following silicone implants; they get written out of the medical literature for all the reasons given in Chapter 1 – no name, no blame and plenty of shame.

CHEMICAL TRIGGERS – CONCLUSION

The important point is that we do have some excellent tests that allow us to identify the chemicals that are causing problems and that have obvious implications for management; we need to put in place the relevant detox regimes to get rid of the cause.

Physical triggers

It is obvious that severe physical stress will cause fatigue. Since the symptoms are so dire (as I have said, they prevent athletes winning gold medals) and the cause so obvious, the diagnosis is easily made. Other physical traumas include:

Unremitting noise: Typically, noisy neighbours

Infrasound from wind turbines (so-called 'wind turbine syndrome'): Infrasound has been shown to disturb sleep in the susceptible up to 14 kilometres distant. This is yet another problem that the Establishment is trying to bury. I reckon it takes about 15–20 years of campaigning to make people realise a problem is real, another 15–20 years for it to become accepted and a further 15–20 years before effective action is taken. This parallels experience with the dangers of tobacco smoking. Professor Richard Doll demonstrated the serious health risks of smoking in 1950 but it was not until 2002 that the Tobacco Promotion and Advertising Act became effective. In the interim period, millions of people died as a result of smoking tobacco, but Government and tobacco companies made billions from tax revenues and sales.

Emotional triggers

The brain is greatly demanding of energy – it accounts for just 2 per cent of body weight but, at rest, consumes 20 per cent of the total energy demands of the body. If the brain is constantly on red alert and hypervigilant, because of emotional stress, then this puts one at risk of chronic fatigue as well as being a trigger.

Post-traumatic stress syndrome/disorder involves a constant reliving of past traumas. In my experience these have included anaesthetic awareness, watching a fellow zoo keeper be mauled to death by a tiger, childhood bullying and sexual abuse, and a young boy, whose father was dying, lost sleep because he was constantly listening out for his father's breathing; there are many other such cases. Bereavements, financial insecurity (including the struggle to get benefits that so many of my CFS/ME patients contend with), sexual orientation and the social opprobrium that may bring, race issues and other such – all have the potential to kick emotional holes in energy buckets.

Other triggers

Chronic insomnia: Shift work is a major risk factor for CFS/ME. Indeed, we are all aware that sleep deprivation is a highly effective form of torture.

Electrical: Intolerance of electromagnetic radiation, typically from wi-fi, cordless phones and mobile phones, is increasingly recognised as a cause of distress. This was highlighted by the case of Jenny Fry who committed suicide aged 15 in June 2015 because wi-fi at her school was making her life a misery. Some small recognition is creeping in for this problem – a French woman recently won a disability case after convincing a court that she suffers from an allergy to electromagnetic radiation from gadgets. Marine Richard, 39, was told she might claim 800 per month for three years as a result.[13]

And doubtless there are many other triggers.

Triggers – interpretation

Often people with CFS/ME come to me and their story starts with the trigger factors. One has to go back and unravel all that went before in order to get the full picture. The sufferers are the best people to do this – they are expert in their own symptoms and history; give them a few clues and patients can do their own detective work.

Catastrophe Theory

As mentioned before, there is a mathematical explanation for the above that Craig Robinson details in his wonderful chapter on such (see Chapter 24, page 271). It explains how we must be careful not to lead life on the edge. I tell my patients, life is like a walk on Beachy Head. Walk well away from the edge so if you trip or get blown over on the green turf it is a small matter to stand up, dust yourself down and continue. But if you live right on the edge then a puff of wind can blow you off the cliff. Not only are you damaged by the fall, but it is a long hard climb to return to the top.

Current symptoms

When CFS patients consult with me, they often come with shopping lists of symptoms. My job is to tease these apart to help us identify the underlying mechanisms which result in those symptoms. It also allows us to prioritise tests and treatments. All those CFS patients by definition have symptoms due to poor energy delivery. In addition, some also have symptoms of inflammation; this clinical picture we call ME (myalgic encephalitis). So, I will divide this section on symptoms into the following three parts:

1. Symptoms of CFS
2. Symptoms of severe CFS
3. Symptoms of myalgic encephalitis (ME – that is, CFS plus inflammation)

Symptoms of CFS

The symptoms of CFS manifest with poor energy delivery, when energy demand exceeds energy delivery.

Every living cell in the body, indeed every living cell in the animal kingdom, requires energy. If that energy supply is switched off, death rapidly ensues. All cells are affected by poor energy delivery mechanisms. If energy delivery mechanisms are impaired, then cells go slow; if cells go slow, then organs go slow – all organs: so the brain, heart, immune system, hormone production, liver, kidney, gut and so on. This explains the multiplicity of symptoms seen in patients with CFS. These symptoms in order of frequency are as follows.

Physical fatigue

CFS patients have poor stamina. They fatigue very quickly, some within seconds of any exertion. This arises because of poor energy delivery to muscles. If they push themselves through they develop post-exertional malaise – often this is delayed by 12–24 hours. This is the one symptom that is common to all CFS sufferers and it is the one symptom that makes 'graded exercise therapy' an oxymoron. Graded exercise is extremely dangerous since one risks major relapse with such.

Mental fatigue

Weight for weight, the brain needs energy 10 times faster than the body. Poor energy delivery to the brain results in 'foggy brain', with poor ability to comprehend, problem solve and multi-task. Short-term memory is often appalling. The clinical picture is of an acute confusional state similar to people who are drunk on alcohol. Indeed, CFS sufferers often say they feel poisoned (actually many are – see more on this in Chapter 7 'The fermenting gut', page 107). Dr Byron Hyde, a Canadian physician, routinely did functional brain scans which looked directly at energy use in the brain.[14] He found the brains of CFS sufferers had large holes akin to those of patients with multiple strokes or vascular dementia. Indeed, CFS sufferers often feel like the unknown author of this quote:

Nothing right in my left brain, nothing left in my right brain!

Mental fatigue can be entirely explained by poor energy delivery mechanisms. As you will read later (Chapter 4, page 51), it is mitochondria which take fuel from the bloodstream and burn it in the presence of oxygen to make the energy molecule ATP. This is the energy molecule that allows neurotransmitters to be synthesised and recycled and electrical signals to pass. Collectively this keeps us alive, thinking and conscious.

Fatigue makes fools of us all – it robs us of our skills,
our judgement and blinds us to creative solutions.

HENRY MACKAY (1864–1933),
anarchist, thinker and writer

However, a further fascinating aspect of energy delivery in the brain has to do with fuel supply. Silvia Raveraa (2009) showed that there were not enough mitochondria in the brain to explain the energy it uses. Essentially, the fatty myelin sheaths which wrap themselves around nerve fibres like a 'Swiss roll' have adopted mitochondrial biochemistry.[15]

This makes great sense; it means that energy production is in close proximity to energy demand. However, the Swiss rolls like to burn fats in the form of ketones as a fuel supply. Ketones are very dense in energy and easy to move around fatty areas – 60 per cent of the brain is composed of fat. It needs modest amounts of long-chain fats to build the Swiss roll membranes to deliver energy, but the fuel comes largely from medium-chain fats – saturated animal fats like lard, dripping and butter; also coconut oil and chocolate fat. Low-fat diets are also a major risk factor for CFS. Incidentally, they are also a risk factor for dementia, cancer and heart disease – but that is another story to be found in my second book, *Sustainable Medicine*.

Dizzy spells and feeling faint

These symptoms too are symptomatic of poor energy delivery to the brain. That can happen when any part of the energy supply chain is impaired, but I suspect poor fuel supply (low blood sugar with inability to keto-adapt – that is, to burn fat) and low blood pressure (because energy delivery to the heart is poor so that it cannot beat powerfully as a pump) are the commonest two mechanisms in CFS.

Feeling of being stressed

This highly unpleasant symptom I suspect arises when the brain knows it does not have the energy to deal with demand; that demand may be in the present or future and be physical, mental, emotional or financial. The demand may be real or 'imagined' – Craig's wife, Penny, was forever telling him 'Not to cross your bridges before you come to them'. The current system of claiming social benefits is a major cause of stress and misery to CFS sufferers – it is partly the stress of not being believed but with potential financial insecurity over and above it. Also, leaving aside these considerable stresses, the physical and mental effort of completing the benefit forms, in ever-shortening deadline periods, is extremely stressful. You almost have to be well to be able to fill in the forms properly within the allotted time span. And additionally, many CFS sufferers, and other sick people, find the process of laying out in black and white just how unwell they are to be a very emotionally draining experience. The fact is that my CFS patients are extremely well adjusted and it always amazes me that more of them don't fall prey to depression and anxiety. Indeed, my CFS patients universally over-estimate what they are capable of, being optimists in the extreme.

We use addiction to cope with this horrible stress symptom. I know – I've used alcohol during stressful times. We know the obvious and dangerous addictions, such as alcohol, smoking, caffeine, cannabis, ecstasy, cocaine and so on. However, the most overlooked but arguably the most dangerous addiction is to sugar and fast carbs (so-called 'junk food'). In the short term it gives us a little energy hit with a calming effect on the brain, but it leads to long-term metabolic disaster. Much more detail on this subject later and also in my third book, *Prevent and Cure Diabetes*.

Low mood, anxiety and depression

Like fatigue, these are also symptoms that protect us from ourselves – they stop us wanting to do things and thereby prevent us spending energy. CFS sufferers tend to procrastinate. Interestingly, the energy molecule ATP multitasks – it is not *just* the energy molecule; it is also a neurotransmitter in its own right. To be precise, it is a co-transmitter. That means other neurotransmitters, such as acetylcholine, GABA, dopamine or serotonin, cannot work unless they have a molecule of ATP. Lack of energy delivery may explain a host of other symptoms, from anxiety and depression to OCD and addiction.

Muscle problems

Muscle power is determined by the quantity of mitochondria (they make up 20 per cent of muscle weight) and muscle stamina is determined by mitochondrial quality. In CFS, muscle power is initially strong but there is rapid loss of power over a few seconds – that is, there is very poor stamina. Of course, in severe CFS, deconditioning and weakness occur since any exercise is impossible. But this is a consequence, not a cause, of CFS.

Muscle pain is common. As energy delivery fails there is a switch from aerobic to anaerobic metabolism, with the production of lactic acid (the acid bit that causes the pain). An athlete recovers quickly from this pain (what is sometimes called a 'stitch') because with rest, lactic acid is rapidly converted back to pyruvate and acetate as a fuel. But this itself requires energy in the form of ATP. (For the biochemists, this occurs via the Cori cycle – see page 187.) CFS sufferers do not have energy in abundance – it takes much longer to clear lactic acid and so the pain is prolonged.

This muscle pain may be part of the clinical picture of fibromyalgia, which often co-exists with CFS. Allergy is another major cause of muscle pain.

Variable blurred vision

Focusing on nearby objects requires the ciliary muscles of the eye to contract to allow the lens to fatten. If these muscles fatigue then the lens cannot focus. Typically this blurring of vision is episodic – worse when the patient is tired. Many need several pairs of glasses to deal with this – like Professor Branestawm! (For those who haven't read the Norman Hunter series of books about Professor Branestawm ['Brainstorm'], then they come recommended. They have the perhaps unique feature that the first title [*The Incredible Adventures of Professor Branestawm*, 1933] was written 50 years before the last title [*Professor Branestawm's Hair-Raising Idea*, 1983).]

Symptoms of severe CFS

People with severe CFS have all the above symptoms and more:

Light intolerance

Weight for weight, the eye needs energy 10 times faster than the brain (so 100 times faster than the rest of the body). This is because the business of converting a light signal that hits the retina into an electrical signal that the brain can read requires huge amounts of energy. Light intolerance is very common in the severely afflicted CFS patient. Many cannot even read or watch TV. Interestingly, light intolerance is also a symptom of severe migraine, which tells me that poor energy delivery is also part of the cause of this problem.

Noise intolerance

The issues are as for light.

Heat intolerance

For the body to lose heat it must pump more blood to the skin. The skin is the largest organ of the body and to do this cardiac output may have to increase by 20 per cent. People with severe CFS do not have the energy available to the heart to achieve this.

Cold intolerance

If energy delivery is poor, then not enough heat is generated to keep warm.

Heart symptoms

Cardiac symptoms in CFS are very common.

Dysrhythmias: With poor energy delivery at the cellular level there may be disturbance of the heart's electrical conductivity, which causes dysrhythmias. Many CFS sufferers complain of palpitations, missed heart beats and the like. This is particularly the case in patients with poisoning by chemicals, especially heavy metals, since these chemicals are also directly toxic to nerve cells. Increasingly, I believe that dysrhythmias are caused by toxic stress.

Chest pain (angina): Again, with poor energy delivery the same problem occurs in heart muscle as skeletal muscle (detailed above, page 36). There is an early switch into anaerobic metabolism with the production of lactic acid, and this is painful. Heart muscle pain due to poor energy delivery is called angina. However, in CFS it is often not diagnosed as such because typically angina clears quickly with rest; where energy delivery is impaired because of poor mitochondrial function (see later, Chapter 4 page 51), recovery is much slower. Again, this is due to the Cori cycle effect. The lactic acid produced is very slow to clear so the pain is much more persistent than typical angina. CFS sufferers are often diagnosed with 'atypical chest pain', but actually this is angina – not angina due to poor blood supply from arteriosclerosis but angina due to poor mitochondrial function. (The Cori cycle occurs in the liver and goes slow for at least two reasons. First, it requires six molecules of ATP to clear one molecule of lactic acid – this is energetically expensive work, something our CFS sufferer cannot afford! Secondly, the liver is already overloaded for the reasons given above [high starch diets, fermenting gut, toxic stress, micronutrient deficiency, etc].)

Low blood pressure: Poor energy supply to cardiac muscle means that the muscle cannot contract powerfully and the heart becomes a weak pump; this manifests with low blood pressure. This is a low cardiac output state bordering on heart failure. (I was heavily criticised once for stating that my CFS patients were in heart failure – this was considered an alarmist statement which scared patients. However, I still maintain they are in heart failure but have to call this 'a low cardiac output state'. The point is that it is a pathologically serious state of affairs.) If blood pressure drops too much, the panic hormone adrenaline is released and this may cause palpitations.

POTs: It is much easier to pump blood on the horizontal so CFS sufferers feel better lying down. (Actually we all feel more rested lying down and do such to sleep, of course.) If the CFS sufferer stands up, then to increase cardiac output the heart has to beat faster (because it cannot beat more powerfully). However, this too is energy demanding and the fast heart rate is not sustainable. Blood pressure may drop precipitously so the patient loses consciousness. This clinical picture has been called POTs (postural orthostatic tachycardia syndrome). POTs is often blamed on the autonomic nervous system which controls the heart rate. However, I think this is to blame the messenger, not the underlying cause.

Patent foramen ovale: Dr Paul Cheney has demonstrated that over 90 per cent of CFS patients have a patent foramen ovale.[16] This is a hole in the heart between the left and right atria (which normally closes as a flap at birth); this means that blood bypasses the lungs and does not pick up oxygen as it should. Strictly speaking it is not a hole but a valve which should snap shut and stick shut at the moment of birth. This converts the single circulation of the foetus to the double circulation of the adult and allows blood to pass round the lungs to collect oxygen. For some people, the valve does not stick – it remains as a flap. This does not matter so long as the higher pressure in the left atrium compared to the right atrium holds the flap shut. But if the heart is weak, as it is in CFS patients because of poor

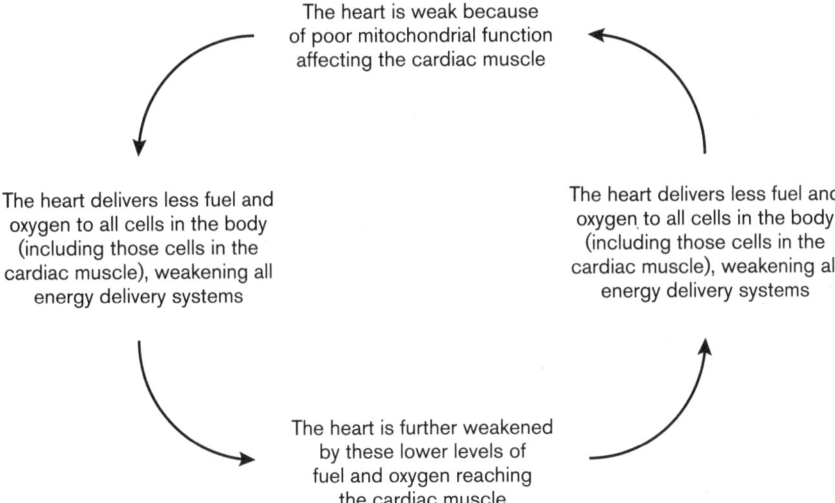
The heart is weak because of poor mitochondrial function affecting the cardiac muscle
The heart delivers less fuel and oxygen to all cells in the body (including those cells in the cardiac muscle), weakening all energy delivery systems
The heart is further weakened by these lower levels of fuel and oxygen reaching the cardiac muscle
The heart delivers less fuel and oxygen to all cells in the body (including those cells in the cardiac muscle), weakening all energy delivery systems

Figure 3.1. A vicious cycle.

mitochondrial function, then the pressure difference is lost and the valve may blow open. If this happens, some blood does not circulate round the lungs; it short cuts back into the left side of the heart. This means oxygen levels in the blood coming from the left side of the heart drop and energy delivery is further impaired because of poor oxygen supply to the tissues. This is a 'lovely' example of one of the many vicious cycles that come into play as energy delivery mechanisms fail. I suspect this explains why some CFS patients can very suddenly deteriorate in a way not commensurate with increased activity.

Pacemaker problems: Poor blood supply to a pacemaker could result in cardiac dysrhythmias.

All the above problems compound all the other symptoms of CFS. The heart delivers fuel and oxygen to all cells in the body and if fuel and oxygen delivery is impaired then this too further impairs energy delivery mechanisms (see Figure 3.1 for further example of a vicious cycle).

Shortness of breath

If energy delivery at the cellular level is impaired, the brain may misinterpret this as poor oxygen delivery and stimulate the respiratory centre to breathe harder. This may result in hyperventilation, which actually makes the situation worse. Hyperventilation changes the acidity of the blood (it becomes more alkali) so that oxygen sticks more avidly to haemoglobin so worsening oxygen delivery. This is yet another example of one of the many vicious cycles that apply in CFS. Remember, shortness of breath may also result from heart failure, respiratory distress and anaemia, and these symptoms need investigating as a separate issue.

Poor immune function and susceptibility to infections

The immune system is like the brain – intelligent, responsive, decision making and active. It is also hugely demanding of energy. As I have said, a generally healthy person given a dose of 'flu will become bedbound within hours. It is a well-recognised fact that when someone is stressed and tired they will be much more susceptible to disease, especially infection.

Poor liver function – intolerance of alcohol and drugs

Poor liver function may result in the symptom of feeling poisoned. Indeed, intolerance of alcohol and prescription medication is extremely common if not universal in CFS. Part of the explanation may be that the liver is working at maximum capacity and does not have the energy to deal with additional foreign chemicals.

The liver is responsible for mopping up sugars from the gut so that they do not pass directly into the systemic bloodstream to cause metabolic syndrome and diabetes. Again, wobbly blood sugar levels are a major cause of fatigue. (Much more information is available on this in my third book, *Prevent and Cure Diabetes*.)

Almost invariably CFS sufferers struggle with:

Alcohol: This is consumed in gram amounts, 10 to 100-fold higher than most prescription drugs.

Statins: They inhibit endogenous production of coenzyme Q10 and therefore energy delivery by mitochondria.

Beta blockers: They slow the heart and reduce cardiac output.

Antidepressants: Often only small doses can be tolerated without side effects – typically, one quarter or less of a normal therapeutic dose.

Both the gut and liver need a large amount of energy to function. As I have said, when the body is resting, the liver accounts for 27 per cent of total body energy consumption. This is more than the heart and brain combined. As detailed above, the liver has a massive job dealing with the products of the digesting and fermenting gut. These are delivered to the liver directly in the portal vein. Interestingly, the least toxic food is fat; it does not even have to go to the liver first but passes straight into the lymphatics and from there directly into the bloodstream via the thoracic duct. It requires no detoxing in the liver and cannot be fermented in the gut. Most people find their energy levels are better on the ketogenic diet (see Chapter 17, page 215), possibly because fat needs so little energy to process it.

Poor gut function

Again, the business of digesting and absorbing foods also requires large amounts of energy. Gut symptoms are common in CFS. However, most symptoms are due to allergy to food and to the upper fermenting gut (Chapter 7, page 107).

Poor hormonal function

Synthesising hormones in glands again requires energy. We know that CFS sufferers have a general suppression of what is called the hypothalamic pituitary adrenal axis (see Chapter 5, page 81) with hypothyroidism (low thyroid function) secondary to this. Poor energy delivery may be part of the reason why.

Poor renal function

The kidneys are greatly demanding of energy. They cannot tolerate even a temporary cut-back in energy without going into failure. So they have evolved a protective series of hormones – the renin-angiotensin system. These maintain energy delivery to the kidneys when all around them is failing. This means that when energy delivery mechanisms are failing, the kidney is one of the last organs to be affected. Indeed, Sophie Mirza, 32, was the first official UK death from CFS (2006) with the immediate cause being renal failure. The coroner stated dehydration, but my guess is that poor energy delivery was a contributing cause.

We can measure kidney function indirectly with blood tests to assess creatinine levels. These levels can vary for different reasons, see Table 3.1 (page 42).

Loss of libido

This is Nature's way of preventing procreation when there is no energy for such. The business of having babies, as any parent knows, is hugely demanding of energy – much more so for the women than the men, which I suspect is why women suffer this symptom much more than men.

Physical degeneration including osteoporosis

This is a longer-term consequence of CFS – part of the reason is simply that bones need exercise to keep them strong and CFS sufferers cannot do such.

Table 3.1. Kidney function test results interpretation

Kidney function result	Possible causes	Comment/treatment
High creatinine (low GFR)	High-protein diet	Fuel the body with fat and fibre, not carbs and too much protein.
	Poor kidney function	Poor energy delivery – concentrate on improving energy delivery (see Chapters 4, 5, 6, 17 and 18)
Low creatinine (high GFR)	Low muscle mass	Creatinine is a breakdown product of muscle – the loss of muscle mass may be caused by reduced levels of 'exercise'
	Low protein diet	Not desirable – do the ketogenic diet (Chapters 6 and 17). This is not a high-protein diet but rather a high-fat, medium-protein, low-carb diet and will address the issue of low creatinine, if caused by low levels of protein in the diet.

They cannot 'use it' so they risk 'losing it'. However, nutritional factors are just as important and good nutrition can reverse osteoporosis – I know because I have collected the figures; see Chapter 23 (page 261).

Symptoms of myalgic encephalitis (ME) and why sufferers have them

The clinical picture of ME is as for CFS plus symptoms of inflammation. ME sufferers have ALL the above symptoms of poor energy delivery *plus* the symptoms of inflammation: infection, allergy and auto-immunity.

Inflammation is characterised by the cardinal symptoms of pain, swelling, heat (redness) and loss of function. Think inflammation with this combination of symptoms. But this begs the question as to the cause of inflammation. We all know the obvious one – infection – but allergy and autoimmunity also result in inflammation and may cause almost any symptom. Historically, syphilis was said to be 'the great mimic', producing almost any symptom and pathology. Lyme disease (Chapter 12, page 161) and suchlike have replaced syphilis in this regard, but allergy too can produce almost any symptom and in the future autoimmunity will be a major player – currently 1 in 20 Westerners has an autoimmune disease.

The living organism that we are is a potential free lunch for others. We fight a constant 'arms race' against invading microbes and parasites. Indeed, it could be argued that all disease processes that involve inflammation are part of this arms race. Some of these invaders we have grown to live with and they now make up an essential part of a healthy body – the gut microbiome (we used to call this the gut flora) is the obvious example. However, viruses have made themselves at home in our body – retroviruses make up at least 8 per cent of normal human DNA!

Many occasional symptoms exist to physically expel or kill invaders. These same disease processes are invoked where there is allergy. Acute symptoms are most likely to be infectious, with chronic or recurring symptoms being allergic or auto-immune.

Symptoms of chronic inflammation: chronic infection, allergy and auto-immunity

Chronic inflammation can produce any symptom. Because inflammation kicks an immunological hole in the energy bucket, these problems also present with symptoms of poor energy delivery.

Whilst inflammation can cause any symptoms (Dr John Mansfield described a case of osteoarthritis of the hip due to allergy to house dust mite)[17], common things are common. Chronologically, inflammation symptoms often start in the nose and throat and extend to the gut, brain and then any other organ. This is because most antigens or infections enter the body through the mouth or nose.

However, if inflammatory insult is via another portal of entry (such as vaccination, tick or insect bite, sexually transmitted disease, needle stick, wound infection, etc) then one may see a different progression.

SYMPTOMS SUGGESTIVE OF ALLERGY – TOGETHER WITH THE COMMONEST ALLERGENS

- All CFS symptoms as above.
- ENT symptoms such as sinusitis, catarrh, deafness, glue ear, snoring and obstructive sleep apnoea, voice changes, cough: allergy to dairy products, yeast (fermenting gut).
- Tinnitus: allergy to food or gut microbes. (I suspect this may also contribute to age-related deafness – Beethoven went deaf following salmonella infection.) Caffeine may cause tinnitus by a toxic reaction.
- Irritable bowel syndrome: allergy to foods and upper fermenting gut problems.
- Inflammatory bowel disease: allergy to foods and upper fermenting gut problems.
- Asthma: allergy to food, biological inhalants and gut microbes.
- Headache: aspartame, dairy. Caffeine may cause a toxic headache.

- Migraine: typical allergic headache, but there are other causes, notably poor energy delivery and toxic reactions from vaso-active amines (see note below).
- Eczema and urticaria: allergy to food and gut microbes.
- Acne and rosacea: allergy to gut microbes and food.
- Interstitial cystitis, chronic prostatitis/epididymitis, vulvitis: allergy to gut microbes, especially yeast.
- Arthritis: allergy to foods and gut microbes.
- Allergic muscles, tendons, connective tissue: allergy to dairy, gluten, and gut microbes.
- Fatigue: allergy to gluten grains.

Note on Causes of Migraines

Vaso-active amines are substances, such as dark chocolate, red wine, cheese, some fish and some food additives, that contain amino groups, such as histamine or serotonin. These act on the blood vessels to alter their permeability or to cause vasodilation. Migraine pain is caused by vasodilation in the cranial blood vessels (expansion of the blood vessels), while headache pain is caused by vasoconstriction (narrowing of the blood vessels). Poor energy delivery can result directly in light sensitivity (a common symptom of migraine). The eyes are very demanding of energy and any drop in the available energy being delivered will result in eye symptoms such as this. Poor energy delivery may also cause poor oxygen delivery and my guess is that this is the mechanism which results in migraine with neurological symptoms such as hemiplegic migraine.

SYMPTOMS SUGGESTIVE OF CHRONIC INFECTION (BACTERIAL, VIRAL, PARASITIC, FUNGAL)

- All CFS symptoms
- Muscle pain or stiffness
- Headache
- Painful or swollen joints, tendon problems
- Fever, shivers, chills, rigors, night sweats
- Swollen lymph nodes
- Numbness of skin, burning, pins-and-needles
- Cough, mucus, shortness of breath

- Other clues: tick bites (indeed, any insect bites) with or without bull's eye rash (think Lyme disease).

Tertiary tissue damage and the cell-free DNA test

- Where there is inflammation there is tissue damage.
- Where energy delivery is poor there is tissue damage.
- A combination of the above results in slow healing and repair.
- The combined effects of these problems can be measured by looking at cell-free DNA, which is a measure of tissue damage.

The significance of the cell-free DNA test

DNA should all be contained within cells. Therefore the level of cell-free DNA is a measure of tissue damage. When tissues are damaged, cells rupture and release their contents into the bloodstream as fragments. Cell-free DNA is raised in all cases of tissue damage, such as sepsis, trauma, cancer, radiotherapy, chemotherapy and other such pathologies. It is also raised in CFS. Dr Norman Booth has graphed the relationship between mitochondrial energy scores and cell-free DNA levels and there is a strong correlation – the worse the mitochondrial energy score, the higher the cell-free DNA level. (We hope to publish the results in a new medical paper.) A high cell-free DNA result therefore tells us something is going very wrong, such as:

The energy equation is in serious deficit – expenditure is above delivery. The patient is not pacing well – in other words, pushing too hard – and this is resulting in cell damage. However, some people who are very disabled have no choice – just the energy required to exist will cause tissue damage. So people with the worst mitochondrial function score often have high cell-free DNAs even though they are doing almost nothing. Here we need to try and improve pacing as best we can, whilst at the same time addressing all other known issues so as to improve energy delivery, as noted at the head of this chapter. (See Chapter 15, page 183.)

There is a very poor mitochondrial function score but the patient is forced to do some muscular activity just in order to live. Here we need to try to do all we can to improve mitochondrial status – see Chapter 18 (page 220) for details of the basic and mitochondrial nutritional packages.

There is poor antioxidant status (see coenzyme Q10, SODase [super oxide dismutase] and GSH-PX [glutathione peroxidase]). Here we need to improve antioxidant status – see Chapter 18 (page 220) for details of the basic and mitochondrial nutritional packages.

There is ongoing toxic stress (such as from pesticides, volatile organic compounds, heavy metals, etc). Here we need to avoid such toxic stress and also detox as best as we can – see Chapter 20 (page 233) for the practical details of detoxing.

There is immune activation (as for example in acute infection). See Chapter 19, (page 226) on avoiding infections, and also the chapters on the immunological hole in the energy bucket (Chapters 9–13).

All these issues need addressing.

The cell-free DNA test tells us when the clinical picture is ME.

The cell-free DNA test puts CFS/ME firmly in the camp of serious organic disorders.

There are major problems with high levels of cell damage:

- It takes time for new cells to be made and this may partly also explain the delayed fatigue in CFS.
- The above business of healing and repair is further demanding of energy and raw materials.
- The immune system may react against these bits of cell floating about, thereby switching on inflammation. Switching on inflammation is a dangerous game because one may not be able to switch it off, especially where antioxidant status is poor. Switching on inflammation can switch on allergy or autoimmunity.
- **These are disease-amplifying effects:** You make yourself worse if you don't pace. Exercise regimes are positively dangerous. Fatigue is the symptom that protects the body from itself.

The importance of symptoms

Remember we have symptoms for very good reasons – they protect us from ourselves and from foreign invaders. Indeed, as I have said, I suspect that heavy use of symptom-suppressing drugs to treat colds and 'flu is contributing to our modern epidemic of post-infection CFS. We need the symptoms of pain and fatigue to make us rest so that the immune system has the energy needed to deal with infection and the stillness to keep infection from spreading. Fever kills all microbes. Cough, sneeze, runny nose, vomiting and diarrhoea all help to expel microbes. Poor appetite prevents us from feeding microbes in the gut and bloodstream. Starvation reduces blood sugar levels very rapidly – sugars are replaced in the bloodstream by ketones which further help to starve out microbes (microbes use sugar as a fuel). Feeding grapes to a sick person is one of the worst things you can do!

Symptoms give us clues as to what is going wrong and why CFS sufferers, especially severe cases, do not have the energy or resources to do everything. Symptoms allow us to prioritise treatments and then the manner in which these symptoms respond to these treatments gives us further clues as to what may be wrong. That is to say, the success or otherwise of the treatments feeds back into our thinking and may either reinforce our first thoughts as to what is wrong or may lead us to consider other sets of possible problems. We have thus begun our detective work.

This is why symptom suppression with drugs is so dangerous. They may allow short-term respite and improved function, BUT the underlying disease processes progress faster and our 'clues' for treatments are 'masked'. Worse still, symptom-suppressing drugs postpone the moment when curative treatment can begin. This makes recovery longer (by definition) and more difficult – more difficult because, by postponing that moment, one risks further problems developing.

To recover from this wretched illness one has to become one's own doctor. The idea of this book is to give you the Rules of the Game and the Tools of the Trade to achieve this. This includes becoming an expert in your own symptoms and your responses to treatments so that you can work out what is going wrong, why it is going wrong and, more importantly, what to put in place to effect a cure.

Knowing yourself is the beginning of all wisdom.

ARISTOTLE (384–322 BC)

The good news is that I am increasingly coming to the view that regardless of whether we are looking at poor energy delivery mechanisms, infection, allergy or autoimmunity, the general approach is the same. Mammal life evolved over 300 million years with these same issues and came to conquer them all – Natural Selection and the Survival of the Fittest ensured that. We must mimic Nature in terms of our diet, sleep, exercise and sunshine – all influences that impact directly on the immune system. We should take advantage of the joys of modern living – security, plentiful food and warmth, and access to great surgeons and antimicrobial medicines when things go wrong. However, when things go *horribly* wrong we now have some very useful tools to help restore normality – we just have to choose wisely what to use.

CHAPTER 3 SUMMARY

The clinical picture of CFS/ME

- People fall ill with CFS/ME because:
  - they are susceptible individuals with predisposing factors;
  - they are subjected to chronic levels of stress;
  - and then there follows a 'trigger' that tips them over the edge.
- Predisposing factors include such things as poor diet, personality type, the Pill and HRT, addiction, allergy, poor mitochondrial or thyroid function, gut problems, toxic environments and so on.
- Stresses that contribute to developing CFS/ME include such things as mental, emotional, financial, immunological or physical 'overload'.
- Triggers can include viral or bacterial infections, exposure to chemical toxins – for example, pesticides or toxic metals, prescription drugs, chemicals created from within the body, such as via a fermenting gut or immune activity – exposure to physical triggers such as infrasound from wind turbines, chronic insomnia, electrical sensitivity and many more.
- A sufferer's current symptoms give clues as to whether the underlying causation of the illness has to do with poor energy delivery (CFS) or inflammation (ME). But also the 'path' into illness, as described above, gives vital clues as to the causation of the particular individual's illness.
- So, having a good clinical history, and a detailed account of current symptoms, allows both the causation and the mechanisms of this patient's illness to be uncovered and this has implications for individually tailored treatment packages.

PART II

The Theory

CHAPTER 4

The mechanisms of energy delivery in the body:

it's mitochondria, not hypochondria

Annual income twenty pounds, annual expenditure
nineteen pounds nineteen and six, result happiness.
Annual income twenty pounds, annual expenditure
twenty pounds nought and six, result misery.

MR MICAWBER in *David Copperfield* (Charles Dickens)

. . . and so it is with energy.

When the gap is positive we have energy.

When the gap is negative we have fatigue.

In treating chronic fatigue we have to maximise energy delivery mechanisms and minimise useless or unwanted energy expenditure in order to create a positive gap.

To repeat my analogy on page 17, in thinking about energy mechanisms it is useful to think of the body as a car. To get it to go we need:

Engine	mitochondria
Fuel	diet and gut function
Oxygen	lungs
Fuel and oxygen delivery	heart and circulation

Accelerator pedal	thyroid gland
Gear box	adrenal glands
Service and repair	sleep
Tool kit	methylation cycle
Cleaning – oil	antioxidants
Catalytic converter	detoxification
A driver	the brain in a fit state

There are three main sections in this chapter:

A. Mitochondria – the engines of our bodies: describing the biochemistry
B. The ATP profiles test: looking at how to measure mitochondrial function and what may be dysfunctional with mitochondria
C. Treating the mitochondrial dysfunction: how to treat dysfunctional mitochondria by way of supplementation and detoxification

A. Mitochondria – the engines of our bodies

Mitochondria are tiny structures ('organelles') found in every cell in the body. Within them the key processes that provide the body's energy take place. This is why I have likened them to the engine of the car/body. All medical students learn about mitochondria at medical school, but then they are forgotten – that happens because conventional medicine ignores them and gives them no clinical application. I loved biochemistry because it was so logical – I cherished the work of Peter Mitchell, a cattle farmer in Cornwall, who won the Nobel Prize in 1978 for his discovery of the mechanism by which mitochondria generate energy (ATP) from fuel and oxygen. In his speech at the Nobel Banquet, 10 December 1978, he said that:

> *The final outcome cannot be known, either to the originator of a new theory, or to his colleagues and critics, who are bent on falsifying it. Thus, the scientific innovator may feel all the more lonely and uncertain.*

And indeed, it took over 20 years to realise that mitochondria are implicated in nearly all disease processes, from cancer and heart disease to autism and dementia. This makes perfect biological sense – if you impair energy delivery to any organ then it will fail. If mitochondria do not work properly, then the energy supply to every cell in the body will be impaired. The varying degrees of failure would explain a wide range of symptoms and pathologies.

I had seen some modest successes treating CFS/ME patients during the first 20 years of my NHS work, from the 1980s to 2000, using all the Tools of the Trade that I knew at that time to be effective, such as diet, supplements, pacing, correcting thyroid function and so on. However, I was left with a hard core of patients who were no better and I was still scrabbling around for answers.

I am eternally inquisitive and hate to be beaten – ask my Team Chase colleagues!* All the time, I felt the need to understand more, and I forever had the words of Robert Boyle, the famous scientist who originated Boyle's Law, ringing in my ears:

> *It is highly dishonourable for a reasonable soul to live in so divinely built a mansion as the body she resides in – altogether unacquainted with the exquisite structure of it.*
>
> R Boyle FRS (25 January 1627 – 31 December 1691)†

In my quest, I had the services of neither Newton nor Boyle to hand but I was extraordinarily fortunate to find an intellectual equivalent in Dr John McLaren-Howard. He was the biochemical genius that I needed to address some of the difficult biochemical questions that I had. Without John's generosity, skill and expertise I would still be stuck in the twentieth century.

Clinically, patients with severe CFS looked like my patients with heart failure – and, indeed, this was subsequently confirmed by work by Dr Peckerman as below:

> *Research by Dr Arnold Peckerman (Peckerman A et al, 2003) shows that cardiac output in CFS sufferers is impaired. Furthermore, the level of impairment correlates very closely to the level of disability in patients. Dr Peckerman was asked by the US National Institutes of Health to develop*

---

* Team chasing is my chosen sport – teams of four riders on horseback race over a cross-country course of about two miles, with about 25 fences to be jumped.

† Sir Isaac Newton (25 December 1642 – 20 March 1726/27) corresponded with Boyle and one such letter, written in 1679, has been put online (www.orgonelab.org/newtonletter.htm). In summary, Newton says of Boyle:

'For my own part, I have so little fancy to things of this nature, that had not your encouragement moved me to it, I should never, I think, have thus far set pen to paper about them.'

Praise indeed!

a test for CFS in order to help them judge the level of disability in patients claiming Social Security benefits. Peckerman is a cardiologist and on the basis that CFS patients suffer low blood pressure, low blood volume and perfusion defects, he surmised they were in a low cardiac output state. To test this he came up with Q scores.

'Q' stands for cardiac output in litres per minute and this can be measured using a totally non-invasive method called impedance cardiography. This allows one accurately to determine cardiac output by measuring the electrical impedance across the chest wall. The greater the blood flow, the less the impedance. This can be adjusted according to chest and body size to produce a reliable measurement. (This is done using a standard algorithm.) It is important to do this test when supine (lying down) and again in the upright position. This is because cardiac output in healthy people will vary from 7 litres per minute when lying down to 5 litres per minute when standing. In healthy people, this drop is not enough to affect function. But in CFS sufferers, the drop may be from 5 litres lying down to 3.5 litres standing up. At this level, the sufferer has a cardiac output which causes borderline organ failure. In CFS, the low cardiac output is caused by poor muscle function and therefore strictly speaking is what is called a 'cardiomyopathy'. This means the function of the heart will be very abnormal, but traditional tests of heart failure, such as ECG, ECHOs, angiograms, etc, will be normal. (Please see here for more on this: www.monkeyswithwings.com/images/DrMyhill-373.pdf.)[18]

My CFS/ME patients were not in heart failure for the usual reasons, such as poor blood supply, death of heart tissue following infarctions, leaky valves or pacemaker problems. There had to be another reason. What about mitochondria? 'Dear John,' went my letter, 'I need a test for mitochondrial function. Please can you arrange this as soon as possible?' Poor man – this must have kept him sleepless for weeks.

Initially, John measured the activity of individual enzymes within mitochondria, including the complexes I to V which drive the process of 'chemi-osmosis' (see page 62). We could not see any clear correlation with the level of energy in my patients. Interestingly, the best correlation was with levels of NAD (vitamin B3 – this is the most important intermediary between Krebs citric acid cycle [see page 63] and chemi-osmosis). I stamped my little foot and pursed my lips in a petulant way. 'I don't care about the complexes. I want a functional test, John. I want something that tells us about how ATP is produced. Get back to that drawing board.' [Editor's note: I feel rather put out that Sarah has never stamped her little foot at me! Craig.]

Thankfully, John's tolerance parallels his brilliance and innovative skills. There are many tests in research biochemistry that are not used clinically because they are perceived to have no medical application. John's forte is to single out and further develop tests which do have clinical application – he ploughs his own furrow. In this respect he has developed a wide range of clinically relevant and applicable tests. But what he developed at this time were the revolutionary mitochondrial function tests which started with 'ATP profiles'.

B. The ATP profiles test

The ATP profiles test is a functional test that looks at how efficiently ATP – that is, adenosine triphosphate (page 62), the universal currency of energy in the body – is made. (ATP is used in all sorts of biochemical jobs, from muscle contraction to hormone production.) There are five potentially rate-limiting steps in ATP production, as follows:

1. How ATP is made from ADP (adenosine diphosphate – see page 62) by the process of 'oxidative phosphorylation' (the metabolic pathway by which fuel is oxidised ['burnt'] with oxygen, inside the mitochondria, to generate the energy molecule ATP).
2. How ATP is moved out of mitochondria into the cytosol of cells (the general body of the cells where energy is needed for the cell to work) by translocator protein.
3. How much ATP is in the cytosol, and
4. How it releases energy in a magnesium-dependent process to form ADP.
5. How ADP is moved back into mitochondria for recycling.

All thc above are measurable steps and if any one step goes slow then the whole process will slow. This allowed us to calculate a mitochondrial energy score by comparing the measured step with the normal range. Effectively this gave us an objective measure which, in those patients for whom other causes of fatigue had been eliminated (and that is a key point), correlated remarkably well with their clinical score. This gave me an objective measure of the level of fatigue. For the first time I could tell my patients how fatigued they were; they did not need to tell me. Indeed, I believe this is the only test in the whole of medicine that can measure a symptom – namely, fatigue. (We do not have direct objective measures of pain, stress, depression, itch, taste, smell, etc.) This test alone has been very helpful in obtaining state and insurance benefits for sick CFS patients who are being treated as hypochondriacs when really they are 'mitochondriacs'. I am currently working hard to find another lab that can replicate this test so that it can be made widely available.

Historical Note

After obtaining 'mito scores' for a number of patients and listing all these out with their ability levels, I sent an unsophisticated spreadsheet of these results to Craig in 2005 – by which I mean three or four rather untidy, handwritten A3 sheets, with more or less straight lines drawn on them. About three hours later Craig emailed me back, saying, 'The correlation coefficient is 0.8, or thereabouts. You've got something here.' This was my 'Wow' moment.

This test allowed us to write and publish peer-reviewed scientific papers. This was a very happy cooperation between Dr John McLaren-Howard of Acumen Laboratories, Dr Norman Booth of Mansfield College, Oxford, and myself. The first paper was an initial study of 71 CFS patients compared with 56 control subjects.

- All had received the Basic Package (Chapter 18, page 220) with respect to diet, supplements, sleep, pacing, thyroid and adrenal function.
- The patient and I (Dr Myhill) agreed an ability score between us.
- Bloods were sent to Acumen who undertook the test 'blind' – that is, McLaren-Howard did not know the ability score.
- The ATP profiles were scored by a third party giving a mitochondrial function score.
- The mitochondrial function score was graphed against the ability score (graphed as energy score).
- The study was written up by Dr Norman Booth and published in the *International Journal of Clinical and Experimental Medicine.*[19]

This initial study, see Figure 4.1, plotted the clinical energy score against the mitochondrial energy score. This clearly showed that those patients with the worst mitochondrial function had the worst levels of fatigue and vice versa.

The very encouraging results of the above study prompted us to continue to collect and analyse the data, and that resulted in our second study, published in 2012. This was an audit of 138 patients undergoing mitochondrial function tests.[20]

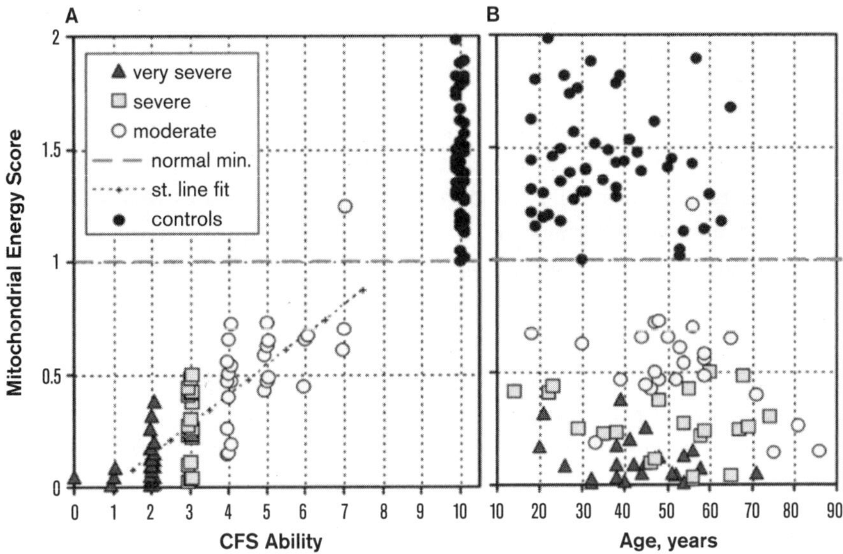

Figure 4.1. Relationship between patients' scores for clinical energy and their scores for mitochondrial energy based on data obtained during the study published as Myhill S, Booth N, McLaren-Howard J. *International Journal of Clinical and Experimental Medicine* 2009; 2: 1–16.

The conclusions of that paper were:

- All patients tested have measureable mitochondrial dysfunction which correlates with the severity of the illness.
- The patients divide into two main groups, differentiated by how cellular metabolism attempts to compensate for the dysfunction. Some switched early into anaerobic metabolism; others employed the 'adenylate cyclase pathway' whereby two molecules of ADP were converted into one of AMP and one of ATP.
- Comparisons with exercise studies suggest that the dysfunction in neutrophils also occurs in other cells. This is confirmed by the cell-free DNA measurements (see page 45) which indicate levels of tissue damage up to three and a half times the normal reference range.
- The major immediate causes of the dysfunction are lack of essential substrates and partial blocking of the translocator protein sites (see page 62) in mitochondria. A substrate is a substance that is needed for the synthesis of another substance, and so, for example, ATP requires the substrate D-ribose for its synthesis – see page 71.

- The ATP profiles test is a valuable diagnostic tool for the clinical management of CFS/ME.

This second paper confirmed the findings of the first paper. Figure 4.2 plots the numbers of abnormal factors (measurements) against the mitochondrial energy score. Since the mitochondrial energy score correlates well with clinical fatigue, it is apparent that those patients with the worst levels of fatigue had the most numbers of abnormalities.

We continued to collect data and were soon able to look at patients who requested follow-up repeat testing. This became the subject of a third paper to address the question as to whether the prescribed regimes were clinically effective. This was published in January 2013.[21]

This study looked at mitochondrial energy scores before and after the treatment regimens detailed below:

1. Eating the evolutionarily correct low-carbohydrate, Paleo diet
2. Ensuring optimum hours of good-quality sleep
3. Taking a standard package of nutritional supplements
4. Getting the right balance between work and rest

Additions to the basic regime were tailored for each patient according to the results of the ATP profiles and additional nutritional tests together with clues

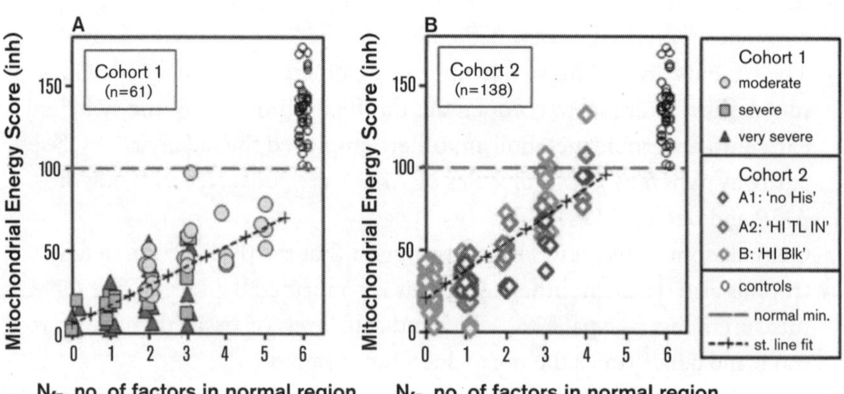

Figure 4.2. Relationship between CFS patients' scores for abnormal factors and scores for mitochondrial energy, based on figures from my paper published in the *International Journal of Clinical and Experimental Medicine* 2012; 53(3): 208–220.

from the clinical history. Mitochondrial function was typically impaired in two ways: either there were deficiencies (in substrates, as described above, or in co-factors – co-factors can be considered as 'helper molecules' in biochemical reactions, such as, for example coenzyme Q10 in the synthesis of ATP) or blockages (inhibition by toxins, exogenous or endogenous [see Chapter 20, page 233]). For the former, additional nutrients were recommended where there was a deficiency, and for the latter, improvement of antioxidant status and selective chelation therapy or far-infrared saunas where appropriate.

Figure 4.3 shows the mitochondrial function scores of 34 patients with their 'before' score in dark grey and 'after' score in pale grey. What was

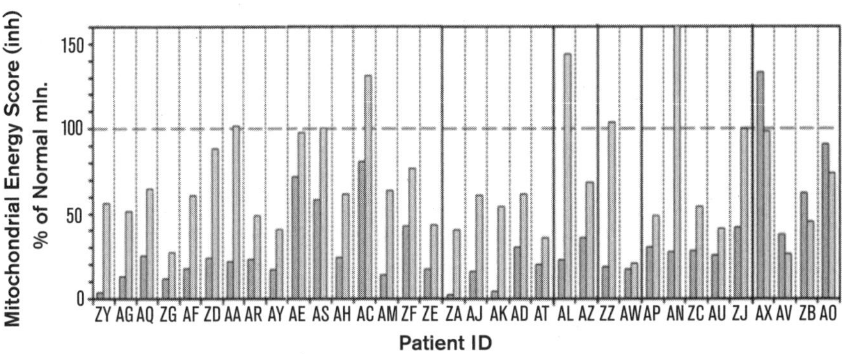

Figure 4.3. CFS patients' mitochondrial function scores before and after a recommended treatment regime. Individual parameters improved where the regime was complied with.

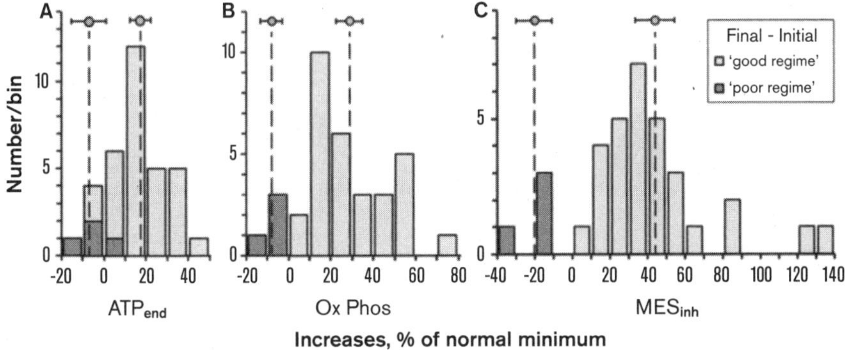

Figure 4.4. Improvements in (A) ATP levels, (B) the rate of oxidative phosphorylation, and (C) mitochondrial energy scores (MES).

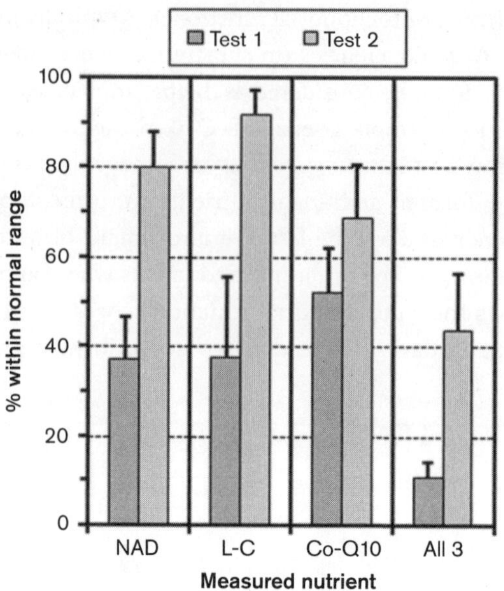

Figure 4.5. Micronutrient levels have improved in the patients who took the relevant supplements.

so significant was that the mitochondrial function scores improved where regimes were complied with (the first 30 patients). Where the regimes were not complied with (patients AX, AV, ZB and AO), there was no such improvement.

We were able to conclude that mitochondrial function tests are a useful tool in managing CFS/ME patients for several reasons:

- They provide an objective measure of the level of clinical disability characterised by fatigue.
- They provide an objective measure of pathology and tissue damage through measuring cell-free DNA.
- They clearly demonstrate that CFS/ME sufferers have serious biochemical pathology.
- They demonstrate that mitochondria go slow because of nutritional deficiencies and that these can be corrected by appropriate nutritional supplements.
- They demonstrate that mitochondria may go slow because of blockages of enzyme systems and that these can be corrected by appropriate detoxification regimes.

A more detailed look at the biochemistry of mitochondria and how this explains some of the symptoms of CFS/ME

It is important to emphasise that in the early stages of mitochondrial failure, the mitochondria look normal; for this reason, a muscle biopsy to look at mitochondria in CFS is rarely helpful. It is a bit like having a car with a spark plug that does not work – an MRI scan of a car would come back completely normal, but if you tried to start it, nothing would work!

The two key symptoms in patients with CFS/ME which I believe reflect the **mitochondrial dysfunction** are:

Very poor stamina (mental and physical): That is, you can do things, but only for a few seconds before tiring. This is due to slow recycling of ATP (see page 62);

Delayed fatigue (mental and physical): That is, symptoms persist for 24 to 96 hours if you overdo things. This is because when mitochondria are stressed, all the energy molecules (ATP, ADP and AMP) are drained out and cells have to wait one to four days for new energy molecules to be made via the 'pentose phosphate shunt' (see page 71).

The molecular mechanisms of energy production in mitochondria

Energy production starts with fuel in the bloodstream. This fuel can come to cells in several forms. I have listed these below in what I suspect is the order of

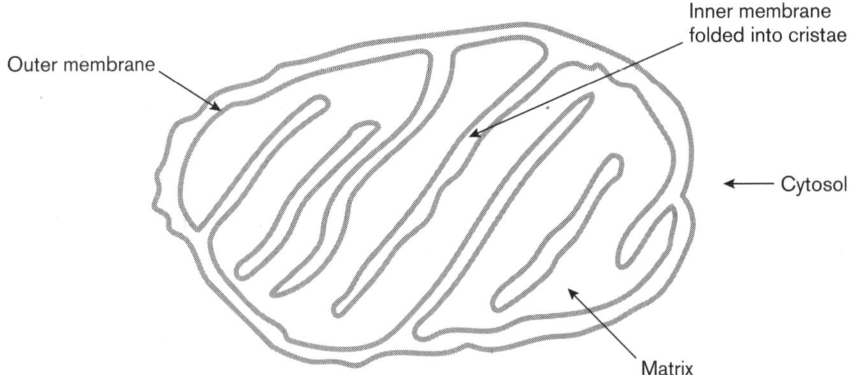

Figure 4.6. What your engine (or many engines) look(s) like. Each mitochondrion is tiny – every heart muscle cell contains 2,000 to 3,000.

preference (by which I mean metabolic ease – the 'cheapest' fuel) for the body. (I could be wrong here!)

Glucose (gut): Directly from the gut when the liver is overwhelmed, as happens when too much sugar is consumed (or absorbed in the mouth, so bypassing the liver)

Short-chain fatty acids: From the fermentation of vegetable fibre by friendly bacteroides in the colon

Pyruvate: When lactic acid is recycled by the Cori cycle (page 187) following an episode of anaerobic metabolism

Glucose (glycogen): Released directly from glycogen stores in the liver and muscle

Glucose from protein stores in the liver: The process by which this is made is called 'gluconeogenesis'

Ketone bodies: From the burning of medium-chain fats, such as our own fat deposits, animal fats, butter, coconut and chocolate fat

Long-chain fats: These are broken down in peroxisomes (organelles in the cell cytoplasm that contain enzymes including catalase and often some oxidases) to medium-chain fats which can be used as fuels; oddly, some CFS sufferers do not seem to be able to do this. Sources of long-chain fats include fish, nut, seed and vegetable oils.

However, all the above fuels have to be converted into acetate, which is what mitochondria like to burn. This is shunted from the cytosol of cells (see Figure 4.6) into mitochondria by a carrier molecule – carnitine. It carries acetate into mitochondria as acetyl L-carnitine, drops off its acetate passenger inside mitochondria and then passes back into the cell as carnitine. Acumen Laboratories measure carnitine routinely in CFS and deficiency is common. I think of carnitine as the nozzle which delivers fuel into the engine.

In the mitochondria, acetate enters Krebs citric acid cycle which generates the intermediary product NADH (nicotinamide adenosine diphosphate). This molecule is used to power chemi-osmosis, which generates ATP (adenosine triphosphate) from ADP (adenosine diphosphate). The raw materials needed for this process include magnesium and coenzyme Q10. Note that NADH is converted to NAD (nicotinamide adenine dinucleotide) in the process of driving chemi-osmosis.

ATP is picked up by translocator proteins, which sit on the surface of mitochondria and move it out into the cell cytosol, where it is needed to energise cell activity. ATP (adenosine with three phosphate groups) is then converted to ADP (adenosine with two phosphate groups) with the release of energy for work. ADP then passes into the mitochondria, courtesy of translocator protein, where it is recycled back to ATP by the process of oxidative phosphorylation.

As I have said, these molecules are the universal 'currency' of energy in the body. Almost all energy-requiring processes in the body have to be 'paid for' with NAD and ATP, but largely ATP. The reserves of ATP in cells are very small. At any one moment in heart muscle cells there is only enough ATP to last about 10 contractions. Throughout a day, the average human generates over 70 kg of ATP! Thus the mitochondria have to be extremely good at recycling ATP to keep the cells constantly supplied with energy.

If the cell is not very efficient at recycling ATP, then it runs out of energy very quickly and this causes the symptoms of weakness and poor stamina. The cell has to shut down and wait until more ATP has been manufactured. Indeed, it is notable from the mitochondrial function tests that levels of ATP are never lower than a critical threshold – I suspect because below this the cell is not viable and cell suicide, or 'apoptosis', results.

As I have said, in producing energy, ATP (three phosphates) is converted into ADP (two phosphates) and ADP is recycled back through mitochondria to produce ATP again. However, if the cell is pushed (in other words, stressed) when there is no ATP about, then it will start to use ADP instead. The body can create energy from breaking down ADP to AMP (one phosphate). This is called the 'adenylate kinase reaction'.

The trouble is that AMP cannot be recycled (or rather, it can, but only very slowly, probably clinically insignificantly, for CFS/ME sufferers – see below). The only way that ATP can be regenerated is by making it from fresh ingredients, but this takes days to do. This explains the delayed fatigue seen in CFS/ME.

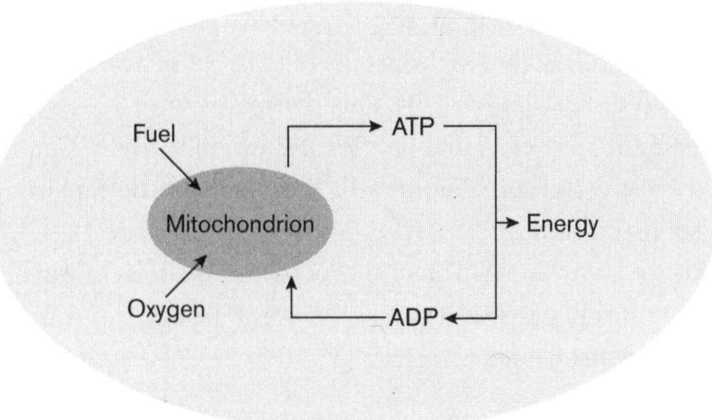

Figure 4.7. Krebs cycle – the process of energy production that occurs in every cell.

So, to summarise, the basic pathology in CFS/ME is slow recycling of ATP to ADP and back to ATP again. If patients push themselves and make more energy demands, then ADP is converted to AMP, which cannot be recycled (but see Figure 4.8) and it is this which is responsible for the delayed fatigue. This is because it takes the body several days to make fresh ATP from new ingredients. When patients overdo things and 'hit a brick wall', this is because they have no ATP or ADP to function. Figure 4.7 is a simplified illustration of that cycle taking place inside every cell.

What happens when you stress the system?

By 'stress the system', I mean when you ask for energy out faster than it can be supplied. There are at least two mechanisms by which the body can make emergency energy. This emergency energy may save you from being caught by a sabre-tooth tiger – or its modern-day equivalent – but both mechanisms have dire biochemical outcomes in the longer term.

1. **The adenylate kinase reaction.** Two molecules of ADP can combine to make one of ATP and one of AMP. Great news about the extra ATP but making AMP is a problem – it can only be recycled very slowly, if at all. This means that the pool of circulating ADP and ATP is rapidly diminished and mitochondria soon start to go slow. The body has to make brand new ATP. ATP can be made very quickly from a sugar called D-ribose, but D-ribose is only slowly made from glucose (via the pentose phosphate shunt for those clever biochemists out there). This takes anything from one to four days. This delay is one possible explanation for the biological basis of delayed fatigue.
2. **Switch into anaerobic metabolism** with the production of lactic acid. Again this is short-term gain and long-term pain. One molecule of glucose, used anaerobically (without oxygen) in its conversion to lactic acid, produces two molecules of ATP. This compares with 32–36 (depending on the efficiency of mitochondria) molecules of ATP when glucose is burned aerobically (using oxygen). Worse still, to convert lactic acid back to glucose requires six molecules of ATP (the Cori cycle – see page 187). CFS sufferers simply do not have the ATP to do this so the lactic acid burn is very persistent. The muscle pain may persist for some hours, often days. Figure 4.8 illustrates these processes.

And now for a bit of good news. AMP *can* be recycled, but it happens very slowly, as I have said. For practical purposes, for patients who are very fatigued,

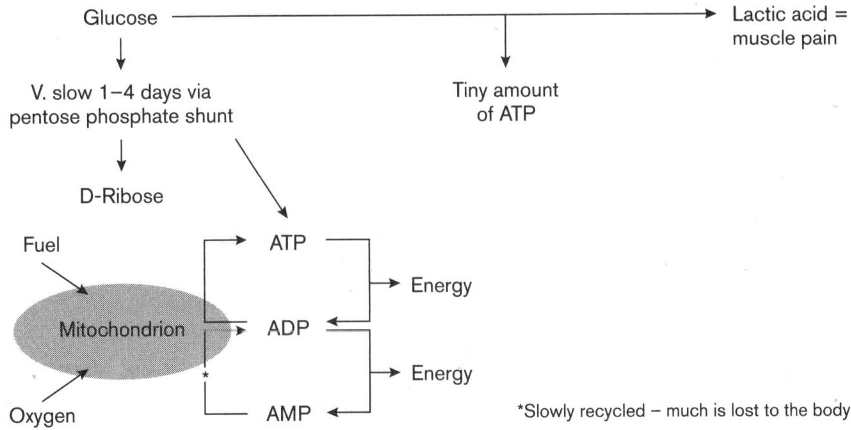

Figure 4.8. What happens when energy (ATP) requirement outstrips energy supply.

this recycling is so slow that it is clinically insignificant. Interestingly, the enzyme which facilitates this recycling ('cyclic AMP') is activated by caffeine. So the perfect pick-me-up for CFS sufferers could be a real black organic coffee with a teaspoon of D-ribose and a large dollop of coconut cream to supply medium-chain fats!

A more detailed look at the ATP profiles test

The ATP profiles test is helpful for three reasons:

1. It is an objective measure of function, and this can be easily calculated, giving us the mitochondrial energy score.
2. It tells us if the patient is deficient in an essential rate-limiting step micronutrient, such as magnesium, coenzyme Q10, acetyl L-carntitine or niacinamide (NAD, or vitamin B3).
3. It tells us if the mitochondria are blocked by something (then other tests can give further clues).

The joy of the ATP profiles test is that we now have an objective test showing that the symptoms of CFS/ME can be explained by poor energy delivery at the cellular level. This test, together with a cell-free DNA test showing tissue damage, clearly shows this illness has a physical basis and that cognitive behaviour therapy, graded exercise and antidepressants are irrelevant in addressing the root cause of this illness. It explains why these treatments have a high failure rate and often make the patient worse – there is no point in beating up the driver of the car if the engine is faulty.

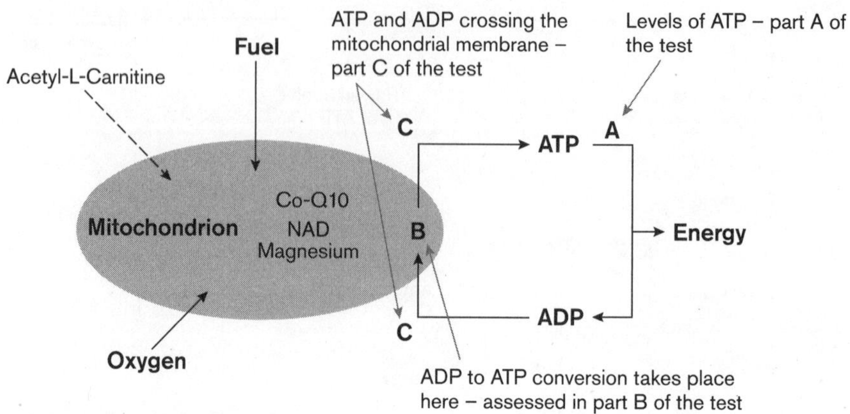

Figure 4.9. Recycling of ATP, relating it to the Acumen ATP profiles test. 'A' corresponds to ATP studies on neutrophils; 'B' to ADP to ATP conversion; 'C' to ADP-ATP translocator protein activity.

To get the full picture, I recommend combining ATP profiles with the following:

Cell-free DNA. This is a measure of tissue damage, as described on page 45. When tissues are damaged, cells rupture and release their contents into the bloodstream as fragments. These fragments include DNA, so when this is found not contained within a cell membrane, it is as a result of tissue damage. Cell-free DNA is raised in, for example, tissue damage due to sepsis, trauma, cancer, radiotherapy, chemotherapy and other such pathologies. It is also raised in CFS/ME and accurately reflects the degree of fatigue. Indeed, Dr Norman Booth has plotted the mitochondrial energy score against cell-free DNA levels and there is a very clear relationship between the two. The lower the mitochondrial energy score, the higher the cell-free DNA. This test alone puts CFS/ME into the category of severe pathology. This is not pathology which can be seen at post-mortem – it is of microscopic quality which potentially affects every cell in the body. A high cell-free DNA therefore tells us something is going very wrong, such as:

- The patient is not pacing well – that is, pushing too hard (athletes call this over-training) and this is resulting in cell damage.
- There is very poor mitochondrial function (see mitochondrial function score, page 130) but patients are forced to do some muscular activity simply in order to live – they have no choice – just the energy required

to exist will cause tissue damage. People with the worst mitochondrial function score often have high cell-free DNAs even though they are doing almost nothing. This emphasises how important good nursing care is in order to protect the patient from him/herself.

- There is poor antioxidant status (see co-Q10, SODase, GSH-PX – in Figure 4.9).
- There is ongoing toxic stress (such as from pesticides, volatile organic compounds, heavy metals, etc).
- There is immune activation (as, for example, infection, autoimmunity or allergy) – the immune system is so compromised that healing and repair go slow.

Superoxide dismutase (SODase) level. SODase is an important antioxidant which mops up free radicals. These free radicals are highly damaging molecules which we all produce in the business of making energy, and may also come from exogenous chemicals and other such. Dr McLaren-Howard measures three types of SODase:

(1) within cells
(2) within mitochondria
(3) outside cells

This gives us a handle on zinc, copper and manganese status. He also looks at the genes which code for the different types of SODase. It is common to find biochemical blockage or 'polymorphisms' (recognised genetic variations) typical of toxic stress.

Glutathione peroxidase level. Glutathione peroxidase is another vital antioxidant, which is selenium dependent. Glutathione multitasks as a molecule essential for liver detox. Deficiency is a common biochemical bottleneck.

Coenzyme Q10 level. I think of co-Q10 as the oil of the engine, allowing smooth passage of electrons within mitochondria to generate ATP. Again almost invariably this is deficient, with some CFS sufferers having appallingly low levels. Indeed, I don't think I have ever seen a normal result in someone not taking supplements.

Serum L-carnitine levels. Carnitine is the fuel pipe/nozzle that allows the fuel of acetate groups to be poured into mitochondria across their membranes. It can be made in the body but is naturally present in meat, hence its name. I suspect this is one reason why vegetarianism is a risk factor for CFS.

Nicotinamide adenine dinucleotide (NAD) level. NAD is a good indicator of vitamin B3 status. Vitamin B3 in this form is the intermediary between Krebs citric acid cycle (see page 63) and oxidative phosphorylation (the metabolic pathway that takes place within the mitochondria by which fuel is 'burnt' in the presence of oxygen to make the molecule ATP). NAD is almost invariably deficient. High doses are needed to correct a deficiency.

One other important co-factor in the production of energy in cells, which I have already mentioned, is D-ribose. It is used up so quickly by cells that measuring levels is unhelpful, but low levels of ATP (from the ATP profiles test) imply low levels of D-ribose.

Examples of some test results

ATP profiles

The patient whose results are shown in Figure 4.10 has low levels of ATP (1), low magnesium (2), poor conversion of ADP to ATP (3) with blockage of the active sites (4), together with poor translocator protein function (5) – no wonder there is severe fatigue.

Please note that TL (translocator protein) 'in' and 'out' refer to the direction in which the TL protein is facing. So TL *in* is looking *in* to mitochondria, picks up ATP and flings it *out* into the cell cytosol. TL *out* is looking *out* of the mitochondria, picks up ADP and flings it *in* to the mitochondria to be recycled. About 80 per cent of mitochondrial membrane is made up of TL protein.

To calculate your mitochondrial energy score ('mito score'), proceed as follows:

- Look at the ATP whole cells with Mg added score. Divide this by the lower of the normal range for this measure (normally 1.6). Call this number A.
- Look at the ratio ATP/ATP^{Mg} added number and divide this by the lower of the normal range figures (normally 0.65). Call this number B.
- Look at the ADP to ATP efficiency ratio number and divide this by the lower range number (normally 60). Call this number C.
- Look at the TL out number and divide this by the lower of the reference range (normally 35 per cent). Call this number D.
- Look at the TL in number and divide this by the lower reference range number (normally 55 per cent). Call this number E.
- Calculate A × B × C × D × E and that is your 'mito score'.

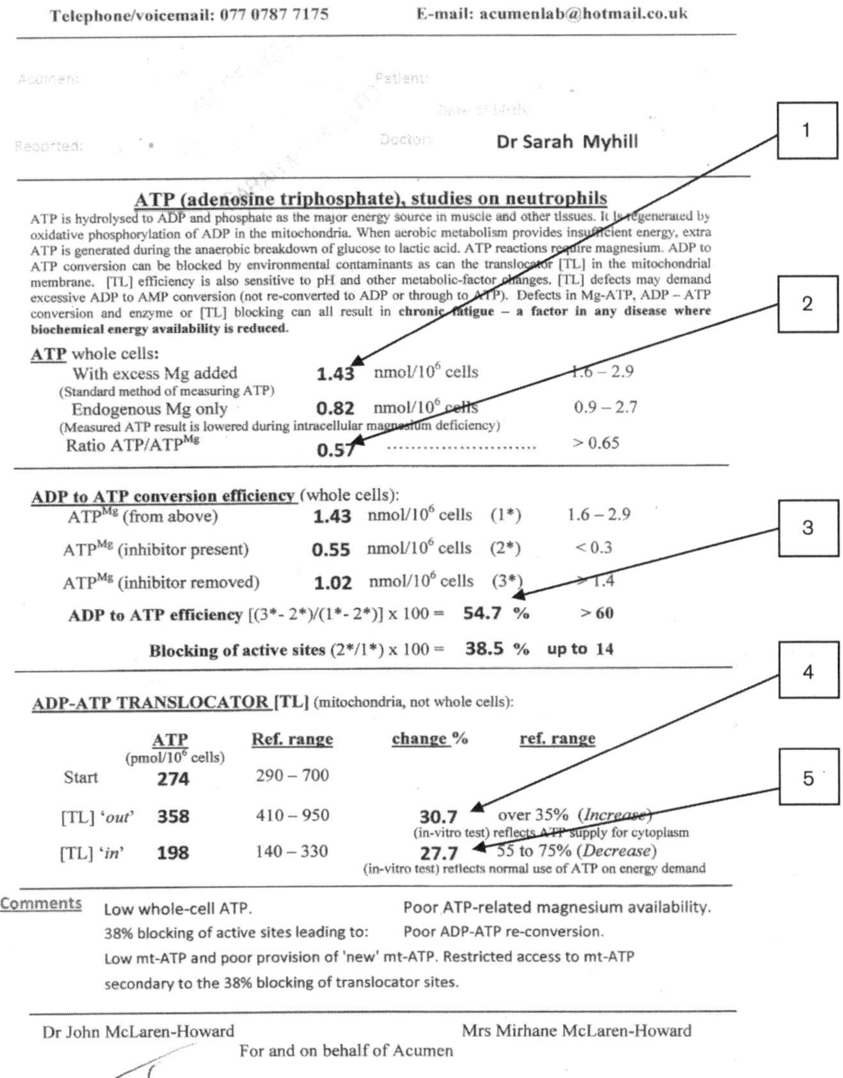

Acumen PO Box 129, Tiverton, Devon EX16 0AJ

Telephone/voicemail: 077 0787 7175 E-mail: acumenlab@hotmail.co.uk

Acumen: Patient:

Date of birth:

Reported: Doctor: **Dr Sarah Myhill**

ATP (adenosine triphosphate), studies on neutrophils

ATP is hydrolysed to ADP and phosphate as the major energy source in muscle and other tissues. It is regenerated by oxidative phosphorylation of ADP in the mitochondria. When aerobic metabolism provides insufficient energy, extra ATP is generated during the anaerobic breakdown of glucose to lactic acid. ATP reactions require magnesium. ADP to ATP conversion can be blocked by environmental contaminants as can the translocator [TL] in the mitochondrial membrane. [TL] efficiency is also sensitive to pH and other metabolic-factor changes. [TL] defects may demand excessive ADP to AMP conversion (not re-converted to ADP or through to ATP). Defects in Mg-ATP, ADP – ATP conversion and enzyme or [TL] blocking can all result in **chronic fatigue – a factor in any disease where biochemical energy availability is reduced.**

ATP whole cells:

With excess Mg added (Standard method of measuring ATP)	**1.43**	nmol/10^6 cells	1.6 – 2.9
Endogenous Mg only (Measured ATP result is lowered during intracellular magnesium deficiency)	**0.82**	nmol/10^6 cells	0.9 – 2.7
Ratio ATP/ATP^{Mg}	**0.57**	....	> 0.65

ADP to ATP conversion efficiency (whole cells):

ATP^{Mg} (from above)	**1.43**	nmol/10^6 cells	(1*)	1.6 – 2.9
ATP^{Mg} (inhibitor present)	**0.55**	nmol/10^6 cells	(2*)	< 0.3
ATP^{Mg} (inhibitor removed)	**1.02**	nmol/10^6 cells	(3*)	> 1.4
ADP to ATP efficiency [(3*- 2*)/(1*- 2*)] x 100 =	**54.7**	%		> 60
Blocking of active sites (2*/1*) x 100 =	**38.5**	%		up to 14

ADP-ATP TRANSLOCATOR [TL] (mitochondria, not whole cells):

	ATP (pmol/10^6 cells)	Ref. range	change %	ref. range
Start	**274**	290 – 700		
[TL] '*out*'	**358**	410 – 950	**30.7**	over 35% (*Increase*) (in-vitro test) reflects ATP supply for cytoplasm
[TL] '*in*'	**198**	140 – 330	**27.7**	55 to 75% (*Decrease*) (in-vitro test) reflects normal use of ATP on energy demand

Comments

Low whole-cell ATP. Poor ATP-related magnesium availability.

38% blocking of active sites leading to: Poor ADP-ATP re-conversion.

Low mt-ATP and poor provision of 'new' mt-ATP. Restricted access to mt-ATP secondary to the 38% blocking of translocator sites.

Dr John McLaren-Howard Mrs Mirhane McLaren-Howard

For and on behalf of Acumen

Figure 4.10. Sample test results for a patient with severe fatigue.

So, in this case we have:

A = 1.43 / 1.6 = 0.89;
B = 0.57 / 0.65 = 0.88;
C = 54.7 / 60 = 0.91;
D = 30.7 / 35 = 0.88 and
E = 27.7 / 55 = 0.50

This gives a 'mito score' of:
0.89 × 0.88 × 0.91 × 0.88 × 0.50 = 0.31 (About 30 per cent of 'normal').

Note: More recent ATP profile tests have a different 'range' for the 'ATP whole cells with Mg added' score. This range is now 2.1–3.4. This is because a different measurement is being taken – namely, mixed leukocytes (all types of white blood cells) rather than neutrophils alone. The calculation would be the same except that one would divide by 2.1 rather than 1.6 to arrive at figure 'A'.

Over the past 10 years I have saved the results of over 800 ATP profiles and Dr Booth is continuing to crunch the numbers. He has spotted an interesting relationship between the rate of oxidative phosphorylation (see page 55) and TL 'in' function – clearly the two are linked, but as yet we do not know the mechanisms of this. Watch this space.

Dr McLaren-Howard has many other innovative tests he uses which are helpful clinically but not yet available generally. Our first step is to find another lab that can do all the above commercially. We are working hard on this. Again, watch this space.

Confirmation of the above findings came from Nicor Lengert and Barbara Drossel (2015) in their paper, 'In silico analysis of exercise intolerance in myalgic and capillary myelitis and chronic fatigue syndrome'.[22] They analysed the energy aspect of the above biochemical pathways and concluded that the highest exertional malaise seen in CFS / ME could indeed be explained as above.

Lengert and Drossel's CFS simulations exhibited critically low levels of ATP, to the extent that an increased rate of cell death would be expected. In order to stabilise the energy supply at these very low ATP concentrations, there is a reduction in the total adenine nucleotide pool and this causes prolonged recovery time.

C. Treating the mitochondrial dysfunction

The ATP profile tests show mitochondria going slow either because they are deficient in raw materials *or* because they are being blocked. (Note, this test does not tell us about the fuel supply, the numbers of mitochondria or their control.)

1 – Mitochondria go slow because of deficiencies

Deficiencies that can lead to mitochondria going slow are principally D-ribose, magnesium, niacinamide (vitamin B3), acetyl-L-carnitine, coenzyme Q10 and vitamin B12.

D-ribose

If the absolute level of ATP present in the cells at any time is low, then this may point to poor production of de novo ATP from its raw material D-ribose. D-ribose in an individual with normal metabolism can be made from glucose via a process called the 'pentose phosphate shunt'. (This is the complex piece of biochemistry which converts six-carbon sugars into five-carbon sugars, which is the starting point for making de novo ATP.) However, this takes time and D-ribose is made slowly. This may explain the delayed fatigue in CFS/ME patients. The treatment is to supplement with D-ribose, starting with three teaspoonfuls daily (15 grams) and adjusting according to response. Sufferers may see changes within a few days. Clinically I expect to see less delayed fatigue and improvement in muscle pain and aching. D-ribose has a very short half-life and ideally should be taken in small doses throughout the day in drinks (hot or cold). Interestingly, caffeine may enhance the effects of D-ribose so I recommend taking it with green tea, coffee, tea or equivalent, so long as these are tolerated. It is worth supplementing D-ribose even with low normal results because I have so much happy feedback from patients taking this supplement.

Some people with a fermenting gut (see Chapter 7, page 107) may ferment D-ribose and worsen the situation. Fermenting gut is very common in CFS. Many CFS sufferers have to reserve D-ribose only for use as a rescue remedy if they really overdo things. The idea is that a low-carb diet used in the treatment of fermenting gut will starve out fermenting microbes so levels become so low that there will not be the numbers to ferment the occasional large dose of D-ribose before it is absorbed.

A few people may not tolerate D-ribose because it is derived from corn and small amounts of corn antigen remain to which they may react allergically. Most will react to preparations on the market that purport to be corn free, so take care!

Very low ATP may mean the patient is not pacing activity well – the moment the CFS sufferer has energy it is all too tempting to spend it because he/she has already missed out on so much. However, pacing is essential to a sustained and substantial recovery. See chapter 15 (page 183).

Magnesium

The release of energy from ATP is magnesium dependent, as is the synthesis of ATP from ADP. Magnesium is of central importance in mitochondria. Magnesium deficiency is one of the knottiest problems I have come across. I think I now know why. Having low levels of magnesium inside cells and mitochondria is a symptom of CFS/ME but also a cause of it. This is because 40 per cent of resting energy simply powers the ion pumps for sodium/potassium (Na/K) and calcium/magnesium (Ca/Mg) across cell membranes (an essential ongoing process for life). When energy supply is diminished, there is insufficient energy to fire these pumps, so magnesium cannot be drawn into cells for oxidative phosphorylation to work. If there is insufficient energy to drag magnesium into cells, then there is a further diminishing of energy delivery. This is just one of the many vicious cycles in CFS/ME.

Sufferers do not simply replete their magnesium levels through taking supplements, although this must be tried. This is because the problem is not just magnesium deficiency but also magnesium in the wrong department. Some CFS/ME sufferers need magnesium by injection to get the desired result. I think this is rather like kick-starting an engine to get it going. CFS/ME sufferers may need a spike of magnesium in the blood to push it into cells to fire up the mitochondria. I suggest patients self-inject say ½ ml of 50 per cent magnesium sulphate subcutaneously daily, usually into the roll of fat round the tummy that we all get when we sit down, using a fine insulin syringe. It astonishes me that such a tiny amount can make a big difference. Such an injection contains about 25 mg of elemental magnesium when the recommended daily amount is at least 300 mg. This is a hypertonic solution and the body does not like that; this means the injection can be painful and may leave small lumps, though with time the lumps do disappear. I also suggest warming the injection to blood heat to make it less painful. What seems to be additionally helpful is to administer the injection very slowly. This gives the magnesium a chance to disperse and dilute so rendering it less of an irritant.

Some people find magnesium by nebuliser (inhaled) works as well. Indeed, nebulised magnesium is an excellent treatment for asthma. (Please see my web page drmyhill.co.uk/wiki/Magnesium_by_nebuliser for instructions on how to make up your solution of magnesium sulphate for nebulising. All you will need is some Epsom salts, to be dissolved in water, and a nebuliser, through which you bubble the dissolved Epsom salts.)

Niacinamide (vitamin B3)

Low levels of nicotinamide adenine dinucleotide (NAD) may be a symptom of poor function of Krebs citric acid cycle (KCA – see page 63). This is because measuring NAD is a functional test and it does not just reflect vitamin B3 levels in the blood. The job of KCA is to take energy from acetyl groups and convert it into NADH (nicotinamide adenosine diphosphate), which is then of course converted to NAD in the process of driving chemi-osmosis (page 62). Therefore, to see normal levels of NAD needs not only an adequate supply of B3 but also a properly functioning Krebs citric acid cycle.

I started off using 500 mg of supplementary vitamin B3, but increasingly I use 1500 mg of slow-release niacinamide. In theory there is potential for NAD to cause liver damage. However, I have never seen this in clinical practice. I believe this is because toxic effects of drugs and vitamins result from micronutrient deficiencies. Where these are being adequately replaced the potential for toxicity is virtually zero.

I recommend using niacinamide, which does not cause flushing. Other forms of B3, such as niacin, can cause a most unpleasant hot flush. I tried it and I actually had to lie down for 10 minutes until the effect passed – most embarrassing and not like me at all!

Acetyl L-carnitine

To get fuel to burn for oxidative phosphorylation (see page 55), it needs to be transported as acetate across the mitochondrial membrane by acetyl L-carnitine. This is normally present in red meat but generally not in large enough quantities to replete the deficiencies found in fatigued states. As a routine I recommend taking supplementary acetyl L-carnitine 1–2 grams daily.

Coenzyme Q10

Coenzyme Q10 ('co-Q10') is also called ubiquinol. Why? Because it is ubiquitously present in all living cells in the animal kingdom. This reflects the fact that mitochondria are ubiquitous and the universal engine that powers all life forms. I often measure levels of co-Q10 but less so now simply because I know what the result will be – low. Indeed, as I have said before, I have never seen a normal level of co-Q10 in someone who is not already taking supplements of such. I recommend using ubiquinol 200 mg daily, often more. Dr Stephen Sinatra, the cardiologist who pioneered the use of co-Q10 in the treatment of all forms of heart disease ('the Sinatra Solution') sometimes uses 1 gram a day. Like the majority of nutritional supplements, it has no known toxicity so over-dosing is virtually impossible. (It is, however, very expensive.)

Vitamin B12 by injection

Vitamin B12 is a big player in CFS/ME. It multi-tasks and is an essential part of the methylation cycle, protein synthesis, energy delivery mechanisms, detoxification and, of course, making new red blood cells. Furthermore, the doses of B12 which work best for individuals vary enormously. This means we have laboratory guidelines that give us a level of B12 in the serum which is sufficient to prevent pernicious anaemia. However, this may well not be sufficient to allow people to function to their full potential. This means we cannot rely on any measurement of B12 to find out if a person has adequate levels.

There are probably epigenetic influences here as well – so, for example, we know that Japanese prisoners of war who suffered severe malnutrition for some years required much higher doses of B vitamins generally in order to remain healthy for the rest of their lives. This is obviously an extreme example, but life may well throw up similar episodes of milder problems. So, for example, being a vegetarian I know is a major risk factor for CFS/ME and vegetarians have a lower intake of B12 than carnivores.

Vitamin B12 is extraordinarily safe stuff – indeed, a colleague of mine commented that the only way you could kill yourself with vitamin B12 would be to drown in it. That means using B12 in high doses is a safe and reasonable thing to do.

We then have the added problem that vitamin B12 is very poorly absorbed – its absorption requires a sufficiently acid stomach and the presence of intrinsic factor in the gastric juice, together with a normal section of terminal ileum. As we age our ability to absorb B12 declines but our requirement for it increases as we become biochemically less efficient. I argue, therefore, that at a certain age – perhaps 50, and certainly 60 onwards – we would all benefit from a monthly injection of vitamin B12.

Dr Patrick Kingsley in his work with patients with multiple sclerosis found that some patients did not respond clinically until they received up to 20 mg (that is, 20,000 microgams) a day by injection. In patients with CFS/ME we know there is a pro-inflammatory tendency. Professor Martin Pall identified a pro-inflammatory cycle which he calls the NO/ONOO cycle; it happens that vitamin B12 is an essential part of damping this down.

I am also aware clinically that for many people, injections are superior to oral supplements. I suspect the reason for this is that an injection really spikes the level of B12 in the blood and, therefore, forces it into the system by the law of mass action – it is a little bit like the Heineken advert: it reaches parts that other beers cannot!

The bottom line is that the only way to ensure good B12 status is a trial of vitamin B12 by injection. Ideally this should be in the form methylcobalamin since this is the one which needs least processing in the body to be effective. We used to be able to get vitamin B12 5 mg/ml but it is much more difficult now, so we have to muddle around with what we can get when the high-dose stuff is not available.

Putting the regime in place

A summary of nutritional regimes to support mitochondria is detailed at the end of this chapter (page 79).

If you are unable to access mitochondrial function tests then these regimes can still be safely put in place with no risk of toxicity problems. Indeed, it is my experience that the abnormalities I see are so predictable that if finances are tight then I would prefer to see money spent on the above treatment regimes than on tests. Having said that, the ATP profiles have been very helpful in getting welfare state benefits for CFS/ME patients because they provide an objective measure of fatigue, and also these profiles do often flag up particular areas of concern – for example, the need for detox regimes if there are blockages caused by toxins (see next section).

2 – Mitochondria go slow because of blocking

Blocking of mitochondria can show up in the synthesis of ATP (conversion of ADP to ATP) or because of poor translocator protein function. We do not know all the causes of blocking but essentially they divide into the following categories:

1. Blockages from toxins from internal metabolism ('endogenous')
2. Blockages from toxins from the external world ('exogenous')

Blockages from internal metabolism

Lactic acid (the acid bit, not the lactate bit). This is what prevents athletes breaking records. When CFS/ME sufferers do not pace activities properly and continue to push themselves, they actually perform less well. It is a bit like athletes in a state of chronic over-training. Telling my patients to do less is difficult.

Sugar. Running a high blood sugar level decreases energy – indeed, I suspect this partly explains the fatigue of diabetes and metabolic syndrome.

Aldehydes. John McLaren-Howard often finds evidence of malondialdehyde stuck onto translocator protein. This is a symptom of poor antioxidant status. I treat this with B12 injections together with nutritional supplements (zinc, copper, manganese, selenium, glutathione and co-Q10).

Products of the fermenting gut. These include bacterial endotoxin, various alcohols, aldehydes and acetones, hydrogen sulphide, D-lactate and many other possible nasties. They do not show up on translocator protein studies, possibly because they are volatile, but it is biologically plausible and fits with my clinical experience that they should block mitochondria. The treatment of course is as per fermenting gut – see Chapter 7 (page 107).

Blockages from chemicals from the external world

These blockages result from toxic metals and volatile organic compounds – see Chapter 20 on detoxing (page 233). They can also come from prescription drugs.

MITOCHONDRIA MAY BE DAMAGED BY PRESCRIPTION DRUGS

A very useful resource produced by 'mitoaction' is their report *Drug-Induced Mitochondrial Dysfunction: An Emerging Model for Idiosyncratic Drug Toxicity*.[23] This concludes that many drugs with organ toxicity have a 'mitochondrial liability'. A screen of more than 550 drugs revealed that 34 per cent of these had mitochondrial liabilities – that is to say that there was potential for mitochondrial harm resulting from their use. The severity of such adverse effects was observed to be idiosyncratic.

The specifics listed next were noted.

MITOCHONDRIAL IMPAIRMENT BY DRUGS RECEIVING A BLACK BOX WARNING*

Liver mitochondria

- Antivirals: abacavir, didanosine, emtricitabine, entecavir, lamivudine, nevirapine, stavudine, telbivudine, tenofovir, tipranavir, zalcitabine, zidovudine
- Anti-cancer: dacarbazine, flutamide, gemtuzumab, methotrexate, pentostatin, tamoxifen

---

* A Black Box Warning is the strictest warning in the labelling of prescription drugs or products by the United States Food and Drug Administration (FDA) when there is reasonable evidence of an association of a serious hazard with the drug.

- Antibiotics: isoniazid, streptozocin, trovafloxacin
- Antifungals: ketoconazole (oral)
- CNS (central nervous system) problems: dantrolene, divalproex, sodium felbamate, naltrexone, nefazodone, valproic acid
- Hypertension: bosentan

Cardiovascular mitochondria

- Anthracyclines: daunorubicin, doxorubicin, epirubicin, idarubicin
- NSAIDs (non-steroidal anti-inflammatory drugs): celecoxib, diclofenac, diflunisal, etodolac, fenoprofen, ibuprofen, indomethacin, ketoprofen, mefenamic acid, meloxicam, nabumetone, naproxen, oxaprozin, piroxicam, salsalate, sulindac, thioridazine, tolmetin
- Anaesthetic: bupivacaine
- Anti-cancer: arsenic trioxide, cetuximab, denileukin, diftitox, mitoxantrone, tamoxifen
- Beta-blocker: atenolol
- Antiarhythmics: amiodarone (oral), disopyramide, dofetilide, ibutilide
- CNS amphetamines: atomoxetin, droperidol, methamphetamine, pergolide
- Diabetes: pioglitazone, rosiglitazone

Conclusion

We have seen that mitochondrial dysfunction is key to the mechanisms that drive CFS and that we now have an objective test, the mitochondrial function profile test, or 'ATP profiles', that gives us a precise measurement of that level of dysfunction. Not only this, but ATP profiles also identify where things are going wrong and why, meaning that we have further clues as to treatments. These treatments essentially fall into two categories:

1. a deficiency in the raw materials, for which the treatment is supplementation
2. a blockage or blockages in the biochemical pathways, for which the treatment is the various methods of detoxification (see Chapter 20, page 233).

In addition, there may have been mitochondrial damage done by prescription medications.

CHAPTER 4 SUMMARY

The mechanisms of energy delivery in the body: it's mitochondria, not hypochondria

For those without the time or energy to digest the full chapter:

- Mitochondria are the 'engines' of our bodies. These 'organelles' (microstructures within cells) are present in the vast majority of cells and are responsible for generating energy.
- Mitochondria are implicated in nearly all disease processes, from cancer and heart disease to autism and dementia.
- This is not surprising because if you impair energy delivery to an organ then that organ will fail.
- The central cause of CFS/ME is mitochondrial failure: 'It's mitochondria, not hypochondria!'
- The ATP profiles test can tell us how well, or badly, mitochondria are functioning.
- This test also identifies the processes in the functioning of mitochondria that are failing, giving highly significant information for the treatment of a patient's CFS.
- Once the extent, and specifics, of mitochondrial failure have been identified in a particular patient, treatments can be applied.
- Mitochondria may be going slow because of deficiencies in 'raw materials', such as D-ribose, magnesium, niacinamide, acetyl L-carnitine, coenzyme Q10 and vitamin B12, all of which can be supplemented. See below for the mitochondrial support supplement package.
- Mitochondria may be going slow because of blocking caused by toxins from either the internal metabolism or from the outside world. Further testing ('translocator protein studies') can identify which toxins are causing these blockages.
- Such blockages can be treated via chelation with DMSA (see page 238), selenium, zinc, clays such as zeolite, high-dose vitamin C and iodine, and suchlike. Heating regimes, saunaing, etc, can also be used to get rid of toxins causing blockages. See Chapter 20 on detoxing (page 233).

- Mitochondria can also be damaged by prescription drugs, and this possibility should also be considered.

The mitochondrial package of supplements is listed in Table 4.1.

Table 4.1.

When	What	Dose	How	Why
With breakfast	Co-Q10	200–400 mg	Swallow	Mops up free radicals
Vital for the smooth running of mitochondria (the oil of the engine)	Niacinamide	1500 mg slow release	Swallow	Essential intermediate between Krebs citric acid cycle (see Fig 4.7) and chemi-osmosis (see page 62)
	Carnitine	1–2 grams	Swallow	The acetate fuel pipe nozzle to get fuel inside mitochondria for burning
	D-ribose	5 grams	In coffee or tea	Raw material to make new ATP. Good for delayed fatigue. Caffeine stimulates cyclic AMP but take care if there is fermenting gut (see Chapter 7)
	Magnesium	½ ml 50% magnesium sulphate	Subcutaneous injection (or by nebuliser – see drmyhill.co.uk)	Kick-starts the mitochondrial engines
	Vitamin B12	½ to 5 mg	Subcutaneous injection	Improves energy delivery. Excellent for fatigue, foggy brain, mood, detoxification, protein synthesis, etc. My favourite prescription!
	Copper	1 mg	Swallow	If SODase is low
	Glutathione	250 mg	Swallow	Vital for glutathione peroxidase and also to detox toxic metals. Arguably we should all be taking this for life

When	What	Dose	How	Why
Lunch	D-ribose	5 grams	In coffee or tea	Last dose of caffeine 2 pm
	Manganese	3 mg	Swallow	If SODase is low
Supper	D-ribose	5 grams	No tea or coffee	Caffeine disturbs sleep
Bedtime	Zinc	30 mg	Swallow	Especially if SODase is low, but arguably for life since zinc deficiency is pandemic
	Selenium	300 mcg	Swallow	Especially if glutathione peroxidase is low, but arguably for life since selenium deficiency is pandemic

NB: 'mg' = milligrams (one thousandth of a gram); 'mcg' = micrograms (one thousandth of a milligram)

CHAPTER 5

Energy delivery mechanisms: thyroid and adrenal function

The thyroid and adrenal glands allow us to match energy delivery closely to energy demands. (In my car analogy in Chapter 4 I likened the thyroid to the car's accelerator pedal and the adrenal glands to the gear box.) To do otherwise is energy wasted which spells evolutionary disaster. It is a spike of thyroid hormones followed by adrenal hormones that wake us up in the morning. Adrenal hormones allow us to go into overdrive in response to stress – the stress of hunting or being hunted. Thyroid hormones decline in winter so that we go into semi-hibernation to conserve energy when food is scarce.

Thyroid gland

The term 'thyroid gland' is derived from the Latin *glandula thyreoidea*. *Glandula* means 'gland' in Latin, and *thyreoidea* can be traced back to the Ancient Greek word θυρεοειδής, meaning 'shield-like / shield-shaped'. The shape and location of the thyroid gland can be seen in Figure 5.1 (page 82).

Hypothyroidism (underactive thyroid) – the under-performing accelerator pedal of our engines

Anybody with CFS could be hypothyroid. Thyroid blood tests are an essential first step, but even a normal test never entirely excludes the possibility of hypothyroidism. That is because of hormone receptor resistance – in other words, the thyroid hormones may be there, but the relevant receptors are not

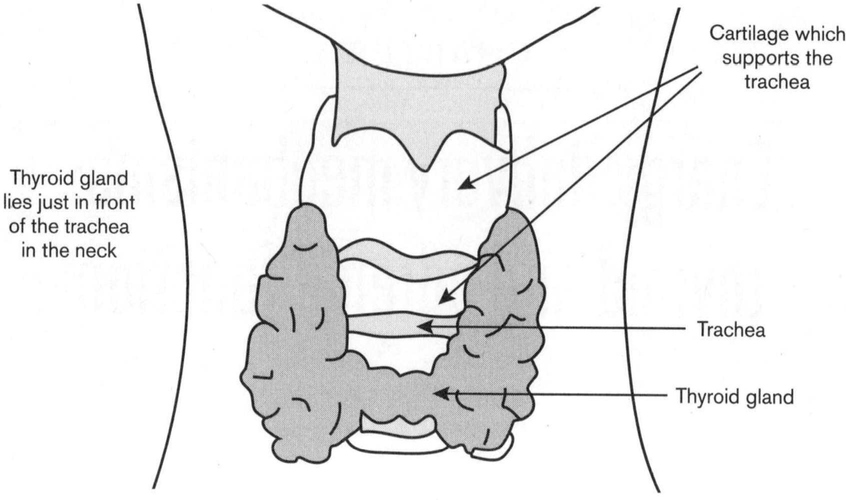

Figure 5.1. Position and shape of the thyroid gland.

responding. This is akin to type 2 diabetes where insulin is high but again there is no receptor response – this is called 'insulin resistance'.

Hypothyroidism is one of the worst diagnosed and worst treated conditions in the UK. Dr Kenneth Blanchard, consultant endocrinologist, reckons that 20 per cent of all Western women are hypothyroid. This concurs with my clinical experience that hypothyroidism is hugely under diagnosed. This is a major source of misery, associated with disease and premature death. How has this situation been allowed to happen?

I consider myself an expert on hypothyroidism for all the wrong reasons. I have received no formal training outside standard medical teachings, but I have been subject to investigation on numerous occasions by the General Medical Council and its Expert Witnesses because of my stance on the prescribing of thyroid hormones. In this respect I have done battle with some of the top endocrinologists in the country – but my practice has not been found wanting. All charges were dropped with no case to answer. I continue to use thyroid hormones as I always have done, through carefully listening to the patient, regularly monitoring blood tests, ensuring the patient remains euthyroid (no signs of under- or overactive thyroid) and, with the patient's consent, keeping General Practitioners informed.

The treatment of hypothyroidism was pioneered by Dr Gordon Skinner. He saw many patients with post-viral chronic fatigue syndrome through his work as a consultant virologist. He found that addressing and correcting thyroid function was an extremely helpful intervention. He recognised that the clinical response of the patient was just as important as the blood tests. Arguably more so. This brought him into conflict with the endocrinologists and he too was subject to GMC investigation. Despite years of burdensome GMC investigation, Dr Skinner continued to practise and in doing so helped thousands of patients. He died unexpectedly and prematurely – I have little doubt that the stress of dealing with the GMC was a contributory factor.

So it is little wonder that doctors stick to the rule book in the treatment of hypothyroidism. No wonder patients cannot find doctors to help them! They have to work it out for themselves.

Symptoms of hypothyroidism

- Poor energy delivery symptoms: all the symptoms detailed in Chapter 3 (page 33).
- Slow metabolism (that is, hibernation mode): weight gain, inability to lose weight, constipation.
- Loss of the circadian rhythm: being an owl, late to drop off to sleep and late to wake.
- Inability to improve physical fitness.
- Metabolic syndrome that does not respond to a low glycaemic-index diet. This results from an inability to keto-adapt – that is, the body cannot switch into fat-burning as opposed to glucose-burning mode, and so is particularly susceptible to low blood sugar.
- Fluid retention: puffy ankles, nerve compression such as carpal tunnel syndrome.
- Hair loss: typically the outer third of the eyebrows. (I would love to know the mechanism of this.)
- Infertility, premenstrual tension, menorrhagia.

Signs of hypothyroidism

- Goitre (abnormal swelling of the thyroid gland that causes a lump to form in the neck): as Figure 5.1 shows, the thyroid gland is shaped like a bow tie and sits where a bow tie should be.
- Fluid retention, which may cause puffy eyes and puffy face.

As I was shopping my daughters used to delight in diagnosing fellow shoppers with hypothyroidism using their embarrassingly strident voices. Another mistake I made was to tell my girls that one symptom of tertiary syphilis was a saddle nose – this meant they kept creeping round the sides of strangers to observe the contours of their nose and try to make a star diagnosis!

- Large tongue: One may see the impression of teeth where the tongue lies against them. Furthermore, if the tongue is protruded, the width of the tongue touches the corner of the lips.
- Hoarse voice, because the larynx is slightly swollen. One patient presented with loss of her usual ability to sing, now happily restored.
- Sleep apnoea, either obstructive (due to oedema – swelling) or central (brain 'forgets' to breathe) – see page 197.
- Slowed Achilles tendon reflex: I suspect all reflexes are slowed, indeed all nerve transmission will be slowed, but it is the Achilles that doctors like to test.
- Dry, poor quality skin and hair.
- Other blood tests showing high cholesterol, enlarged red blood cells (macrocytosis), anaemia.

Doctors do not listen to patients

Doctors ignore the patient's story. Patients will paint a classical clinical picture, listing many of the above symptoms, but that seems to cut no ice with their physician. Many patients have actually tried thyroid hormones that they have purchased online and felt considerably better as a result. Again this cuts no ice. The only thing the doctors are interested in are the blood tests – and they even get the interpretation of those horribly wrong.

Misinterpretation of blood tests

The common reasons for this misinterpretation of thyroid tests are as follows.

The upper reference range for thyroid-stimulating hormone (TSH) is set too high

When levels of thyroid hormones in the blood start to fall, the pituitary gland increases its output of thyroid-stimulating hormone (TSH), which kicks the thyroid into life and increases the output of thyroid hormones. If the thyroid gland starts to fail, this is reflected by levels of TSH rising. The question is, at what point should the prescription of thyroid hormones begin?

The reference range for TSH in the UK varies enormously from one laboratory to another. This means that in some locations a thyroid prescription would not be given until the TSH rises above 5.0 mIU/l (milli-International Units per litre). As a result of research, the reference range for TSH in the United States has now been reduced so that anybody with a TSH above 3.0 mIU/l is now prescribed thyroid hormones. This research has shown that people with a TSH above 3.0 mIU/l are at increased risk of arterial disease (a major cause of death in Western culture), insulin resistance (and therefore diabetes), inflammation and hypercoagulability (sticky blood). Indeed, there is a recommendation afoot in America to further reduce the threshold for prescribing to 2.5 mIU/l.

What is completely illogical is that in the UK the target TSH level for patients on thyroid replacement therapy is often stated as being less than 2 mIU/l, and sometines even less than 1.5 mIU/l. This is a ridiculous anachronism given that prescription is not recommended until levels exceed much higher levels, say, 5.0 mIU/l. So, someone could have a level of 4.0 mIU/l and not be receiving thyroid replacement therapy (because their level is not above 5.0 mIU/l), whereas if someone was on thyroid replacement therapy, a level of 4.0 mIU/l would be considered much too high and would need to be brought down to below 2.0 mIU/l or even 1.5 mIU/l.

We should amend the threshold for prescribing thyroid hormones in the UK to 3.0mlU/l, or better still 2.5 mIU/l.

There is a further inconsistency in BTA (British Thyroid Association) guidelines. The level of thyroid hormones in pregnancy is critical for foetal development. For pregnancy, the target for TSH is a level below 2.5 mIU/l. Furthermore, requirements during pregnancy increase, so thyroid function should be checked every three months. What is the logic of only prescribing thyroid hormones to a non-pregnant woman when her TSH is above 5.0 mIU/l but if pregnant prescribing them when levels exceed 2.5 mIU/l? Indeed, research has shown that the IQ of the child is inversely proportional to the TSH of the mother in pregnancy – low TSH results in clever children. Again, I was subject to GMC investigation for pointing this fact out to an NHS GP and prescribing thyroid hormones to our mutual patient. The astonishing outcome was that my actions were fully supported by the GMC Expert Witness, but the GP was also exonerated. I can only infer that clever kids are not desirable in that practice.

Dr Kenneth Blanchard states that he considers reliance on a test for TSH level to diagnose hypothyroidism to be the biggest single medical error of modern times. It has resulted in millions of people missing out on this safe, life-transforming, disease-preventing treatment.

The reference ranges for thyroid hormones are falling

Reference ranges are based on the average levels in the general population. The problem is, the general population is no longer normal – micronutrient deficiencies are pandemic (especially of iodine), and we are all poisoned by pollution (especially fluorides, bromides, mercury and radioactivity from pollution and radiological investigations, such as mammography. [Yes, sigh, thanks to the GMC I am also an expert in mammography.]) All our thyroid glands are slightly under-functioning. As a result, the reference ranges for normal levels are falling. The private lab that I use has a normal range for 'free T4' of 12–22 picomols (pmol, an SI unit of amount of substance equal to 10^{-12} moles) per litre. In contrast, some NHS labs have a reference range of 7–14 pmol per litre. Furthermore, in the first edition of the British Medical Association book, *Understanding Thyroid Disorders*, consultant endocrinologist Dr Antony Toft stated that some people do not feel well until their free T4 is running at 30 pmol/l.[24] (In more recent editions Dr Toft changed his advice and so you may not find this comment in newer versions of this book. Please see www.drmyhill.co.uk/wiki/Thyroid_disease_-_how_to_persuade_your_GP_to_diagnose_and_treat#UNDERSTANDING_THYROID_DISORDERS_by_DR_ANTHONY_TOFT for further discussion.) Note: T4 is the (relatively) inactive form of thyroid hormone and needs to be converted into T3, the biologically active form in order to be used by the body.

Population reference range versus individual reference range – they are not the same

The population reference range for levels of thyroid hormone in the blood is not the same as the individual normal range. We differ as individuals in our biochemistry as we differ in our looks, intelligence and morphology. This biochemical variation should be taken into account when it comes to prescribing thyroid hormones.

The population reference range for free T4 is 12–22 pmol/l. A patient, therefore, with blood levels of 12.1 would be told they were normal because they are within the population reference range, but actually that person's personal normal range may be high. They may feel much better running a high T4 of say 22 – that is, nearly twice as much but still within the population reference range.

Research done originally in the UK, and now repeated in America, clearly shows that the individual normal range of thyroid hormones is not the same as the population reference range.[25]

In order to find out who the individuals are with high or low normal range, patients have to be assessed clinically as well as biochemically. In actual UK clinical practice this is rarely done except by a few physicians conversant with this issue. I suspect the nub of the matter is that it is much easier in terms of time and intellectual challenge to treat a blood test than a patient.

Some people feel better on different preparations of thyroid hormones

In theory, if a patient has been shown to be hypothyroid, then all his/her symptoms should improve with synthetic sodium thyroxin (T4). In practice, this is not always the case – there is no doubt that clinically some patients feel very much better taking biologically identical hormones, such as natural thyroid (a dried extract of pig thyroid gland which is a mix of T4 and T3). Indeed, before synthetic thyroid hormones became available, all patients were routinely treated with natural thyroid. The purity and stability of these preparations have been long established – indeed, much longer established than synthetic thyroxin.

Part of the reason why people feel better taking natural bio-identical hormones is that some people are not good at converting T4 (which is relatively inactive) to T3 (which is biologically active). However, this does not explain the improvement in every case. It is difficult to explain why there should be an additional effect, but for many people it is the difference between drinking cheap French plonk and good quality Spanish Rioja. The alcohol content is the same, but the experience completely different! It may well be there are other thyroid hormones (such as T1 and T2) which have a hitherto unrecognised benefit.

Timing of dosing

I have learned much more from consultant endocrinologist Dr Kenneth Blanchard's book, *The Functional Approach to Treating Hypothyroidism* (2012). He makes many useful clinical points, including:

- Thyroid hormones should be taken with food – he observes that cravings can be triggered by thyroid hormones taken on an empty stomach.
- T4 (thyroxin) is slow acting and 'base loads', meaning that there will be a time lag between taking (inactive) T4 and it being synthesised into (active) T3 that the body can use. The body needs a constant level of T4 'ready to be converted' into T3 – the 'base load'. T4 is termed the 'night hormone' (in contrast to T3, the 'day hormone') – we should split our daily dose of it into two. The evening dose should be taken with supper, which should be at least four hours before bedtime. For some people, this improves sleep quality. Many find it impossible to remember to take half the dose this way

and in this case they should go back to once-daily dosing – better to take all at once than forget half the dose.
- By contrast, T3 is the day hormone that wakes us up. Our circadian rhythms are determined by light, via the pineal gland (melatonin) and enacted by the pituitary gland, the conductor of the endocrine orchestra. TSH levels rise sharply at midnight and this is followed by spikes of T4 at 4 am and of T3 at 5 am. Cortisol also spikes in the morning. As they come together, they trigger wakefulness. Some people are improved by taking a morning dose of T3 at 5 am.
- Our requirements change with the seasons – in Nature TSH falls in the winter, and so levels of T4 and T3 fall; this puts us into semi-hibernation and allows energy conservation by causing mild fatigue and depression, with greater need for sleep. The reverse is true for the summer. In modern times, with food and warmth aplenty, the imperative to do this has declined. However, some people need more thyroid hormones in winter to prevent severe fatigue and depression. In this event, Dr Blanchard suggests 'jump starting' followed by a different maintenance dose – so, for example, in the autumn someone taking 100 micrograms (mcg) of T4 would have a jump start of 150 mcg for three days, then a maintenance dose of 110 mcg. In the spring one would do the reverse – stop T4 for three days, then return to the usual 100 mcg per day.

This may or may not be important but it emphasises the importance of giving patients all the information they need in order to tweak the dose for best effect. Some of my patients take a little more thyroid if they have a busy day ahead, and less on holiday. Remember, the word 'doctor' comes from the Greek meaning 'to teach'. We need to teach patients the rules, give them the tools and let them get on with their lives independently.

Some people only feel well using pure T3

This fact can only be explained by thyroid hormone receptor resistance. The idea here is that the T3 receptor is blocked. Sometimes very high doses of T3 are required to overcome that resistance and restore normal clinical function.

At present we do not have biochemical tests to predict who these people are. A 'reverse T3' test may help but may not. If symptoms are typical of hypothyroidism but the patient does not respond to T4 or T4/T3 mixes, then a trial of pure T3 may be in order. T3 is short acting and must be taken at least three, possibly five, times daily. The smallest size tablet is prescription-only tertroxin 20 mcg (equivalent to 100 mcg of T4). A starting dose would be 10 mcg split into three doses, which is tricky. I suggest crushing half a tablet, and using a wet finger-tip to take a third of the powder three times daily. One may know within a few days if this is making a difference but a proper trial would be a few weeks. For details, see Paul Robinson's excellent book on the subject, *Recovering with T3: My Journey from Hypothyroidism to Good Health Using the T3 Thyroid Hormone.*[26] (For more detailed discussion see www.nahypothyroidism.org/thyroid-hormone-transport where the importance of pure T3 is explained in terms of the transport of T3 across cell membranes.)

I have had one patient who required 180 mcg of T3 to recover completely from her CFS. As part of the treatment, she also went on to a strict ketogenic diet. Not only did she lose weight and look wonderful, but she was able to reduce her dose of T3 to a more physiological level. This experience I have repeated with others; this may be explained by the other interventions I routinely make, such as improving micronutrient status and detoxing. However, there is something about metabolic syndrome that I suspect also leads to thyroid hormone receptor resistance. Indeed, in practice I very often see this 'unholy trinity' of metabolic syndrome, hypothyroidism and allergy.

Blood tests for hypothyroidism

The bare minimum of testing that is required is to measure levels of TSH, free T4 and free T3. This we can now do on a finger-drop sample of blood – a very useful DIY test. Table 5.1 shows how to interpret the results.

Remember that thyroid hormones manifest through kicking mitochondria into action. If your mitochondria are down, then taking thyroid hormones may make things worse – it is like pressing on the accelerator pedal when the engine cannot respond; it may scream at you but you cannot go any faster! Even if you cannot access tests for mitochondrial function you should at least take the package of supplements to support mitochondria (Chapter 4, page 51) and perhaps consider some detox regimes, as noted in Chapter 20 (page 233).

Trialing thyroid hormones

A trial of thyroid hormones would be:

- Thyroxin 25 mcg with breakfast for two weeks. If all is well, go to . . .
- Thyroxin 50 mcg with breakfast for two weeks. If all is well, go to . . .

Table 5.1. How to interpret the results of the thyroid finger-prick test

TSH: range 0.15–3.0 mIU/l	Free T4 (fT4): range 12–22 pmol	Free T3 (fT3): range 0.1–6.8 pmol/l	If clinically hypothyroid then trial of:	Comments
More than 3.00	Irrelevant	Irrelevant	Thyroxin 25–75 mcg then re-check blood	Also check thyroid antibodies for auto-immunity
In range	Below 16	In range	Thyroxin 25–75 mcg then recheck blood	May feel better running fT4 at top of range
In range	In range	Below 4 – could be poor converter of T4 to T3	Trial of natural thyroid ½ grain to 1½ grains (30 mg to 90 mg)	May feel better running fT3 at top of range
Below range	Above range	Above range		Could be thyrotoxic i.e. overactive – URGENT REFERRAL
In range	In range or high	High or above range	Possibly T3 receptor resistance	Address all other causes of fatigue before considering trials of T3

- Thyroxin 50 mcg with breakfast plus 25 mcg with supper (at least four hours before bedtime). If all is well, then wait four weeks (it takes this long for the TSH to readjust), then re-check all the bloods.

This gives us two points to plot on the graph of your blood TSH, T4 and T3 levels and, together with the clinical information, an idea of whether there is scope to increase the dose further. Most people need at least 50 mcg and some up to 300 mcg; a typical average dose is 50–150 mcg depending on size, age and activity.

Natural thyroid hormones

With respect to natural thyroid, this is a mixture of T4 and T3. Roughly speaking, one grain of natural thyroid is equivalent to 75 mcg of thyroxin.

Are you clinically 'euthyroid'?

Clinically 'euthyroid' is to say, are there any symptoms or signs of an overactive thyroid? This is not as easy as one might think, simply because the symptoms of too much thyroid hormone are the same as too much of the stress hormone adrenaline. Indeed, in the body they have similar effects. Sometimes it is impossible to distinguish, especially if the patient is chronically stressed and constantly pouring out adrenaline.

The main symptoms and signs of too much thyroid hormone would be:

Short term (hours to days). Irritability and anxiety, loss of sleep, fine tremor, palpitations, fast pulse (regularly more than 90 bpm) and high blood pressure. (All these can also be caused by adrenaline. I know – I experience them every time I go team chasing!)

Longer term (days to weeks). Weight loss (because of too much fat burning), bulging eyes (usually associated with an autoimmune thyrotoxicosis).

Initial improvement followed by decline

Dr Blanchard observed that some patients improved on thyroxin and then worsened. He describes a 'sweet spot' of optimal levels of T4. He believes the reason for this is that TSH is partly responsible for converting T4 to T3, so if levels of these hormones are too high, TSH is switched off and with that comes a switching off of T4 to T3 conversion. T3 is the day hormone that fires us up and because T4 is slow-acting there may be a delay in noticing this 'switch off' of T4 converting to T3, and this can be clinically very confusing.

Another explanation may be that, having been underactive for some years, the thyroid hormone receptors have become more sensitive; this sensitivity then normalises with treatment. One may have to increase the dose in order to get a result.

Monitoring treatment just by using a TSH level can be misleading

It is vital to measure levels of free T4, and ideally free T3 as well, and assess the patient clinically – that is, how does he/she feel – in order to achieve and maintain the optimum dose of thyroid hormone. Are there any clinical symptoms of under- or over-dosing?

It is my experience that the above approaches are invariably scowled at by doctors, especially endocrinologists (with a few notable exceptions). Doctors do not realise what power they wield over patients. I have seen so many people who have stopped treatment and given up their quality of life simply because 'the doctor was not happy with me and the blood tests are normal.' Poppy cock! Worse than that, they tell patients they will get heart disease and osteoporosis if they continue to take thyroid supplements. Whilst this advice holds for patients with thyrotoxicosis (overactive thyroid), it is also true for people with underactive thyroids!

It is all about balance. Get this right, for quality and quantity of life.

The current state of affairs

I no longer have the time to see and treat the many people who contact my office. Worse still, there are very few other doctors who treat thyroid disorders in the above way. This is resulting in epidemics of disease and misery. What to do?

Many people, quite understandably, take control of their health without resorting to doctors. Now people can access tests directly without needing doctor referral. Furthermore, we have excellent, inexpensive devices for home monitoring of blood pressure and pulse. I hope the above advice will give people the confidence and knowledge to do such, safely and effectively.

Adrenal glands

The term 'adrenal' comes from *ad-* (Latin for 'near') and *renes* (Latin for 'kidney'); the location of the adrenal glands can be seen in Figure 5.2.

The adrenal glands – the gear box of our engines

The adrenal glands are responsible for the body's hormonal response to demand, when above normal energy use is required to deal with an extraordinary

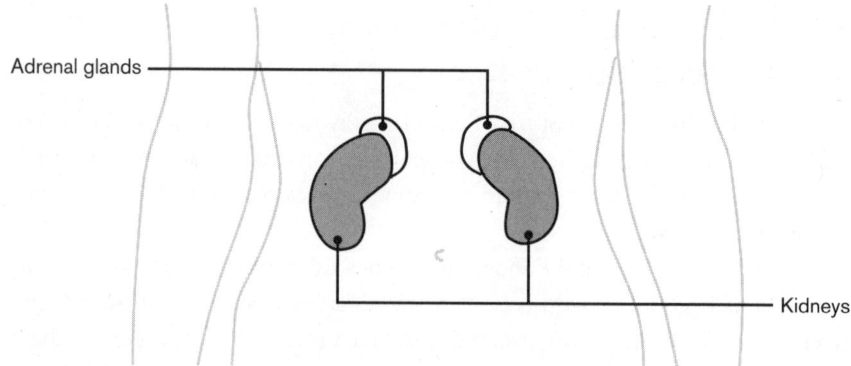

Figure 5.2. Location of the adrenal glands.

situation. The immediate stress response is to secrete adrenaline, which produces the fight-or-flight reaction. The medium-term response hormone is cortisol, together with DHEA making up the long-term stress hormone response. Cortisol suppresses the immune system, breaks down tissues and has a generally catabolic effect. However, these effects are balanced out by DHEA, which has the opposite (anabolic) effect, activating the immune system and building up tissues. All adrenal hormones are anti-inflammatory; that makes sense – it means energy can be diverted into the necessary departments to deal with stress.

All these hormones are made from cholesterol. It may be significant that the first biochemical step from cholesterol to pregnenolone (see Figure 5.3) takes place in our mitochondria – the very department which is malfunctioning in many CFS/ME sufferers.

There is a one-way flow of hormone production that starts with cholesterol upstream – as shown in Figure 5.3.

Both cortisol and DHEA are essential for life – too little cortisol causes the life-threatening condition Addison's disease (see page 98); too much causes the debilitating condition Cushing's syndrome. The name of the game is to get the right balance. To achieve this, both hormones must be measured. This can be done with the adrenal stress profile (ASP) test (see the next section). By measuring and supplementing within the physiological range, with biologically identical hormones, one is not going to get any unpleasant side effects – in other words, we are trying to copy Nature and restore normality.

The ASP test looks at cortisol and DHEA levels over 24 hours. It entails taking salivary samples through the day (yippee, no needles). Indeed, salivary sampling is felt to be the most accurate way of assessing steroid hormone levels because this gets round the problem of protein binding, which can distort blood results.

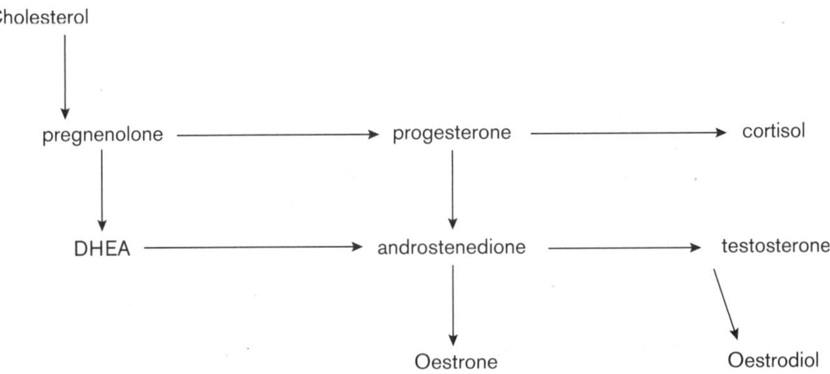

Figure 5.3. The sequence of adrenal hormone production, starting with cholesterol.

An abnormal result may be a symptom of other problems or it may cause problems in its own right. The response of the body to stress (any stress – infectious, nutritional, emotional, physical) is to increase the output of stress hormones. This gears the body up for action by raising blood pressure, increasing heart rate, improving mental alertness (which can cause anxiety), increasing energy supply and so on. This gearing up is metabolically very inefficient because it uses up lots of energy, but totally desirable if one has to fight for one's life. This reaction is essential for short-term stress, but unsustainable in the long term. So time for rest and recovery is equally essential.

Problems arise when the stress is unremitting because eventually the output of the adrenal glands will fall, making one far less able to tolerate stress. This is in addition to other energy-delivery mechanisms also being exhausted. Indeed, this is often a complaint of my CFS/ME patients – they simply do not tolerate stress at all well.

This pattern of stress response was beautifully described by the Hungarian endocrinologist Dr Hans Selye in his 'general adaptation syndrome'. This describes the body's response to shock and stress in terms of adrenal function and adrenal fatigue. Indeed, it was Selye who coined the term 'stress'. His book *The Stress of Life* is essential reading for any therapist. Selye has been described as the 'Einstein of Medicine'. As he pointed out, we are all constantly immersed in stress; some of it is joyful stress – many enjoy the adrenaline buzz of a serious, potentially dangerous, challenge. Problems arise when we cannot adapt to a stressor and we end up with disease and unhappiness. Pathological stress is the clinical picture we see when we do not have the energy to deal with demands.

The diagnosis of stress is clinical and usually self-evident. However, an adrenal stress profile test, as available from Genova Diagnostic Labs, gives us a further handle on this. The pattern of the result from the adrenal stress profile test gives some idea as to where one is along the stress-response time-line.

Interpretation of the adrenal stress index test for DHEA and cortisol levels

Levels of DHEA and cortisol vary according to the level of stress and for how long that stress has been applied. Increasing cortisol production is the normal response to stress and is highly desirable, so long as the stress is removed and the adrenal glands can recover. Ongoing, unremitting stress means the adrenal glands and the whole body are in a constant state of alert, do not get time to recover and eventually fatigue. So, there are several stages of declining adrenal function gradually leading to failure:

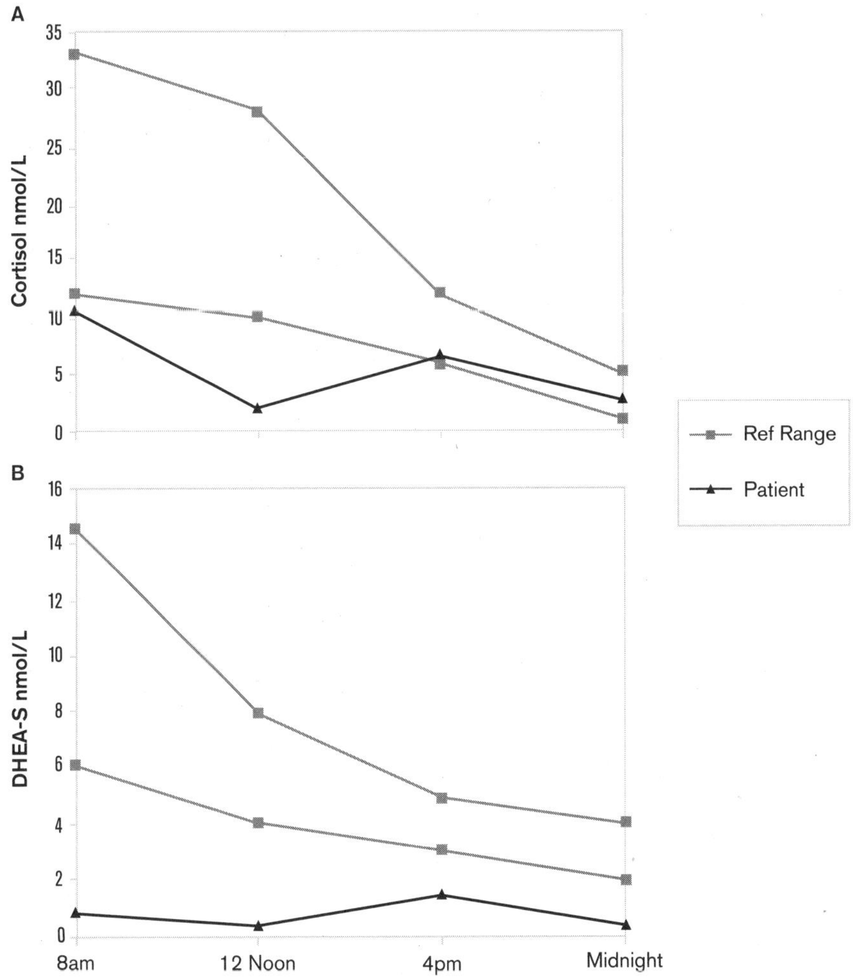

Figure 5.4. A typical CFS/ME adrenal stress profile test result showing low levels of (*a*) cortisol and (*b*) DHEA. (The DHEA stated reference range is age and gender related – as shown here it is for females aged 55–64 years).

1. Normal levels of total cortisol and DHEA. Normal result. Normal adrenal function.
2. Raised levels of total cortisol and normal DHEA. This indicates a normal short-term response to stress.
3. Raised levels of total cortisol and DHEA. The adrenal gland is functioning normally but the patient is chronically stressed. So long as the stress is removed, the adrenal gland will recover completely.

4. Raised total cortisol, low levels of DHEA. The body cannot make enough DHEA to balance cortisol. This is the first sign of adrenal exhaustion. The patient needs a long break from whatever that chronic stress may be – an important part of a package of recovery that addresses the root causes.
5. Cortisol levels low, DHEA levels low. The glands are so exhausted that they can't make cortisol or DHEA. By this time patients are generally severely fatigued. I often see this picture in my severe CFS patients. At this moment, Dr Selye's lab rats were close to death. To attempt physical activity in these circumstances is a case of beating a dead horse! Don't laugh – doctors recommend this for CFS; it is called GET (graded exercise therapy). See comments about PACE, CBT and GET in Chapter 1 (page 3).
6. Cortisol levels low, DHEA borderline or normal. This may represent the gland beginning to recover after a long rest.
7. A flat cortisol with no morning peak of cortisol or DHEA – could point to hypothyroidism.
8. A spike of cortisol in the morning followed by absolutely low and flat levels later may point to sleep apnoea.
9. Any spike of cortisol in the day means an acute stressor in the day, commonly low blood sugar in someone who cannot keto-adapt – that is, they cannot switch from glucose burning to fat burning to provide their energy.

Treatment of adrenal fatigue

There should be a two-pronged approach.

1: Identify the cause

This is not the place for a list of all possible stressors, not least because one person's stress is another's joy. However, a greatly overlooked cause of stress, and I suspect, the most common, is a tendency to hypoglycaemia due to an inability to keto-adapt. This occurs in people with metabolic syndrome.

2: Use pregnenolone

I think pregnenolone may be particularly pertinent in the treatment of CFS/ME, and indeed the ageing process, for two reasons:

1. **Poor mitochondrial function.** As described above (Figure 5.3, page 93) pregnenolone is the precursor of all the adrenal hormones and immediately downstream from cholesterol. The conversion of cholesterol to pregnenolone takes place in the mitochondria and so one can easily see how poor

mitochondrial function could result in poor output of pregnenolone and, therefore, adrenal hormones.

2. **Pregnenolone steal.** If the body becomes stressed, for whatever reason, then the production of adrenal hormones is moved away from the anabolic building, healing and repair hormones to the catabolic stress hormones, such as cortisol. In essence, when sufficiently stressed, pregnenolone is diverted away from making anabolic hormones (such as DHEA) to making catabolic hormones (essentially cortisol). Consequently, less hormone is available for healing and repair. People with CFS/ME are permanently stressed by many factors, not least of which is their inability to live up to their potential. Hence, CFS/ME sufferers will likely suffer from pregnenolone steal. This is bad news not only because this will mean that there is less hormone available for healing and repair but also because pregnenolone steal worsens the problems of low pregnenolone production in CFS/ME sufferers, as already described above, resulting from their poor mitochondrial function. I used to treat DHEA deficiency with DHEA. However, I believe pregnenolone is more physiologically appropriate because it is upstream of all adrenal hormones, including progesterone and cortisol.

Cholesterol is the raw material from which steroid hormones are made in the body. The next biochemical step is pregnenolone. As I have said, it is the mother and grandmother of all steroid hormones. Starting off with pregnenolone means that all steroid hormones can be naturally synthesised in the correct physiological balance. In theory, this should greatly simplify the business of prescribing and monitoring hormones because the body can do its own natural balancing act. A physiological dose of pregnenolone is 25–50 mg, depending on body weight, but the dose is not critical. I suggest taking it under the tongue. This works because sublingual doses bypass the liver – the so-called 'first pass effect'. Pregnenolone has been dubbed 'the memory hormone' and is highly concentrated in the brain. It is also protective against osteoporosis.

In patients in which the adrenal stress profile (ASP) test shows a deficiency of cortisol it may be worth trying 1 per cent hydrocortisone cream. This can be purchased over the counter. It is the biologically identical hormone and if given in small doses (5–10 mg in the morning – that is, ½–1 ml of cream) it has no side effects and induces no suppression of the adrenal gland. There are no long-term side effects, there is no need to carry a steroid card, and no need to tail the dose off when stopping the course.

Hydrocortisone should be seen as a crutch to the adrenal gland. Use of it allows the adrenal gland to rest a little and, in time, resume normal production, at which point the hydrocortisone can be stopped. This removal of the hydrocortisone support should only happen once the patient feels considerably better, which may take several months or even years. There is no need to re-check levels of cortisol once on treatment.

It may be that pregnenolone will be more effective as a cortisol replacement; time will tell. I am in the throes of collecting the results of the ASP test in patients before and after taking pregnenolone. I only have four results so far but in all cases the ASP test result has normalised. Watch this space.

Addison's disease

In Addison's disease there is complete failure of the adrenal gland, not because of chronic stress but because of autoimmunity. This is a life-threatening disorder and the patient is severely ill. The main clinical symptoms are severe postural hypotension (low blood pressure when standing) and hypoglycaemia (low blood sugar). Addison's disease is tested for by a 'short synacthen test' in which cortisol levels are measured before and after an adrenal gland stimulant, ACTH. Many patients with CFS/ME undergo this test, which is found to be normal. They are then told that their adrenal gland is fine and no action is required. Oh dear – WRONG! The problem with this test is that it only shows where the adrenal gland is completely non-functioning; it does not diagnose partial adrenal failure or adrenal stress, and no measurements of DHEA are made. This test can be potentially misleading in CFS patients.

Any person with Addison's would be diagnosed with an adrenal stress profile test (ASP) because it would show either an extremely low level of cortisol or none.

CHAPTER 5 SUMMARY

Energy delivery mechanisms: thyroid and adrenal function

THYROID FUNCTION

- Anyone with CFS can be hypothyroid – the symptoms are very similar but for hypothyroidism look also for:
    - Low metabolism (in other words, hibernation mode): weight gain, inability to lose weight, constipation.

  - Fluid retention: puffy ankles, nerve compression such as carpal tunnel syndrome.
  - Hair loss: typically, the outer third of the eyebrows.
  - Infertility, premenstrual tension, menorrhagia.
  - Large tongue.
  - Hoarse voice.
  - Goitre: an abnormal swelling of the thyroid gland that causes a lump to form in the neck.
  - Dry, poor quality skin and hair.

- Doctors don't listen to patients' clinical histories or look at the signs and symptoms – they will be guided by NHS test results, which are inadequate.
- Reference ranges for a 'normal' TSH result are set too high.
- So, many hypothyroid patients will be missed by NHS tests and doctors.
- At the very least, have a thyroid panel blood test of TSH, free T3 and free T4 – TSH is 'thyroid-stimulating hormone' and T3 and T4 are two types of thyroid hormone.
- Some hypothyroid patients do well on T4 (thyroxin) prescriptions, whereas others need natural thyroid or T3.
- Table 5.1 is a guide to prescribing based on a thyroid panel test of TSH, free T3 and free T4. All patients on these drugs need regular careful monitoring.

ADRENAL FUNCTION

- Many CFS/ME patients have poorly functioning adrenal glands.
- The best way to check adrenal status is to do the 'adrenal stress profile' (ASP) test; this is a saliva test and is done at home.
- This test measures the levels of two hormones – cortisol and DHEA – at points throughout the day.
- If this test suggests that treatment is needed then there are three treatment options:

  - Address any hypoglycaemic tendencies as these will stress the system and can cause adrenal problems.
  - A physiological dose of pregnenolone is 25–50 mg, depending on body weight, taken under the tongue. Pregnenolone is the

precursor of all adrenal hormones (all others originate from it) and should re-balance the adrenals naturally.

- In patients where the ASP test shows a deficiency of cortisol it may be worth trying 1 per cent hydrocortisone cream. This can be purchased over the counter. This is the biologically identical hormone and if given in small doses (5–10 mg in the morning – that is, ½–1 ml of cream) it has no side effects and induces no suppression of the adrenal gland.

- Once again, the situation must be monitored regularly and carefully, by reviewing clinical sign and symptoms and possibly re-testing using the ASP test.

CHAPTER 6

Diet: the fuel in the tank

One cannot think well, love well, sleep well,
if one has not dined well.
VIRGINIA WOOLF (25 January 1882 – 28 March 1941)

I spend more time talking about diet than all other subjects put together. This is in direct proportion to its importance. It may be the most difficult thing I ask people to do, but also the most vital. People want me to be prescriptive about diet and tell them exactly what they can and cannot do, but there is no such universal prescription – we are all so very different with respect to allergies, likes, dislikes, gut function, deficiencies, ethnic background and so on. Choosing the right diet for oneself is like playing cricket – I can give you the rules (whoops, 'laws') of the game, but everyone has to develop their own style within those laws. Geoffrey Boycott was as effective a cricketer as Ian Botham (I mean, Sir Ian), but they were completely different players.

Metabolic syndrome (that is, loss of control of blood sugar levels and all its attendant problems – see my third book *Prevent and Cure Diabetes* for much more detail) is a major risk factor for CFS/ME and part of the reason why we are seeing epidemics of that condition. I read recently that 3 per cent of school children were off school because of CFS/ME.

In the early days of treating CFS/ME, I used to pussy-foot around with diet, negotiating what each patient was and was not allowed to eat. I used to do deals with patients – 'OK, cut out the dairy products but you can have butter'; 'OK, cut out the wheat but you can have rice'; 'OK, cut out the sugar but you can have honey.' However, I now know that those deals just postponed recovery. As I cruelly say to my patients now, my job is to get you better, not to

Table 6.1. Rules of the diet game – order of priority

Food type	Comments and reasons
No alcohol – 90% of CFS/ME sufferers are alcohol intolerant.	Directly toxic to brain and liver. Suppresses the immune system, increasing the risk of infection and cancer.
	Stimulates insulin and inhibits glucagon (the hormone that increases glucose levels in the bloodstream), worsening metabolic syndrome; this switches on other cravings such as for sugar and snacks.
	Uses up micronutrients and causes deficiencies.
Increase intake of fat and fibre	The body should be powered by fat and fibre, not starch and sugar. Switching to such is called keto-adapting – it may take two to three weeks to convert. Please note, our epidemics of cancer, heart disease and dementia are driven by starch- and sugar-based diets. Fat is protective. Fibre is fermented by friendly microbes to produce short-chain fatty acids – a useful fuel. Much more detail in *Prevent and Cure Diabetes.*
No sugar No fruit sugar – fructose is even more pernicious than the white stuff No honey Nothing ending in -ose	Triggers wobbly blood sugar levels and metabolic syndrome. Directly toxic to brain and liver. Suppresses the immune system, increasing the risk of infection and cancer. D-ribose is a 5-carbon (as opposed to a 6-carbon) sugar. It is a highly desirable raw material. However, I suspect it too can be fermented so should only be used if the rest of the diet is truly ketogenic.
	Sugars are easily fermented in the upper gut to produce alcohols, including D-lactate. Sugar feeds unfriendly gut microbes, including yeast. See fermenting gut section – Chapter 7 (page 107).
No artificial sweeteners – but stevia and xylitol are fine to use in moderation	Aspartame and other such are toxic to the liver. Artificial sweeteners keep alive the psychological craving for sugar. Xylitol is a low GI prebiotic (feeds the gut flora) and therefore anti-microbial.
Low-starch diet (care with all grains, root vegetables and pulses)	Starches may be rapidly digested and spike blood sugars, further driving metabolic syndrome. Starches may be fermented by unfriendly gut microbes (see fermenting gut, Chapter 7, page 107).

Food type	Comments and reasons
Starches to be eaten just once a day and then in modest amounts	Reverse metabolic syndrome. Squeeze the liver glycogen-sponge dry*. (More in Prevent and Cure Diabetes.)
No snacking	Reverse metabolic syndrome. Squeeze the liver glycogen sponge dry*. More in *Prevent and Cure Diabetes*.
All foods to be eaten within a 10 hour window of time – for example, breakfast at 8 am, supper finished by 6 pm	A 14-hour window of time for fasting reverses metabolic syndrome and encourages fat burning. Squeeze the liver glycogen sponge dry*. More in *Prevent and Cure Diabetes*. Encourage the body to be fuelled by fat.
Cut out all foods containing gluten, dairy and yeast	These are major allergens – allergy kicks a hole in the energy bucket. If you suffer headaches or bowel symptoms then this is a priority.
No milk protein either	Milk protein is also a growth promoter and a risk factor for cancer.
No hydrogenated fats, such as margarine. Do not use nut, seed, fish or vegetable oils for cooking. Make sure cold pressed oils really are cold pressed.	Heating or hydrogenation of long-chain cis (left-handed) oils flips them into toxic, trans (right-handed) oils. Cook with medium-chain fats, such as lard (from beef, pig, lamb, poultry) or coconut oil. Goose fat is gorgeous! These tough saturated fats are not denatured by heat.
Avoid added chemicals	One can be allergic to anything, including chemical additives. Many require detoxification in the liver and so add to its burden.
Caffeine	If tolerated then use at breakfast and lunch. Avoid after 2 pm or you risk disturbing sleep. Maximum three cups a day.
Chocolate	Most people are addicted to the sugar and the milk of a chocolate bar. If you can enjoy a square of 70 per cent and not scoff the whole bar then you are not addicted.
Other addictions – nicotine, cannabis, social highs, etc	You can't have an upper without a downer. One addiction leads to another. To recover you must give them all up. Ouch! But I did, so you can too.
Eating organic	This of course is highly desirable, but for many, unaffordable and impossible. Do your best.

* Excess glucose is stored as glycogen in the liver and is the first source of fuel when glucose in the blood runs low.

entertain you. For that to happen we have to have as much in place as we know we can do. All the elements of the car have to be working to get it to go. Once you are recovered, then you can, as I call it, do a deal with the Devil and allow yourself to relax the regime, so long as you stay well. Interestingly, most of my patients having recovered stick to the rules that allowed that recovery. Having been ill they never want to go there again. To repeat an earlier quotation:

> *Health is like wealth – you don't know*
> *you've got it until you've lost it.*
>
> Popular saying

One of my philosophies is that I never ask my patients to do anything that I cannot do. I had to write a book to fully convince myself of the importance of not just the Paleo but also the ketogenic diet. I am not going to repeat all the arguments iterated in that book here – you will have to buy *Prevent and Cure Diabetes*; both it and *Sustainable Medicine* cover this in detail. Indeed, most of my ill CFS/ME patients would not have the energy to read and digest either book, so what follows are the simple Rules of the Game followed by a suggested daily menu. Yes, it may sound boring, but as I say above, my job is not to entertain . . . (By popular demand, I am also working on a cookery book at the time of the second edition going to press. Again, watch this space!)

Suggested daily menu

Breakfast

- Bacon, eggs, fried tomato
- Smoked fish (kippers, mackerel with lemon juice)
- Nuts and seeds with soya yoghurt or coconut yoghurt

Lunch

- Cold meat, fish (tinned fish in olive oil is fine), prawns, salami, smoked fish, rusk-free sausage (i.e. 100 per cent meat), avocado
- Salad (lettuce, cucumber, tomato, celery, peppers, etc), French dressing
- Green vegetables with nut/seed oils
- Home-made soup (made from meat stock, not cubes, only with allowed vegetables)

- Nuts and seeds with soya yoghurt or coconut yoghurt
- Linseed bread

Supper

- Meat, fish or eggs, green vegetables
- Berries, soya yoghurt, coconut yoghurt, coconut cream
- Nuts, seeds

Initially, be careful with root vegetables such as potato and parsnip, which are relatively high in carbohydrate. Whether to include them in the diet later depends largely on whether there is a fermenting gut problem. Most people can introduce some; others not at all.

Always remember: breakfast like an emperor, lunch like a king and sup like a pauper!

The *full* details of what you are going to eat can be found in the last section – the practical details of how to recover; see Chapter 17 (page 215) in particular.

Don't dig your grave with your knife and fork.

OLD ENGLISH PROVERB

CHAPTER 6 SUMMARY

Diet: the fuel in the tank

- Metabolic syndrome – loss of control of blood sugar – is a major risk for CFS/ME patients.
- A palaeolithic/ketogenic diet is the prescription.
- If you need convincing of this, then please do buy and read my other books, *Sustainable Medicine* and *Prevent and Cure Diabetes,* where I discuss the scientific justification for such diets in much more detail.
- Table 6.2 shows my summary guidelines for diet. (More detail is given in Chapter 17 (page 215) and the justification for these rules is in Table 6.1 on page 102).

Table 6.2. Summary guidelines for diet

No alcohol – 90 per cent of CFS/ME sufferers are alcohol intolerant
Increase intake of fat and fibre
No sugar
No fruit sugar – fructose is even more pernicious than the white stuff
No honey
Nothing ending in -ose! (except D-ribose)
No artificial sweeteners
Low-starch diet (take care with all grains, root vegetables and pulses)
Starches to be eaten just once a day, and then in modest amounts
No snacking
All foods to be eaten within a 10-hour window of time – for example, breakfast at 8 am, supper finished by 6 pm
Cut out all foods containing gluten, dairy and yeast
No milk protein either
No hydrogenated fats, such as margarine. Do not use nut, seed, fish or vegetable oils for cooking. Make sure cold-pressed oils really are cold pressed!
Avoid added chemicals

CHAPTER 7

The fermenting gut

And let me adde, that he that thoroughly understands the nature of Ferments and Fermentations, shall probably be much better able than he that Ignores them, to give a fair account of divers Phænomena of severall diseases (as well Feavers and others) which will perhaps be never thoroughly understood, without an insight into the doctrine of Fermentation.

ROBERT BOYLE FRS
(25 January 1627 – 31 December 1691)

I make no apology for discussing the issue of gut fermentation at length because the fermenting gut is almost universal in my CFS/ME patients. Without good gut function we cannot extract the goodness from food; indeed – worse – we end up feeding the unfriendly microbes which then make us ill. This occurs for at least two reasons – they ferment foods to toxins which poison us, and, perhaps worse, they spill over into the bloodstream, the immune system sensitises to them and this drives inflammatory reactions elsewhere. But as usual with me, enthusiasm is getting ahead of logic. I need to start with the basics as my lovely editor, Craig, tells me . . . so here goes.

Research on the gut microbiome is currently progressing at an exponential rate – there is so much I need to know. The simplistic state of affairs as I detail it below is what you and I need to know for biological plausibility and clinical relevance.

A. The normal state of affairs

The human gut is almost unique amongst mammals – the upper gut is a near-sterile, digesting carnivorous gut (like a dog's or a cat's) evolved to deal with meat and fat, whilst the lower gut (large bowel or colon) is full of bacteria and is a fermenting, vegetarian gut (like a horse's or cow's) evolved to digest vegetables and fibre. From an evolutionary perspective this has been a highly successful strategy – it allows people who live in Northern Canada, such as Inuits and Yupiks, to live on fat and protein, and people in other parts of the world to survive on pure vegan diets.

Problems arose when humans learned to cook and to farm. This allowed them to access new foods – namely, pulses, grains and root vegetables – all of which need cooking to be digestible and are high in carbs. From an evolutionary perspective this has, again, been a highly successful strategy and has allowed the population of humans to increase at a great rate. However, carbohydrates have the potential to be fermented in the upper gut with problems arising as detailed below. CFS/ME sufferers can be viewed as evolutionary carnivorous relics. You are in good company – I am a relic too. [Editor's note: Me too! I'm pre-Google. Craig.]

The stomach, duodenum and small intestine (collectively, the upper gut) should be almost free (it is impossible to be entirely free) from micro-organisms (bacteria, yeasts and parasites – collectively referred to as microbes hereinafter). This is normally achieved by eating a low-carb 'Stone Age' or 'Paleo' diet and having an acidic stomach which digests protein efficiently and kills the acid-sensitive microbes, followed by a relatively alkali duodenum, which kills the alkali-sensitive microbes; then via bile salts (which are also toxic to microbes) and pancreatic enzymes to further digest protein, fats and carbohydrates. The small intestine does more digesting and also absorbs the amino acids (building blocks of proteins), fatty acids (building blocks of fats and oils), glycerol and simple sugars that result. All these products pass into the portal vein and directly to the liver to be sorted out; the only exception is fat, which passes into the lymphatic system and directly into the bloodstream via the thoracic duct – I think this is a lovely illustration of how non-toxic fat is. Like me, you must become a lover of fat!

The overwhelming majority of bacteria are in the final section of the gut – that is, the large bowel. Oxygen levels here are very low, which encourages oxygen-hating bacteria to flourish, such as bacteroides (see the next section).

The main types of microbe that we need to be aware of are as follows.

Bacteroides

The bacteroides are, or should be, by far and away the most abundant gut bacteria. The human body is made up of 10 trillion cells, whereas in our gut we have 100 trillion microbes or more – that is, 10 times as many microbes as cells. They do much good:

- They ferment vegetable fibre to produce **short-chain fatty acids** (SCFAs): this is the main source of food for the cells lining the bowel, and if low, atrophy of the colon results.
- Short-chain fatty acids are a useful fuel for the body. If blood sugar runs low the body can switch to burning SCFAs. It is estimated that up to 500 Kcal per day may be generated via the production of SCFAs by bacteroides fermenting soluble fibre – a very significant source of energy.
- Bacteroides are essential for the recycling of bile acids (otherwise useful fats would be unnecessarily lost in faeces).
- Bacteroides occupy the surface of the gut, thus preventing pathogenic species (such as salmonella, shigella and clostridia) from adhering to it and causing infection.

There is no probiotic on the market which contains bacteroides, simply because these organisms cannot exist outside the human gut; oxygen kills them quickly. We just have to feed the gut with the right food (prebiotics), found in beans, peas, lentils, nuts, seeds and vegetables, so as to encourage bacteroides. In a stool test sample it is very unusual to see no bacteroides – indeed, such a state would be accompanied by severe gut pathology, such as ulcerative colitis, *Clostridium difficile* or pseudomembranous colitis. In all three conditions the perfect treatment is *faecal bacteriotherapy*, which gives an excellent chance of permanent cure. The idea here is to take a small sample of fresh faeces from someone with normal gut microbes, most importantly with good numbers of bacteroides and free from pathological strains, and instil this by enema into the prepared gut of the recipient. Having low numbers of bacteroides is a major risk factor for colon cancer. (The bacteroides in the 'transplant' do not survive more than a few minutes outside the gut. Full details of how the infusion is carried out can be accessed via my web page: drmyhill.co.uk/wiki/Faecal_bacteriotherapy.)

Aerobic bacteria

There are three strains of aerobic (oxygen-using) bacteria which ideally should all be present – namely:

- *E. coli (Escherichia coli)*, which ferments vegetable fibre and fucose (present in chick peas, hazelnuts and figs – care with figs, I can easily eat too many!) to produce:
  - Folic acid
  - Vitamin K2 (protects against osteoporosis)
  - Coenzyme Q10 (essential for mitochondrial function)
  - Three amino acids – namely, tyrosine and phenylalanine (these are pre-cursors of dopamine, lack of which results in low mood) and tryptophan (this is the pre-cursor of serotonin, which is responsible for gut motility as well as positive mood)
- Lactobacilli and bifidobacteria. I suspect the main benefits of these two bacteria are that:
  - They occupy the gut and so physically displace unfriendly bacteria.
  - Any sugars or starches can be rapidly fermented before the unfriendlies get them.
  - They programme the immune system. I think of this as an immunological boot camp – the immune system needs constant training to remind it what is good and what is bad. A constant presence of goodies means that anything else is a baddie.

Probiotics

Given the wrong substrate, probiotics can do harm. So, for example, lactobacilli ferment sugars to lactic acid; this can be a problem for some patients because two forms are produced – namely, L-lactate, which can be broken down, and D-lactate which can't; it is a toxin! Humans do not have the enzymes to break down D-lactate. Neither do cattle. Indeed, D-lactate acidosis cannot be distinguished clinically from BSE (bovine spongiform encephalophy). Lactobacilli therefore have the potential to do good, but if there is too much table sugar and fruit sugar in the diet, then there is potential for great harm – all the more reason to consume a low-carb, no-sugar ketogenic diet.

The best results from probiotics come from fermented foods (see Appendix 8 'Growing your own probiotics', page 327). If stomach acid is working as it should, then probiotics should not survive the stomach and pass dead into the small and large intestine. However, this does not mean they do no good – even dead bacteria fulfil many of the above functions.

Unfriendly gut microbes

High-carbohydrate Western diets lend themselves to the development of the upper fermenting gut. The best example of an unfriendly microbe is *Helicobacter pylori* (see page 116), but yeast is a common offender too. We used to be able to test for this by measuring blood alcohol levels before and after a glucose load, and indeed, my dear friend and colleague Dr Keith Eaton spent much of his life researching this and producing seminal papers. He established beyond reasonable doubt that candida is a common and major upper gut fermenter.

B. The problems created by the fermenting upper gut

1. Unpleasant symptoms

(a) Wind, gas and bloating

Vegetable fibre in the large bowel is fermented by friendly bacteria to produce hydrogen and methane – these farts do not smell. They are flammable – but I do not recommend testing this with a lighted match! This is the only 'normal' wind there is. Burping means you are fermenting in the upper gut and that is clearly abnormal. Farting foul wind means that foods are not being digested efficiently upstream and are available for fermentation downstream. We all do this when we eat too much food and overwhelm our ability to digest it.

(b) Reflux and heartburn

We are seeing epidemics of this pair of symptoms. The problem is the drug-prescribing, symptom-suppressing doctors turn to acid-blocking drugs like PPIs (proton pump inhibitors, such as omeprazole, or any '-azole'). This makes the fermenting gut worse since stomach acid is wiped out. (No acid means that the acid-sensitive gut microbes are not killed.) This iatrogenic hypochlorrhydria (low stomach acid) is a major risk factor for cancer (see page 116), osteoporosis (we need acid to absorb minerals) and infection (acid is a frontline defence against microbes).

(c) Foul-smelling breath and halitosis

The products of bacteria fermenting include hydrogen sulphide (stink bomb material). Halitosis may also be symptomatic of chronic infection in the mouth, sinuses, upper airways and chest (such as bronchiectasis).

(d) Disturbances of normal gut movement

These lead to constipation or diarrhoea.

(e) Foggy brain

The products of fermentation, such as alcohol, esters, aldehydes and other lipid-soluble substances, have a general anaesthetic-like effect on membranes of the brain. This probably manifests by inhibiting energy delivery mechanisms to the brain. See in the Glossary, 'Anaesthetic action', page 348.

(f) Night sweats

Dr Henry Butt suggests that night sweats result from microbes or endotoxin spilling over into the bloodstream to trigger such.

(g) Being apple-shaped

Dr Caroline Pond (1998) asked the question, 'Where does the body first dump fat when it comes available?' The answer is, 'Where the immune system is busy'.[27] Keeping the gut microbes at bay requires a lot of energy and the immune system (like the brain) likes to run on fat. Altogether, 90 per cent of the immune system is gut associated. The immune system is our standing army and standing armies are demanding of raw materials and energy – especially as they are constantly being trained by gut microbes. Gut fermenters carry their fat round their gut; non-fermenters are pear shaped. I am pear shaped; a younger version would be hour-glass shaped! Perhaps that is the biological basis of beauty, the hour-glass figure being the picture of feminine health and so the best bet for child rearing?

(h) Fatigue

The business of dealing with all these microbes (see above) and toxins requires energy – and a lot of it. I was fascinated to discover that at rest the liver uses up 27 per cent of all the energy available to the body, compared with the brain at 19–20 per cent and the heart at 7 per cent. Much of this energy is for detoxification. In CFS/ME, where energy delivery is impaired, one may expect detoxification also to be impaired – yet another vicious cycle. These unwanted toxins from microbes have to be detoxified by the liver's cytochrome P450 detox system. In summary, these phases, or stages, comprise:

Stage 1 – Conversion of a toxic chemical into a less toxic one, although this stage may sometimes result in a more toxic chemical.

Stage 2 – Adding a substance to render toxins less harmful.

In theory, the above toxins should all be detoxified by the P450 cytochrome system, but in practice, especially when liver function is already compromised, some of these can spill over into the systemic circulation with production of free radicals and inhibition of mitochondria (*ergo* more fatigue).

Indeed, this may explain why Gilbert's syndrome (see Glossary, page 357) is a major risk factor for CFS/ME – over 80 per cent of Gilbert's sufferers complain of fatigue. Essentially they are poor detoxifiers and so are much more susceptible to the toxic stress produced by the fermenting gut (and, of course, toxins from the outside world).

Examples of unwanted toxins include, but are not limited to:

- Alcohols such as ethyl alcohol, propyl alcohol, butyl alcohol and possibly methyl alcohol. These would be metabolised by stage 1 into acetaldehyde, propylaldehyde, butylaldehyde and possibly formaldehyde. Alcohol and acetaldehydes result in foggy brain, 'toxic brain', feeling 'poisoned' and so on. Alcohol also upsets blood sugar levels. This makes the sufferer crave sugar and refined carbohydrates – the very foods bugs need in the upper gut to ensure their own survival. This is arguably a clever evolutionary ploy by microbes to ensure their own survival.
- Noxious gases, such as hydrogen sulphide, nitric oxide, ammonia and possibly others. Hydrogen sulphide is known to inhibit mitochondria and block the oxygen-carrying capacity of haemoglobin. It also greatly increases the toxicity of heavy metals by enhancing their absorption.
- Odd sugars such as D-lactate. As I explained above, this right-handed sugar (see Figure 7.1, page 114) cannot be detoxified by lactate dehydrogenase, a liver enzyme that can detoxify L-lactate. With serious overproduction, patients typically present with episodic metabolic acidosis (usually occurring after high-carbohydrate meals) and characteristic neurological abnormalities, including confusion, cerebellar ataxia, slurred speech and loss of memory. In a review of 29 reported cases, for example, all patients exhibited some degree of altered mental state. They may complain of, or appear to be, drunk in the absence of ethanol intake. Interestingly, this phenomenon is much better described in the vet world. D-lactate is a recognised cause in cattle of neurological manifestations. Furthermore, products of fermentation are thought to be a cause of laminitis in horses. Indeed, the encephalopathy of liver failure can be treated by gut-only antibiotics to wipe out unwelcome overgrowth of fermenting gut flora. D-lactate is fermented from sugars, including fruit sugars. This is a further reason to cut out sugar and fruit

strictly from the diet. One molecule of sugar generates two molecules of D-lactate.

- Other products of fermentation I don't yet know about!

Biochemical Note: Sugars can be 'left-handed' or 'right-handed', according to their biochemical shape. For example, see what L-lactate and D-lactate 'look' like in Figure 7.1.

---

2. Bacterial endotoxin

This is a lipopolysaccharide from bacterial membranes which is markedly pro-inflammatory – that is, it switches on the immune system. I suspect this explains the Herxheimer 'die off' reactions that so many patients suffer with when making interventions to change gut microbiome. Friendly bacteria displace unfriendlies and reduce levels of endotoxin.

3. Bacterial translocation

Microbes in the gut are miniscule compared with human cells and all too easily spill over into the bloodstream. They are excreted in urine and, indeed, normal human urine can contain up to 10,000 microbes per millilitre (ml) before it is declared to be infected. This is very confusing for women with allergic cystitis (and possibly men with prostatitis); they sensitise to these microbes and get all the symptoms of inflammation (pain, frequency and urgency, and sometimes

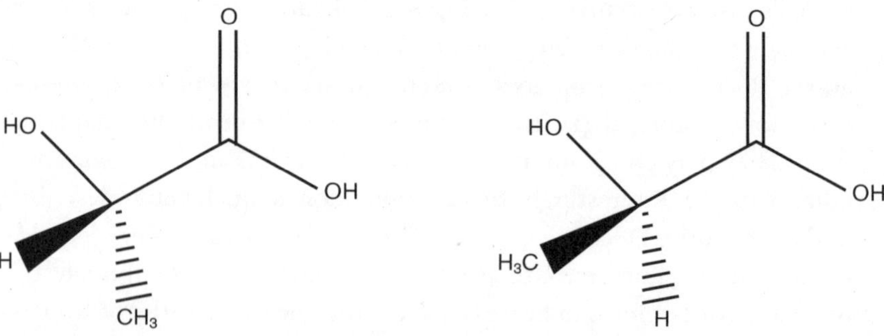

Figure 7.1. The comparative structures of D-lactate and L-lactate.

even blood in the urine) when the bacterial counts in their urine are less than 10,000 microbes per ml. I think of this as bacterial allergy; it also responds to antibiotics because these greatly reduce the allergic load.

Numbers of bacteria spilling over by bacterial translocation are not sufficient to cause septicaemia, but the immune system could sensitise to them, especially if they get stuck elsewhere in the body. I suspect many modern diseases can be explained by allergy to gut flora – namely, irritable bladder (interstitial cystitis), prostatitis, arthritis, asthma, temporal arteritis, polymyalgia rheumatica, skin problems (urticarial, venous ulcers, rosacea, psoriasis, etc) and many other possibilities. Furthermore, this unnecessary inflammation is wasteful of immune energy, thereby causing fatigue.

4. Fermenting gut may lead to fermenting brain

It is possible that some psychiatric conditions are caused by gut microbes getting into the brain and fermenting neurotransmitters to create amphetamine- and LSD-like substances; this is not my idea but that of a Japanese researcher Katsunari Nishihara, presented in his paper 'Disclosure of the major causes of mental illness – mitochondrial deterioration in brain neurons via opportunistic infection' published in the *Journal of Biological Physics and Chemistry*.[28] This hypothesis further explains the gut-brain connection that is so obvious in clinical medicine and, indeed, everyday life.

5. Malabsorption of micronutrients

Microbes in the gut are as hungry for micronutrients as you are!

6. Susceptibility to infections

For the reasons given above. Travellers are routinely recommended probiotics which are of proven benefit against 'travellers' diarrhoea'.

7. Leaky gut

An abnormal microbiome may result in low-grade inflammation and that causes leaky gut. Products of protein digestion – viz, short-chain polypeptides – may leak into the bloodstream and act as hormone mimics. For example, a strip of amino acids Ser-Tyr-Set-Met would mimic ACTH, the hormone which stimulates the adrenal gland. An eight-amino acid fragment could act like glucagon and so deplete glycogen (sugar) stores in the liver; this would mimic diabetes.

8. Where there is upper fermenting gut there will be fermenting mouth

Bacteria fermenting in the mouth will cause a furry tongue (the tongue should be pink and scum free), gum disease (you get long in the tooth) and tooth decay. Dental plaque is one example of biofilm – that is, a protective shield which bacteria throw up and hide behind. Indeed, the mouth is a good indicator of a sufficiently low-carb diet – teeth should feel glassy smooth (as if they have just been polished by your dentist). Dental health is a strong predictor of other degenerative conditions, such as arthritis and heart disease.

9. Friendly bacteria ferment to produce lactic acid

Lactic acid reduces the numbers of microbes and protects against infection. This is a positive!

10. Long-term disease – cancer

I suspect fermenting gut is a risk factor, possibly the *major* risk factor, for cancers of the oesophagus, stomach and large bowel. This is biologically plausible – many tumours are driven by inflammation. *H. pylori* infection is a known risk factor for stomach cancer, as is hypochlorhydria (low stomach acid), which is also a risk factor for fermenting upper gut. Barrett's oesophagus is a premalignant condition – I have now seen four patients who have got rid of their Barrett's through interventions to tackle their upper fermenting gut. When these patients pointed out to their conventional doctors that their supposedly irreversible Barrett's had been cured, the response, in all cases, was, 'Oh dear, we must have got the diagnosis wrong in the first place'!

C. Tests for the abnormal fermenting gut

Clinical tests

- **Look at the tongue.** The tongue should be clean and pink with no fuzz or fur; any fuzz or fur represents colonies of bacteria and yeast hiding behind biofilm.

- **Feel your teeth.** Your teeth should feel like they do after a polish at the dentist – glassy smooth. Any roughness results from bacterial colonies – dental plaque, in other words (another example of biofilm).
- **Bicarbonate challenge test.** Hypochlorhydria is a major risk factor for upper fermenting gut. Mix ¼ teaspoon of baking soda in a cup of water first thing in the morning before eating or drinking anything. This should react with acid in the stomach and you should burp (carbon dioxide) within three minutes. If you do not burp within that time, then there is a lack of stomach acid – in other words, hypochlorhydria.
- **A good clinical test** indicating upper gut fermentation is that one produces wind or gas (belching, bloating, feeling full, noisy gut, etc) after eating carbohydrates.
- **Tenderness in the right iliac fossa** (lower right side of tummy half way between the groin and the tummy button). Tenderness here may reflect inflammation in the lower ileum where microbial numbers start to rise exponentially.
- **Burning sensation in the rectum** or on passing a stool may reflect the acidity of the stool as a result of abnormal fermentation.
- **Use your nose.** Gibson, a food microbiologist from Reading, divides people into 'smellies' and 'inflammables' – normal gut fermentation produces hydrogen and methane, which allows one to 'light one's own flatus', hence 'inflammables'. I would not like to recommend this as a routine clinical test! Normal fermentation should be odourless. However, with sulphate-reducing bacteria present in the gut, hydrogen sulphide is produced giving the rotten eggs smell and a positive test for hydrogen sulphide in urine. This situation (that is, the 'smellies') indicates abnormal gut fermentation. Indeed, Professor Kenny de Meileir,* a specialist in treating

---

* Professor de Meileir still treats CFS/ME patients and has published more than 80 papers, mostly related to CFS/ME. In the paper 'Research on Extremely Disabled M.E. Patients Reveals the True Nature of the Disorder',[29] the researchers compared totally bedridden patients (Karnofski score 20–30 [the Karnofski score is an index of functional impairment]) with less ill ME patients (Karnofski score 60–70), family controls, contact controls and non-contact controls and found that plasma LPS (lipopolysaccharide) level distinguished the groups, with the highest values in the bedridden patients. LPS is a strong activator of the immune system, and high plasma concentrations suggest a hyper-permeable gut. There are many

CFS/ME, reported using a hydrogen sulphide urine test as a marker test for the condition.

Laboratory tests

- There is no point in doing expensive laboratory tests unless they change management in some way. Furthermore, they need proper interpretation; Biolab, for example, can measure D-lactate. However, a negative test does not mean there is no gut fermentation. With respect to the fermenting gut, the clinical picture is much more useful than expensive laboratory tests. Knowing what I now know, I would rarely start with tests. I would go with the clinical information as detailed above, put in place the relevant treatments as detailed below, and see what happens. This may be all that is needed. However, if we got stuck then I would consider a 'comprehensive digestive stool with parasites test' (see next section). This test is much easier to interpret when the dietary regimes have been established.
- D-lactate can be measured by a blood test following a carbohydrate meal. The snag is that postal samples are not completely reliable and in order to have the test, the patient either needs to go to Biolab to have blood taken and processed straight away or he/she has to find a laboratory where they will spin and separate blood immediately and freeze it so that a frozen sample can be sent to Biolab. This is quite difficult to organise and I rarely recommend this test – see Appendix 1 (page 291).
- Hydrogen sulphide can be tested for with a urine test from Red Laboratories, but again it is technically difficult to organise and so I rarely

---

possible causes for this, but a lack of 'local' energy production is one of them. In a separate study (*In Vivo*, in press) the same researchers observed intestinal overgrowth of Gram positive D/L-lactate-producing bacteria which are also known to produce H_2S (hydrogen sulphide) in the presence of certain heavy metals as a survival defence mechanism. They therefore hypothesised that the urine of the bedridden ME patients would contain more H_2S derived metabolites than the less ill and the controls. Using a proprietary simple colour change urine test this hypothesis was confirmed. (For a listing of all Dr Meileir's research go to: cris.cumulus.vub.ac.be/portal/en/persons/kenny-de-meirleir(36717038-46d0-452d-a187-c786872383bc)/publications.html.)

request it. The sniff test is much less sensitive but cheaper. Not my nose but yours!

Comprehensive digestive stool analysis with parasites (Genova Laboratories)

I am painfully aware of the problems of testing stool samples, not least of all because the most abundant microbe, namely bacteroides, do not survive outside the gut. (One can do microbial ecology profiles which look for the DNA.) However, one can get a reasonable grip on gut function and microbes present. Clinically I find these accord reasonably well with symptoms and have implications for treatment interventions which afford benefits and allow one to hone treatment.

INTERPRETATION OF THE GENOVA COMPREHENSIVE DIGESTIVE STOOL ANALYSIS

Remember that in interpreting any test, high normal or low normal may also be a significant result – the individual normal range is not the same thing as the population reference range. (see Tables 7.1 and 7.2)

D. Treatment of the fermenting gut – the principles of treatment

Diet

- **Low-carb/high-fibre/ketogenic diet.** Feed the friendly microbes and starve the rest out. This is the single most difficult but also the most important intervention. Indeed, it may be all you need to do. All sugars and starches have the potential to be fermented. Fibre feeds the friendly fermenters in the lower gut. Fat starves them all because it cannot be fermented. How do I know this? I can leave a bottle of olive oil in my pantry for months without it going off! I can leave a lump of lard in my fridge – with time it may oxidise and go rancid but it does not ferment. Indeed, I suspect fat is a vital defence against infection, and modern high-sugar/starch diets are largely responsible for our growing need for antibiotics. Interestingly, and I am not sure of the mechanism of this, low-sugar/starch diets are also protective against viral infections.
- **Do not snack.** Give the stomach a chance to empty, become fully acid and kill any residual microbes that may be there. Ideally, have 14 hours in every 24 when there is no food in the stomach.

Table 7.1. Interpretation guidelines for Genova Comprehensive Digestive Stool Analysis test

Measurement of	Too high and what it indicates	Too low and what it indicates	Action
Putrefactive short-chain polypeptides	Poor protein digestion Too much protein in the diet overwhelming digestion? Intestinal hurry? Low stomach acid? Poor pancreatic function?	Normal is zero	Reassess diet Assess gut transit time by eating beetroot or sweetcorn Check for hypochlorhydria Consider pancreatic enzymes
Meat fibres in stool	As above	Normal is zero	Ditto above
Fat in stool	Poor fat digestion Too much fat in diet overwhelming digestion? Intestinal hurry? Poor pancreatic function Low-level bile salts (needed to emulsify fats)		Reassess diet Assess gut transit time as above
		Low-fat diet	Eat more fat!
N butyrate and SCFAs	Can't be too high! Indicates good levels of friendly bacteria in the large bowel		Carry on
		Low-fibre diet Intestinal hurry?	Eat more fibre
High-beta glucuronidase often with low N butyrate	Fermentation of fibre in the upper gut. Not desirable!		Restore normal digestion with acid, enzymes, bile salts and carbonates page 122. Consider two weeks of the GAPs diet.

- **Use foods which are already partly digested** (such as well-cooked meats and broths) or are full of enzymes to assist the process (raw vegetable juices) or have the fats within in an emulsion of tiny globules (smoothies, coconut cream).
- **Spicy foods,** if tolerated, may be helpful because these are naturally antimicrobial. I wonder if this explains why the most popular British dish is now curry. Curry is delicious and medicinal.
- **Tea** contains tannins which are mildly toxic to microbes. But tannins also chelate minerals, so I recommend drinking tea outside meal times.
- **Chewing gum.** The parotid salivary gland provides a rich source of endothelial growth factor (indeed, this is what John McLaren-Howard

Measurement of	Too high and what it indicates	Too low and what it indicates	Action
Inflammatory markers high or blood present	Could represent serious bowel pathology		Urgent referral to gastro-enterologist for further investigation. Faecal calprotectin is an additionally helpful test
Lactobacilli		Absent	Grow and consume probiotic cultures such as kefir
E. coli		Absent	Grow and consume probiotic cultures such as Mutaflor
Bifidobacteria		Absent	Grow and consume probiotic cultures from bifidobacteria
Additional bacteria	**I suspect a normal result should be very low or zero. But I have not seen enough results from enough people doing ketogenic diets to be sure**		
Alpha, gamma and beta strep	High sugar/starch diet		Reduce sugar and starch Increase fat and fibre Restore normal digestion
Any other microbes	High sugar/starch diet		Ditto above
Pathogenic bacteria	High sugar/starch diet		Ditto above May need herbal or antibiotic prescription
Yeast	High sugar/starch diet		Ditto above
Parasites	High sugar/starch diet		Ditto above

measures in his hypochlorhydria test) which stimulates growth of the lining of the gut. Chew, because this stimulates flow of saliva. Sugar-free, additive-free gum please! A preparation containing xylitol seems sensible because xylitol further helps kill microbes.

Restore normal digestion by copying Nature

- Take acid supplements with food, such as the juice of a whole lemon, a dessertspoon of cider vinegar (care if you are allergic to yeast), or betaine hydrochloride 220 mg × 1–5 capsules depending on the size of the meal and individual tolerance of such.

- Then 60–90 minutes later take pancreatic enzymes, magnesium carbonate (one heaped teaspoonful – take care as it can cause diarrhoea) or sodium bicarbonate (2–3 grams/ ½ teaspoonful) possibly with bile salts such as bile acids, 1 gram.

Displace the little wretches with probiotics

There is much to be learned about the use of probiotics so watch this space. But the general principles are:

- It is a simple numbers games: probiotics do not colonise the gut – they are killed by stomach acid. However, even the dead microbes do much good. Live, actively fermenting cultures get the best results and are very cheap. The principles of growing them are the same. Start with a culture that you can purchase, such as kefir or Mutaflor, mix it in to a tolerated substrate (such as coconut milk), keep it warm (it likes to be at body heat) for at least 24 hours, possibly longer, then drink it. (See Appendix 8, page 327, for details).
- There is no probiotic on the market which contains bacteroides – that is because, as I have explained, they are killed by oxygen. We acquire bacteroides from our mother during childbirth and retain those bacteria for life. Not only do we inherit our mother's mitochondria but also her gut flora.

Care with nutritional supplements (at least initially)

Nutritional supplements could make things worse. Microbes are just as hungry for nutritional supplements as we are. Instead of nourishing you, your precious supplements might be feeding the microbes. Indeed, from an evolutionary perspective mitochondria are derived from bacteria. It is biologically plausible that what mitochondria like, bacteria will also thrive on. Perhaps this explains why the fermenting gut is a particular problem for 'mitochondriacs' because their gut microbes are nicking mitochondrial raw materials.

Kill the little wretches

- The fermenting gut starts with the fermenting mouth. Neem mouth wash and neem tooth paste are good at killing *Streptococcus mutans*, the major cause of dental decay and gum disease.

- Saliva is high in amylase. Although this is held up to be important for digesting starch, I do not buy that idea. Saliva is an excellent antiseptic (an injured animal can lick its wound and that will keep it free from infection). I think it much more likely that amylase is present to kill microbes (in addition to SIgA, lactoferrin, etc). Again, this is further reason not to snack.
- Vitamin C at night. Vitamin C kills all microbes. It is poorly absorbed which, for our purposes, is ideal. The idea is to take sufficient vitamin C to reduce the thousands of microbes in the upper gut but not to kill the billions, nay trillions, in the lower gut. When this happens there is diarrhoea. This is called taking vitamin C to bowel tolerance. It is an excellent treatment for any gut infection. Take a sub-diarrhoeal dose. Most people need at least 2–3 grams, some up to 10 grams, to achieve this. I keep my vitamin C next to the toothbrush and that reminds me.

Occasionally antimicrobials are required. There is no point in killing microbes if one is feeding them at the same time, so all the above must be done first and, indeed, this may be all that is necessary. Treatments may have to be

Table 7.2. Prescription medications and herbals to treat gut microbes

Microbe	Medication/herbal	Notes
Yeast	Itraconazole 100 mg daily OR Fluconazole 100 mg daily AND nystatin powder AND any herbal preparation as indicated by the CDSA*	Expect to get 'die off' Herxheimer reactions
Blastocystis hominis	Paromomycin 15 mg/kg three times daily for two weeks AND Doxycycline 100 mg twice daily for two weeks AND Metronidazole 400 mg three times daily for two weeks AND artemisia 500 mg three times daily – continue for 1–2 months.	A real pig to get rid of; this is the only regime I have seen to be effective.
Entamoeba	Metronidazole 400 mg three times daily for two weeks Artemisia 500 mg three times daily for 1–2 months	This works reliably well.
Other microbes	Antibiotics according to sensitivity tests from the CDSA* OR herbals according to sensitivity tests from the CDSA*	The clinical response is as useful as retesting.

* CDSA = comprehensive digestive stool analysis

prolonged – certainly for weeks, possibly months. As a rule of thumb I reckon to continue treatment for at least one month after symptoms have cleared. The commonest regimes I use are listed in Table 7.2, page 123.

CHAPTER 7 SUMMARY

The fermenting gut

In essence, our game plan here is to get our gut microbiome back to what used to be normal for humans. To do this we have to do some detective work, via clinical symptoms and sometimes laboratory tests, to understand in what ways out individual guts are not normal. Once we have decided upon this, we can then embark on treatment, which broadly consists of starving out or killing the bad bugs. This is a very tough part of what you have to do to get better because temptation is all around you and so easy to access in the form of sweet, sugary and high-carb cheap food. However, once you have changed your diet, you will never look back; it becomes a good habit and one that will serve you for life.

We are what we repeatedly do. Excellence, then, is not an act, but a habit.
ARISTOTLE (384–322 BC)

- The fermenting gut is almost universal in the CFS/ME patients that I have treated over the past 30 years.
- If gut function is not good, then the body cannot extract what it needs from food and then we end up feeding unfriendly microbes, which can make us ill in their own right.
- This happens in two ways:
  - The unfriendly microbes ferment foods into toxins which poison us.
  - The unfriendly microbes spill over into the bloodstream where the immune system sensitises to them and this drives inflammatory reactions elsewhere.
- The normal state of affairs in the human gut has been upset by Western diets which are high in carbohydrates and sugars.

- There are many clinical signs and symptoms of a fermenting gut and these include:
  - Wind, gas and bloating
  - Reflux and heartburn
  - Foul smelling breath and halitosis
  - Constipation or diarrhoea
  - Fermenting brain – for example, foggy brain
  - Night sweats
  - Being apple-shaped
  - Fatigue
  - Malabsorption of micronutrients
  - Susceptibility to infections
  - Leaky gut
  - Fermenting mouth – for example, furry tongue
- You can test for a fermenting gut by looking for the signs and symptoms as above and, in addition, by looking for these features:
  - If your gut is healthy then your tongue should be clean and pink with no fuzz or fur.
  - If your gut is healthy then your teeth should feel like they do after a polish at the dentist's.
  - If you belch, feel bloated or full, or have a noisy gut, etc after eating carbohydrates, then this indicates a fermenting gut.
  - Tenderness in the right iliac fossa (lower right side of tummy half way between the groin and the tummy button).
  - Burning sensation in the rectum or on passing a stool.
  - Smelly farts.
- You can also test for a fermenting gut with the 'Comprehensive digestive stool analysis with parasites' test from Genova Laboratories. See page 119 for an interpretative guide to this test's results.
- You treat the fermenting gut using a multi-pronged approach:
  - Low-carb / high-fibre / ketogenic diet, with no snacking – see Table 6.1 on page 102 for more detail.

- Restore normal digestion by taking acid supplements with food and then 60–90 minutes after food, taking pancreatic enzymes and magnesium carbonate.
- Take probiotics – make your own kefir or Mutaflor.
- Kill the unfriendly microbes with neem and vitamin C, and sometimes prescription drugs will be needed.

CHAPTER 8

Holes in the energy bucket

As I have said repeatedly, fatigue occurs when energy demand exceeds energy delivery. Remember the energy equation:

Available energy = Energy delivery – Energy expenditure

The name of the game is to maximise energy delivery and minimise the controllable elements of the energy expenditure side of the equation in order that there is a surplus of energy that can be used for repair, renewal and recovery. For an overview see Appendix 7.

Certain elements of energy expenditure are unavoidable. We must 'spend' this energy in order to stay alive; this is the energy needed for basic house-keeping duties within the body.

Energy expenditure in the body

In fact, two thirds of all energy spent goes on staying alive. This is the basic metabolic rate (BMR). This always strikes me as being a lot of energy. Having insufficient energy for BMR presents a particular problem for people with severe CFS/ME because these sufferers do not even have the energy for basal metabolism. Hence, they can suffer mild multiple-organ failure, simply due to a lack of energy. Essential organs, such as the kidneys, are relatively protected. My clinical guess is that as the energy equation goes into negative territory (that is, expenditure exceeds delivery), then organs fail, and give rise to symptoms in the order shown in Table 8.1 on page 128.

After having spent two thirds of our energy on BMR, this leaves one third to spend physically, mentally and on the essential evolutionary reason that we are

Table 8.1. The effects of inadequate energy

Body system	**Symptoms in the short term**	**Pathology in the long term**
The body as a whole	Accelerated ageing	Suffer degenerative disease before our time
Brain–intellectual	Foggy-headed, poor concentration, difficulty multi-tasking, poor short-term memory	Dementia
	Migraine (note this may also be an allergy symptom)	
Brain–emotional	Anxiety, depression	Suicide
Brain–primitive	Poor pituitary function	
Hormonal function	It may be that the poor thyroid and adrenal function so often seen in CFS can be explained by poor energy delivery mechanisms	Increased risk of all above and below
Immune system	Susceptibility to infection	Upper respiratory tract infections Chest infections Urinary infections
	Susceptibility to autoimmunity and allergy	Autoimmune conditions
	Susceptibility to cancer	Cancer
Heart	Low cardiac output: low blood pressure, fatigue, pallor, cold hands and feet, feel better lying down Postural hypotension and POTs Chest pain – this is the angina of lactic acid burn Pacemaker problems – heart does not beat regularly	Heart failure
	Risk of patent foramen ovale opening up and greatly worsening heart function*	
Muscle	Muscles are not wasted as much as one would expect in CFS/ME patients who must rest. I suspect lactic acid protects from severe muscle wasting. This is because lactic acid is a powerful stimulus to make new mitochondria. Mitochondria make up 20 per cent of muscle bulk.	Muscle loss
Bone	All CFS sufferers are at risk of osteoporosis because they cannot exercise	Osteoporosis

* Dr Cheney has done much work on this aspect. In essence, the idea here is that if mitochondria go really slow, the heart does not beat strongly so there is little pressure differential between the left and right atria. This can result in the flap, which normally closes the foramen ovale (and which should have sealed up at birth), blowing open. This means that blood passes directly from the right atrium to the left atrium, bypassing the lungs and not picking up oxygen as it should. This means arterial oxygen levels will drop precipitously and CFS/ME patients suddenly dive into a much worse state. The interested reader can find more information on page 375 (Glossary).

Body system	Symptoms in the short term	Pathology in the long term
Gut	Poor digestion – increased risk of fermenting gut, malabsorption, etc	Bowel cancer
Pancreas	Increased risk of metabolic syndrome and malabsorption	Diabetes
Liver	Poor detoxification – increased susceptibility to toxic stress from the outside world and endogenous toxins	Increased risk of all above and below
Bone marrow	Tendency to anaemia, which of course reduces the oxygen-carrying capacity of the blood which in turn worsens any fatigue and increases the work of the heart	The anaemia which accompanies many chronic diseases
Fertility	The evolutionary imperative to procreate is so powerful that fertility is often maintained even when health is failing	
Kidney	This is probably the last organ to fail – it may be significant that the terminal event in some people dying from CFS/ME has been renal failure	

alive – to reproduce. In CFS/ME, even this one third can be further reduced by two significant holes. These holes reduce the energy left for the sufferer to spend on repair, renewal and recovery and also on the pleasant things in life too, such as reading, socialising and (in my case) team-chasing. It is a serious point and anything that one can do to close up or at least reduce the size of these holes will improve things, often quite dramatically.

Two significant holes in the energy bucket

The two potential holes in the energy bucket are the emotional hole and the immunological hole. The latter is a major problem – many cases of CFS/ME have an infectious trigger. Remember, the immunological hole embraces not just chronic infection but also allergy and autoimmunity. This helps us with the naming of the disease since names should reflect the underlying causes – as noted before, ME is CFS plus symptoms of inflammation, and inflammation has causes rooted in infection, allergy and autoimmunity. So, if a sufferer has a large immunological hole, then this indicates an ME clinical picture.

Regarding the two holes in particular:

Emotional. For very good reasons, many CFS/ME sufferers do not welcome discussion of this subject simply because it is leapt upon by doctors as the only cause of their fatigue – they are labelled as psychiatric patients, given inappropriate and often damaging therapies, such as CBT and GET, and all other causes are ignored. The ignoring of other causes is severely detrimental as this limits the chances for recovery. Also see Chapter 21, 'The emotional hole in the energy bucket' (page 245).

Immunological. Inflammation: allergy, fermenting gut, infection, healing and repair, autoimmunity.

Please see Appendix 7 (page 325) for the overall plan.

The energy equilibrium in CFS/ME

Dr John McLaren-Howard of Acumen Laboratories points out that it is vitally important for treatment to recognise that all patients with CFS/ME are in some sort of energy equilibrium. This equilibrium can be a very delicate and critical one. Indeed, it is quite shocking from the results seen so far how critical that situation is. It is a marvel of human metabolism and the human spirit that patients with these very severe results manage to exist at all. For example, the cell-free DNA results (see page 45) are similar to those of patients on cancer chemotherapy, and everyone knows how ghastly these patients feel and how little they can do. Remember, two thirds of all energy production goes into housekeeping duties. Most CFS/ME sufferers I see have a mitochondrial energy score of 0.6, or considerably less, meaning that they have less than 60 per cent of the energy available compared with the lower limit of normal reference range. This means that any physical or mental activity will be at the expense of housekeeping duties. This is potentially a dangerous situation since vital organs will be starved of the energy supply needed to allow them to function normally. One would expect the most energy-demanding tissues to be most affected, such as immunity, liver, brain, gut function and heart, as noted in the table on page 128.

CHAPTER 8 SUMMARY

Holes in the energy bucket

- The energy equation is: Energy delivery minus Energy expenditure.
- About two thirds of energy expenditure is on basic metabolism – the basic metabolic rate or BMR.
- This leaves very little energy for other things, and in fact some sufferers don't have enough energy even for the BMR.
- These sufferers can face multiple mild organ failure as a result of not having enough energy for basic body 'housekeeping tasks' (see the table on page 128).
- Whatever the situation regarding energy delivery, all sufferers face two significant 'holes' in their 'energy bucket' – these will further worsen the situation vis à vis the energy equation. These two holes are:
  - The emotional hole (see Chapter 21, page 245)
  - The immunological hole
- Dealing with the immunological hole is discussed in detail in Chapters 9–13 (starting on page 132) and may include testing for chronic viral presence (such as EBV) or chronic bacterial presence (such as Lyme) and trying therapies such as enzyme potentiated desensitisation so as to switch off allergies.

CHAPTER 9

The immunological hole in the energy bucket – Inflammation: the general approach

Remember:

- Chronic fatigue syndrome (CFS) = poor energy delivery mechanisms
- Myalgic encephalitis (ME) = CFS + inflammation (from healing and repair, infection, allergy, autoimmunity)

The immune system is greatly demanding of energy and therefore has huge potential to punch an immunological hole in our energy bucket. We all know this – give a healthy person a dose of 'flu and they will be bed-bound. A 175-pound man (12½ stone or 79 kilos) would require more than 250 calories daily to maintain a fever of approximately 39° C (102°F). To put that expenditure in context, the same man requires 373 calories daily for his brain and 168 calories daily for his heart.[30]

Other immune activities that require energy (and raw materials) include producing proteins and generating new immune cells in order to fight infection.[31]

Inflammation occurs when the immune system is active. This may be the inevitable normal inflammation that results from normal life, with healing and repair, or abnormal inflammation induced by Western diets and lifestyles.

Normal inflammation

- Healing and repair – bruises, fractures, tissue tears, and lacerations all need to be healed by the immune system. When CFS/ME sufferers (and, indeed, athletes) overdo things, there is minor tissue damage which has to be repaired.
- Dealing with 'friendly' microbes in the gut and keeping them in the right department – that is, in the gut.
- Infection – dealing with unfriendly microbes that breach our frontlines of defence (skin, eyes, airways, perineums).

Abnormal inflammation

- Allergy – This is an abnormal, irrelevant and energy-sapping immune activity against non-life-threatening exposures, such as pollen, animal danders, foods and gut microbes. Allergy causes serious symptoms; indeed, anaphylaxis kills people.
- Autoimmunity – This is an abnormal, irrelevant, destructive and energy-sapping immune activity against the body's own tissues – an immunological disaster! It amounts to civil war. We now know much autoimmunity is driven by pollutants, vaccination and infection, especially viruses.
- Chronic infection – We now know many cases of fatigue are driven by low-grade infection which may be viral (typically Epstein-Barr virus), bacterial (such as Lyme disease) or fungal.

Inflammation explains many of the deeply unpleasant and distressing symptoms that CFS/ME sufferers experience. Local inflammation is characterised by pain, heat, redness, swelling and loss of function. Systemic inflammation is characterised by severe fatigue with a dramatic decrease in activity and decreased interest in pleasurable pursuits, such as food, socialising and sex. These are energy conservation measures. Systemic inflammation is also characterised by malaise (feeling ill), illness behaviour, lymph nodes swelling, sore throat and tender muscles and joints.

CFS/ME sufferers often ask me for supplements to 'boost' the immune system. That question shows a misunderstanding of the above underlying principles. Stimulating the immune system which is acting inappropriately may be disastrous. Conversely, suppressing the immune system, which should be active in fighting infection, may be equally damaging. We need just the right amount of appropriate inflammation for optimum health.

The immune system is our standing army – keep it standing and not fighting!*

The immune system has a difficult job to do. It has to recognise those things which are good for us (such as food) from things that are bad for us (such as unfriendly microbes). Sometimes it has to swing into action to fight infection; this involves inflammation (pain, heat, swelling, redness and loss of function). Although short-term inflammation is vital to prevent death from infection, it is a dangerous tool – there is great potential for damage to self through 'friendly fire'. But worse, we may sensitise the immune system to things that are not dangerous to us – things like grass and tree pollen, animal danders, house dust, foods, gut microbes, our own tissues (autoimmunity), chemicals and even electromagnetic radiation. Once switched on, the immune system continues to fight (inflammation) and this may cause any symptom in any part of the body.

I think of the immune system as a 'mobile brain' in that it displays common features to those of the brain but can act anywhere in the body. Both the brain and immune system are intelligent, capable of making decisions, holding memory and solving 'problems'. They are both susceptible to, and employ, the same hormones and neurotransmitters. Just like brain cells, cells of the immune system are soft (they are contained within the bony 'skull' of long bones) and they love fat – bone marrow and brain matter are both delicate, friable materials. What is good for the brain is good for the immune system.

---

* **Historical Note:** In Great Britain, and its erstwhile colonies in America, there was distrust of a standing army not under civilian control. In England, this led to the Bill of Rights 1689, which gives authority over a standing army to Parliament, and not to the monarch. In the United States, this led to the US Constitution (Article 1, Section 8) which reserves by virtue of 'power of the purse' similar authority to Congress, instead of to the President. We need an equivalent Bill of Rights, or a Power of the Purse, for our bodies to ensure that our standing armies *stay* standing and only fight where and when absolutely necessary, and then only for as long as required – they must stand down when the job is done.

The immune system has to be clever, just as most brains have to be. The immune system's cleverness is not demonstrated through its ability to solve algebraic equations though, but rather through its ability to distinguish between 'good' and 'bad' and mount an appropriate response – a much trickier and more finely balanced task. However, just like the brain, the immune system can learn the wrong thing and this may cause life-long distress.

The normal state of affairs

How our immune cells are programmed to learn what is right and what is wrong

We imagine our bodies to be completely free from other microbes (infection). But this is not the case. Firstly, the gut is teeming with bacteria, yeasts and viruses. Indeed, if we were to add up all the cells in the body, then bacteria would outnumber human cells by 10 to 1. These bacterial cells are constantly leaking into the bloodstream and this process is called 'bacterial translocation'.[32] Even human DNA is not pristine. The human genome carries about 100,000 pieces of DNA that come from retroviruses (see Glossary, page 379), known as endogenous retroviruses. All told, these add up to an estimated 5–8 per cent of the entire human genome – that is, several times more DNA than makes up all 20,000 of our protein-coding genes.[33]

The immune system cannot 'kill' all these microbes. It would end up killing the host – that is, you and me. It has to do deals with them: 'You leave me alone and I will leave you alone.' I suspect many CFS/ME sufferers have inappropriate ongoing reactions against gut flora and viruses when their immune systems should really be doing deals with these microbes. One example we all know about is the chicken pox virus – once infected with this, the virus lies dormant, causing no trouble, for years. However, it can flare as shingles. Typically this happens if our immune system becomes less vigilant or 'gets its wires crossed'. Possibly for the same reason, I suspect Epstein-Barr virus (EBV, otherwise known as glandular fever or infectious mononucleosis, or 'mono') can cause a low-grade chronic reaction that makes people ill.

I suspect that the immune system learns, just as all other biological systems learn, on the apprenticeship system. The immature immune system that we are born with is initially programmed by our mother. It is programmed to accept whatever she offers her baby as being safe. The biggest two factors in this are diet and gut flora. Mother should be eating a Paleo-ketogenic diet, meaning that those food antigens spill over into breast milk and the baby learns to accept those as the norm. The same is true of gut microbes – the foetal gut starts to be inoculated even across the placenta whilst in utero and then there is a further large inoculation at the moment of birth. Indeed, we know these first 24 hours after birth are a critical window of time for this immune education to take place. These microbes are then fed friendly foods from human breast milk and so the gut is colonised with the mother's friendly bacteria. In its plastic (in the sense of something you can change) learning state, the baby's immune system accepts all this as the norm.

We know that 90 per cent of the immune system is associated with the gut and these mature, grown-up cells at the 'coal face' know what they must and must not react to. Immature adolescent immune cells are released on a daily basis from the bone marrow into the bloodstream and I think that they learn from the 'grown-ups' (that is, the mature immune cells working at the coal face, largely in the gut). They learn to tolerate the status quo. They too then become mature cells and so immune memory is passed down through the generations and maintained in this way. This explains the mechanism of ongoing immune tolerance to gut microbes and food – that is, most of the time the immune system can ignore these antigens and does not react against them as if they were viruses. The baby, toddler, teenager and adult has learnt not to.

In a past generation I would have been born and bred in Llangunllo, where I now live, eating the local meats and vegetables, acquiring my gut microbes from my mother, who would of course have eaten the same local diet. The rest of my life would have been spent eating the same foods that my mother had done. I might have met the odd traveller from Hereford; very occasionally such a traveller would bring in a virus. My brain and taste buds would have been bored stiff, but my immune system would have been awfully pleased with me.

Western diets and lifestyles interfere with normal immune programming and tolerance

The problem with modern life is that it is pro-inflammatory and there are many factors which tend to switch the immune system on. By the time people get to see me they have switched on their immune system for many possible reasons.

Things that are directly immunogenic – that is, a tiny dose of them can switch on the immune system – include:

Viruses. We are exposed to viruses more than ever before and more quickly than ever before because of population numbers and world travel. Furthermore, we are seeing more new viruses, perhaps with climate change, such as Ebola, bird 'flu and Zika virus.

Vaccination. This is a two-edged sword. There is clearly potential for good but also potential for harm. Vaccination may switch on the immune system to allergy to foods, to self (autoimmunity) and to gut flora. Many of my CFS/ME patients find their condition triggered or worsened by vaccination. I wonder if polio vaccination may have unleashed our epidemics of post-glandular-fever (EBV or 'mono') CFS/ME. I wonder if getting full-blown polio conferred some immunity to other enteroviruses so we 'swapped' polio for post-viral CFS, as people did not acquire immunity to, say, EBV because they were never exposed to polio. If Judy Mikovits is correct (see page 24), and she has yet to be disproved, vaccines may well be contaminated with mouse retrovirus XMRV and that may be immunotoxic.[34]

Toxic metals, such as mercury and aluminium, switch on the immune system. We know this because they are added to vaccinations. Without these adjuvants the vaccine is ineffective.

Silicone. I have seen over 250 women with CFS/ME largely due to allergies and autoimmunity following silicones used in surgery as part of depot contraceptive implants, surgical mesh for hernia repairs and other such.

Outdoor air pollution, such as small particulate matter, that is inhaled. The best example of this is particulates from diesel engines. Combined with grass pollen, they can switch on hay fever. A Japanese study showed that hay fever was more common in towns than the countryside, despite pollen counts being lower in the towns. As a result of this, approximately 25 million people (about 20 per cent of the population) in Japan currently suffer from seasonal hay fever. A dear friend and colleague, the late Dr Dick van Steenis, flagged up the very serious problems of air pollutants from industry and how well they switched on inflammation, leading to increasing rates of lung disease, heart disease and cancer.

Social and prescription drugs. These can be immunotoxic – that is, the immune system learns to recognise things which are poisonous to the body, as being 'bad' – this results in allergies PLUS multiple chemical sensitivity, i.e. allergy to chemicals

The upper fermenting gut. A recent paper by Dr Carl Nathan demonstrated how gut microbes have the potential to switch on inflammation, describing how a transient infection can trigger a chronic disease. He described the example of *Yersinia pestis* infection in mice which switched on an inflammatory reaction that persisted for 42 weeks (equivalent to 28 years in humans).[35]

Pesticides and volatile organic compounds. I have seen many patients with CFS/ME following exposure to chemicals. They suffer from such problems as sheep dip 'flu, Gulf War syndrome, aerotoxic syndrome, 9/11 syndrome and sick building syndrome. Almost invariably they have allergies to chemicals and foods, and often there is autoimmunity as well. Many develop electromagnetic sensitivity. Dr Martin Pall has suggested the mechanism of damage is that EMF (electromagnetic frequency) disrupts voltage-gated calcium channels across cell membranes, allowing calcium to flood into cells, where it is toxic.[36]

Cosmetics. It is little short of criminal that cosmetics are not assessed for toxicity. Hair dyes are known carcinogens, well absorbed through the skin, and often show up on tests of toxicity. Aluminium is used daily as a deodorant, and again easily migrates through the skin and is immunotoxic and neurotoxic. Nickel is a common allergen and carcinogen but widely used in piercings. Tattoos contain phthaltes (one of the World Health Organisation's 'Dirty Dozen'), toxic metals and hydrocarbons.

Evolutionarily incorrect foods. The commonest food allergies are to dairy products, gluten grains and yeast.

Treating inflammation

Having established the causes of inflammation, this allows us to treat it. There is a two-pronged approach:

- First, we must put in place the general interventions that apply to all cases of inflammation, not only to try to re-programme the immune system but also to prevent new inflammations developing – our 'Bill of Rights'.
- Second, we can use specific interventions to target specific problems – our 'Power of the Purse'.

The general approach to treating any condition associated with inflammation

Thankfully we have many interventions which protect the immune system from switching on inappropriately but sadly many of us are lacking in these. There is much more detail on this in my book *Sustainable Medicine*. Essentially, there is what I call the Basic Package of treatment and the Bolt-on Extras.

The Basic Package

1. **Paleo-ketogenic diet.** Staple foods: meat, fish, eggs, vegetables, nuts, seeds, salad, berries. Occasional treats: fruit.
2. **Multivitamins, minerals, essential fatty acids.** Good nutritional status (particularly antioxidants such as those detailed in Chapter 4 on mitochondria [page 51]). Anyone not taking supplements will have deficiencies simply because of Western agriculture. We all need a 'Basic Package' of nutritional supplements (see Chapter 18, page 220).
3. **Sleep.** Good quality sleep for healing and repair (see Chapter 16, page 196).
4. **Pacing** and the right sort of exercise. See Chapter 15 (page 183) and Appendix 2 (page 301).
5. **Sunshine and light.**
6. **Reduced chemical burden.** Attention to avoiding the immune stressors described above.
7. **Sufficient physical and mental security** to satisfy our universal need to love and care, and be loved and cared for. We need love, happiness and security. Upset, angry, stressed people are inflamed people. We know this because of the railway worker who suffered a terrible abdominal injury. He recovered but was left with a hole in his abdomen so that the lining of his stomach could be seen. When he became angry (as indeed I might with a nosey doctor poking around) the lining of his gut also became inflamed.
8. **Avoid infections** and treat aggressively. Try to make good choices about sexual partners and travel. I always think that going to university is particularly dangerous: there is a toxic cocktail of stressful work, disturbed sleep, crap diets, sexually transmitted diseases, the Pill, vaccinations and foreign travel.*

The Bolt-on Extras

Probiotics (such as *Lactobacillus rhamnosus, Lactobacillus plantarum*). These have proven anti-inflammatory effects in the gut.

Vitamin D. Westerners are all deficient because we do not get enough sunshine. We need at least 5000 IU daily.

Vitamin C. All humans are deficient because, along with guinea pigs and fruit bats but unlike other mammals, we cannot make our own vitamin C. We need at least 2 grams daily.

---

* **Editor's note:** But sometimes you learn a few useful things and meet wives and husbands to be!

Vitamin B12 by mouth or injection. I usually start with ½ mg (500 mcg) daily subcutaneous injection, then adjust the frequency according to response, or 5,000 mcg by sublingual spray or 1000 mcg chewable tablet daily. B12 is very benign – a colleague of mine once said, 'The only way you could kill yourself with B12 would be to drown in the stuff'!

Low-dose naltrexone (LDN). Naltrexone is an opiate-blocker used in high doses, such as 50 mg, to block the effect of opiates. However, LDN can be used in tiny doses, such as 1–4 mg at night. The idea is to slightly block the action of the body's own endogenous opiates (endorphins), which results in an increase in endogenous production. Endorphins are naturally anti-inflammatory. This property gives LDN wide clinical application for the treatment of any condition associated with inflammation. See www.lowdosenaltrexone.org for detailed information.

Alkalinisation. The use of bicarbonates and carbonates has long been recognised as a way to switch off allergy reactions, especially to foods. I suggest magnesium carbonate 500–2,000 mg last thing at night, or at least away from mealtimes. We need a window of time – at least 90 minutes after food – to achieve an acid stomach to allow normal gut function. Magnesium carbonate may be additionally useful if acid supplements are being used to treat hypochlorhydria. Where there is hypochlorhydria, one may take additional acid with food (as ascorbic acid or betaine hydrochloride). The stomach normally takes one to two hours to empty; at this point take magnesium carbonate 1–2 grams, which neutralises stomach acid and assists digestion in the duodenum.

Specific interventions to target specific problems

Having got the general approach in place, we can then look to specific interventions to tackle abnormal inflammations. Essentially these divide into:

The fermenting gut – see Chapter 7 (page 107)
Allergy – see Chapter 10 (page 143)
Chronic infection – see Chapters 11 (page 151) and 12 (page 161)

CHAPTER 9 SUMMARY

The immunological hole in the energy bucket – Inflammation: the general approach

- Inflammation, caused by the immune system, can be useful or destructive.
- Useful forms of inflammation include dealing with infections and cuts and bruises, etc.
- Destructive forms of inflammation include allergy, autoimmunity and chronic infection.
- Inflammation explains many ME symptoms.
- Inflammation uses large amounts of energy.
- So, reducing destructive inflammation reduces wasteful expenditure of energy and assists with the recovery process.
- Things which cause destructive inflammation include:
    - Viruses
    - Vaccinations
    - Toxic metals
    - Silicone
    - Outdoor pollution
    - Upper fermenting gut
    - Pesticides
    - Cosmetics
    - Evolutionarily incorrect foods
- Treatment to avoid generalised destructive inflammation includes:
    - Paleo-ketogenic diet
    - Basic package of nutritional supplements
    - Good sleep and pacing
    - Reducing the chemical burden
    - Avoiding, and aggressively treating, viruses
    - Probiotics
    - Vitamin C – at least 2 grams at night
    - Vitamin D – at least 5000 IU daily

  - Vitamin B12
  - Low-dose naltrexone (LDN) – 1–4 mg at night
  - Alkalinisation – 500–2,000 mg magnesium carbonate last thing at night

- Treatment to deal with specific causes of destructive inflammation:

  - The fermenting gut – see Chapter 7 (page 107)
  - Allergy – see Chapter 10 (page 143)
  - Chronic infection – see Chapters 11 (page 151) and Chapter 12 (page 161)

CHAPTER 10

The immunological hole in the energy bucket – Inflammation: allergy and autoimmunity

Allergy is the inflammation which results from response to substances (called antigens) from outside the body. Some of these present no threat to the body. Examples include pollen, house dust mites, animal dander and foods. Some antigens do pose a threat in high doses, such as metals (lead, mercury, arsenic, nickel), toxic chemicals (pesticides, solvents) or electromagnetic radiation (wi-fi, mobile phones, cordless phones, etc).

Allergy has been known about for centuries. For example, 5–10 per cent of people with asthma are also allergic to sulphites.[37] Pliny the Elder wrote of this when he reported the case of an asthmatic patient (rare for his times) who died from a bronchospasm in 79 AD after the eruption of Mount Vesuvius. The patient had lived a 'normal life' but for this 'one incident'.

Autoimmunity is the inflammation that results from responses to tissues within the body. I suspect most autoimmunity is switched on by pollutants (toxic metals, pesticides, volatile organic compounds and silicone), viruses or vaccination.

Allergy

Allergy is the great mimic and can produce almost any symptom. Furthermore, one can be allergic to anything under the sun, including the sun!

Allergy is common – at least 30 per cent of the population are allergic to some foods. However, by the time allergy has produced fatigue it has usually caused other problems beforehand. Suspect an allergy problem if any, or a combination, of the following are present:

The onset of fatigue is pre-dated by or there is a long history of:

- asthma, sinusitis, rhinitis, eczema or urticaria
- irritable bowel syndrome with wind, gas, bloating, abdominal pain, alternating constipation and diarrhoea
- migraine or headaches
- joint (arthritis) and muscle pain
- mood swings, depression, anxiety, PMT
- almost any unexplained, recurring, episodic symptom

Childhood problems. This would include being a sickly child with recurrent 'infections', such as tonsillitis (actually probably allergy). Indeed, a colleague who is a consultant paediatrician considers it medical negligence to surgically remove tonsils without first doing a dairy-free diet. Rhinitis, sinusitis, catarrh and colic are typical dairy allergy symptoms.

Symptoms change with time. Often the allergen is the same but the symptom changes through life. Allergy to dairy products typically starts with colic and projectile vomiting as a baby, followed by toddler diarrhoea, catarrh and glue ear, recurrent infections (tonsillitis, croup, middle ear infections) and 'growing pains'. Teenagers develop headaches, depression, irritable bowel syndrome, PMT and asthma. In adult life, muscle, tendon and joint pain (arthritis). Any of the above may be accompanied by fatigue.

Positive family history. I have yet to find a patient who is dairy allergic who does not have a first-degree relative (parent, sibling, child) who also has symptoms suggestive of allergy to dairy products. Allergy to gluten grains also runs in families.

Tendency to go for a particular food. One of the interesting aspects of allergy is that sufferers often crave the very food to which they are allergic. This was illustrated by one patient who told me that when he died he wished to take a cow to heaven with him. It was dairy which was his main problem! If wheat appears with every meal, then allergy to such is likely.

Symptoms of fermenting gut. Microbes from the gut are minuscule and easily spill over into the bloodstream. This is called 'bacterial translocation'. These bacteria do not cause septicaemia (blood poisoning), but they may cause allergy reactions at distal sites. I suspect many clinical pictures can be explained by this, including irritable bladder, interstitial cystitis, intrinsic asthma, chronic urticaria, chronic venous ulcers, polymyalgia rheumatica and arthritis (osteoarthritis, rheumatoid arthritis, ankylosing spondylitis and so on). See Chapter 7, 'The fermenting gut' (page 107).

Tests for food allergy

I never do tests for food allergy because they are unreliable. False negatives are common – so, for example, many people who are intolerant of gluten will test negative for coeliac disease. Often, when the test is negative, they are told by their doctor that it is safe to eat that food – not so! There are many tests for food allergy on the market, but again I find positive results can be misleading, not least because the patient believes absolutely in the accuracy of tests and ends up avoiding foods unnecessarily or eating foods which are causing them symptoms.

The only reliable way to diagnose food allergy is by an elimination diet. The key is to cut out those foods that one is consuming daily. The reason that reactions may be prolonged or delayed is that daily consumption masks the link between exposure and symptom. Western diets include daily consumption of grains, dairy products and often yeast. If in addition one is eating other foods, such as potato, soya or tomato, or drinking regular tea, coffee or whatever on a daily basis then this too should be excluded. One should stay on this diet for at least one month before reintroducing foods to the diet – this should be done cautiously since reactions can be severe. Dr John Mansfield developed a practical, easy-to-follow elimination diet that is described in his last book, *The Six Secrets of Successful Weight Loss*.[38]

The Paleo-ketogenic diet is a 'best guess' diet and a useful starting place. If it transpires that there are multiple allergies, then these days I do not put people on a more restricted diet – that is because some people get completely stuck on two or three foods and are unable to bring in new foods because of the above severe reactions. Instead, I put in place the interventions as detailed in Chapter 9 (page 132) (the general approach to inflammation), together with specific desensitisation techniques to switch off allergy (see page 168).

Increasingly I am finding that one does not have to be perfect to reduce allergy and allergy symptoms. Simply reducing the total load is helpful – attention to the general approach is as important as specific desensitisation.

Multiple chemical sensitivity (MCS)

The twentieth century has brought a plethora of new chemicals to which humans have never previously been exposed. Largely speaking, the body is able to ignore these as if they were not there. However, some people become sensitive to them and react in an allergic way – for example, with sneezing, runny nose, itching eyes, brain fog, headache or fatigue. A recent survey of a normal population suggested that over 38 per cent of 'normal' people reported adverse reactions to chemicals. For most people, thankfully, this chemical intolerance is no more than a nuisance and symptoms are avoided by avoiding that chemical. However, some people become multiply allergic to many chemicals and have major problems with avoidance. In these cases, health can sometimes be severely affected.

Professor Claudia Miller, in her book *Chemical Exposures: Low Levels and High Stakes*, describes the important phenomenon of chemical sensitivity.[39] Many sufferers have their chemical sensitivity triggered by overwhelming exposure to some sort of toxic chemical, such as organophosphates or other pesticides, silicone, carbon monoxide or prescription drugs. This phenomenon is called 'toxicant-induced loss of tolerance' (TILT). Once sensitised to one chemical, patients often go on to sensitise to other unrelated chemicals and this is called the 'spreading phenomenon'. Those patients who recognise their problem with chemicals avoid them strictly in order to avoid symptoms. MCS is very common in patients I see whose CFS/ME has been triggered by chemical exposure – notably Gulf War veterans (organophosphates and other chemicals), sheep dip 'flu farmers (organophosphates), aerotoxic pilots, 9/11 syndrome (organochlorine poisoning from burnt plastics) and so on. Appendix 4 (page 312) gives a list of common toxins, all of which I have seen within my clinical practice to have switched on MCS.

Treatment for MCS

Treatment of MCS is always difficult and the priorities are:

- Avoidance – do your best to do a good chemical clean-up (see Appendix 5, page 315).
- Detoxify, to reduce the endogenous load (see Chapter 20, page 233); this helps to reduce the total exposure to chemicals. With allergy, much is about reducing total load.
- The general approach to treating inflammation (see Chapter 9, page 132).

Electrical sensitivity (ES)

Electrical sensitivity (ES) is a real phenomenon. I have had too many people affected by electromagnetic radiation (EMR) to think otherwise. Clinically, I nearly always see electrical sensitivity in people who are already suffering from chemical sensitivity.

It's hardly surprising that one can be electrically sensitive – high doses of EMR can kill and EMR is a known cause of cancer. The body can detect it, and if it can detect it, it can sensitise to it – there are obvious parallels with chemical sensitivity.

There are many symptoms that can be switched on by electrical sensitivity and it appears that almost any electromagnetic frequency (EMF) can cause this. These are emitted by all sorts of electrical pieces of equipment, such as mobile phones, cordless phones, internet connections, computers, microwaves, baby listeners, microwave room sensors, burglar alarms, mobile phone masts, television sets, strip lighting and many other gadgets.

Thanks to Professor Martin Pall (see page 138) we have a biochemical explanation for ES, viz, EMF disrupts voltage-gated calcium channels across cell membranes. So in a susceptible individual, ES will allow calcium to leak into cells. Calcium is toxic inside cells – the normal concentration gradient of calcium outside to inside is a 14,000-fold difference. Since all cells have voltage-gated calcium channels, ES can present with any symptom.

As always, diagnosis is difficult and good detective work is needed – one needs a high index of suspicion. Of course, symptoms arise and worsen when one is exposed and resolve when one is not exposed. However, we now have some gadgets that can help to diagnose the electrical sensitivity. One can buy an electro-smog detector, which tells one if there is EMR pollution. This converts the EMR into an audible signal so one can easily tell where the hot spots are. This is available from Healthy House (see page 385).

Recently (August 2015), as I mentioned in Chapter 3 (page 32), a French court awarded a woman a disability grant for 'allergy to gadgets', as it was phrased. The court recognised that Marine Richard, 39, suffers from electromagnetic hypersensitivity to everyday devices, such as mobile phones.[40]

How to protect yourself from electromagnetic radiation (EMR)

I am grateful to Sarah Dacre, who has put me in touch with some organisations which help further – namely, Detect & Protect, and Powerwatch; also Electric Forester (see page 384).

It is also possible to get shrouds that one can wear like a sort of cloak which block out all EMR. This, for example, allowed Sarah to attend a meeting at the House of Commons recently. These are available from Powerwatch's product site, EMFields (see page 386). She showed me how the detector howled with noise outside the shroud and went almost silent inside it. This convinced me!

Finally, do contact Electrosensitivity UK (see page 384). They have a freely available helpline staffed by volunteers.

For protection from radiation emitted by mobile phones and computers, visit SaferWave (see page 386).

Earthing is often helpful to reduce the electrical charge load. The idea here is for the body to come in direct contact with the ground via a conducting medium – for example, walking barefoot on grass, earth, rock, etc. Wearing rubber-soled shoes or boots blocks this effect.

There is some evidence that in electro-sensitivity (ES), production of melatonin is reduced and this impacts on sleep. Try melatonin 1–9 mg at night to counter this.

Toxic metals may worsen ES

We are all conductors of EMR – I can greatly improve the reception of my wireless by holding the aerial! Toxic metals will make us better conductors and therefore better receivers. Since humans have been mobilising minerals from the Earth's crust, more have appeared in our food, water and air and so we all have a toxic metal load. Indeed, I suspect this is what is contributing to our current epidemics of cardiac dysrhythmias, such as atrial fibrillation. I recommend measuring urine for toxic metals after taking the oral chelating agent DMSA (see page 355). The metals that most commonly come up are mercury, lead, arsenic and nickel. See Chapter 20 (page 233) on detoxing to see how to rid the body of toxic metals.

Autoimmunity

Autoimmunity is essentially allergy to self. It is self-evident that this is a completely useless and destructive immune process. One can be 'allergic' to any tissue within the body or, indeed, any cell organelle within the body. One possible mechanism by which this may arise is called 'molecular mimicry'. The idea here is that the immune system reacts to an antigen, such as a food or microbe, in the gut. Through pure chance this antigen is the same shape as a cell type in the body. Autoimmunity is switched on because the body 'sees' the cell type as an antigen. Perhaps the best example is ankylosing spondylitis. In this condition there is molecular mimicry between klebsiella bacteria in the gut and the spinal ligaments of people who are HLA B27 positive. So, in essence the body makes antibodies against klebsiella bacteria in the gut and then these antibodies cross-react with spinal ligaments and cause the condition of ankylosing spondylitis. A ketogenic diet is a highly effective element in treating this condition because klebsiella organisms are starved out of the gut. Gluten has been associated with autoimmune thyroiditis, autoimmune hepatitis, vitiligo, rheumatoid arthritis and many other conditions. Please see www.glutenfreesociety.org/gluten-and-the-autoimmune-disease-spectrum.

As I have said already, the human body has several hundred cell types and so there is potential for several hundred different autoimmune conditions and each one has a different name. However, the approach to treatment is the same as allergy – first the general and then the specific. Unlike with allergy to antigens, we do not have any specific tools to switch off autoimmunity. However, many autoimmune conditions are driven by microbes, of which there is much more in Chapters 11 (page 151) and 12 (page 161).

CHAPTER 10 SUMMARY

The immunological hole in the energy bucket – Inflammation: allergy and autoimmunity

- Allergy is inflammation caused by exposure to external substances – 'allergens'.
- Autoimmunity is inflammation caused by a reaction against tissues within the body.
- Allergy is the great mimic and can cause almost any symptom.
- Allergy can be suspected if there is evidence of:
  - A history of:
    - asthma, rhinitis, eczema or urticaria
    - irritable bowel syndrome with wind, gas, bloating, abdominal pain, alternating constipation and diarrhoea
    - migraine or headaches
    - joint (arthritis) and muscle pain
    - mood swings, depression, anxiety, PMT
    - almost any unexplained, recurring, episodic symptom
  - Childhood problems
  - Symptoms changing with time

  - Positive family history
  - Tendency to go for a particular food
  - Fermenting gut

- Tests for food allergy are unreliable and so the best way to diagnose is to do an elimination diet.
- Multiple chemical sensitivity (MCS) is a real condition. The principles of treatment are:

  - Avoidance – do your best to do a good chemical clean-up (see Appendix 5, page 315).
  - Detoxify, to reduce the endogenous load (see Chapter 20, page 233); this helps to reduce the total exposure to chemicals. With allergy much is about reducing total load.
  - The general approach to treating inflammation (see Chapter 9, page 132).

- Electrical sensitivity (ES) is a real condition and almost always associated with MCS.
- Professor Martin Pall has shown that any electromagnetic frequency (EMF) disrupts voltage-gated calcium channels across cell membranes, bringing too much calcium into cells; this could be the physiological basis for ES.
- Treatment for ES is based on protecting yourself from electromagnetic radiation (EMR) and also testing for and chelating toxic metals which may worsen the problem (see page 353 for more detail).

CHAPTER 11

The immunological hole in the energy bucket – Inflammation: chronic infections – Viral

Life is an arms race. You and I are a free lunch for microbes which try every possible ploy to make themselves comfortably at home within our delicious bodies. (Much more of this in my book *Sustainable Medicine*). Prevention is better than cure, but most of us ignore the 'prevention' side of things until we become ill, or maybe until we see someone we love become ill. And so, like the old Irish joke, when asked the way to Dublin the traveller was told:

Well, if I were you I wouldn't be starting from here.

I would love to start my work with well people and that way we could keep them well, but people only come to me when they are ill (or, to complete the analogy, when they are 'lost' like the traveller on his way to Dublin) and so here we are.

Many patients with CFS/ME have an infectious burden and the commonest offenders arise from:

1. The fermenting gut (see Chapter 7, page 107)
2. Chronic viral infection (this chapter)
3. Chronic bacterial infection (see Chapter 12, page 161)

Chronic viral infection

I have learned so much from the work of Dr Martin Lerner (see Appendix 6, page 319). I also know from my own clinical experience that the interventions he recommends are very often effective. We know many viral infections are associated with fatigue, with the obvious offenders being hepatitis and HIV. The treatment of these conditions is to reduce the viral load so that clinical benefits result. The principle in CFS/ME is exactly the same, but I suspect it is more a case of allergy to virus rather than total viral load. I may be wrong here

Table 11.1. The normal person with normal, appropriate immune reactions; this person is tolerant

Low numbers of antigen	Medium numbers of antigen	High levels of antigen (e.g. pneumonia)
No threat to the body	Modest threat to the body	Immune system alerted and appropriately switched on
No symptoms	Immune system can ignore	Severe symptoms, possibly life threatening

Table 11.2. The slightly sensitive, mildly allergic person (38 per cent of the population)

Low numbers of antigen	Medium numbers of antigen	High levels of antigen (e.g. pneumonia)
No threat to the body	Modest threat to the body; immune system alerted and inappropriately switched on	Immune system alerted and appropriately switched on
No symptoms	Allergy symptoms: catarrh, cough, asthma, headache, IBS, arthritis, etc	Severe symptoms, possibly life threatening

Table 11.3. The very sensitive person

Low numbers of antigen	Medium numbers of antigen	High levels of antigen (e.g. pneumonia)
No threat to the body; immune system alerted and inappropriately switched on	Modest threat to the body; immune system alerted and inappropriately switched on	Immune system alerted and appropriately switched on
Allergy symptoms: catarrh, cough, asthma, headache, IBS, arthritis, etc	Severe symptoms, possibly life threatening	Severe symptoms, possibly life threatening

– it may be that the virus is tucked away in the immune system and brain so it does not appear in the bloodstream – this would make it difficult to measure total viral load. Not that this matters greatly for practical purposes.

The only difference between allergy reactions and infectious reactions is the load of antigens (in this case, the number of microbes) and the immune system's reaction to such. I think of this as a spectrum of activity. We start with the normal person with appropriate immune reactions (Table 11.1), then the slightly sensitive, mildly allergic person (Table 11.2), then the very sensitive person (Table 11.3).

Herpes viruses are notoriously persistent in the body. The best known example is chickenpox – that virus may lie dormant in the body for decades and emerge as shingles later. We know herpes viruses drive many cases of autoimmunity (probably by molecular mimicry) and these viruses also drive cancer, although the process of this occurs without symptoms. Where inflammation is a major player we see the ME clinical picture and not just CFS – remember, ME equals CFS plus inflammation (see page 42).

I think the herpes virus family is particularly implicated in post-viral CFS/ME for the reasons listed below and expanded in Table 11.4 (page 154):

1. Martin Lerner reckons Epstein-Barr virus (EBV) is causally involved in over 80 per cent of cases of ME.
2. All these viruses infect the brain, peripheral nervous system and immune system – all areas affected by ME.
3. ME is often triggered by these infections, especially EBV (also known as glandular fever, mononucleosis, infectious mononucleosis and 'mono').
4. Neurological symptoms are common in ME and are known to be associated with herpes viruses; these include pain (what I think of as allergic nerves), numbness, tingling and weakness. Indeed, many of the symptoms of multiple sclerosis are very similar to ME.
5. Immunological disorders, like allergy and autoimmunity, are common in ME.
6. Vitamin B12 by injection is often very helpful. Dr Patrick Kingsley, who treated over 5,000 patients with multiple sclerosis (MS), used B12 injections routinely and to good effect – he too reckoned herpes viruses were causal in ME.[41] Since at least 1961 there has been evidence of the efficacy of B12 against herpes viruses.[42] MS has also been linked with herpes viruses in many studies, for example that by Hawkes et al (2006), 'Seroprevalence of herpes simplex virus type 2 in multiple sclerosis'.[43] This may explain the efficacy of B12 in MS patients too.

Table 11.4. The relationship between herpes viruses and other conditions

Herpes virus	Infection with
HHV 1 Herpes simplex	Mouth ulcers Whitlow Encephalitis Contact with an infected area of the skin during reactivations of the virus (as a result, this was a common affliction of dental surgeons prior to the routine use of gloves)
HHV 2	Genital herpes Meningitis
HHV 3 *Varicella zoster* virus	Chicken pox Shingles
HHV 4 (EBV)	Glandular fever Gets into immune cells
HHV 5 (cytomegalovirus)	Glandular, fever-like illness Infects every organ of the body, including brain eye immune system Hepatitis Pneumonia
HHV 6 herpes virus	Acute febrile illness with rash (roseola) Encephalitis
HHV 7 herpes virus (HHV 7 has been shown to reactivate HHV 6 infection)	Similar to above
HHV 8 (KSHV)	

Please see Alibek et al (2014), 'Implication of human herpes viruses in oncogenesis through immune evasion and suppression', for more detail on the possible mechanisms involved.[44]

Autoimmunity	Cancer	Other
Myasthenia gravis	Oral cancer HHV1 has been detected in benign and malignant thyroid tumours and melanoma	Alzheimer's disease Mollaret's meningitis Herpes simplex encephalitis
	Cervical cancer Cancer of the penis, anus, vagina, vulva	
	Leukaemia, lymphoma, skin cancer, benign and malignant breast tumours	Encephalitis Pneumonia Post-herpetic neuralgia Mollaret's meningitis Ramsay Hunt syndrome
At least 33 different conditions: lupus, rheumatoid arthritis, MS and Sjögren's syndrome	Burkitt's lymphoma Nasopharyngeal cancer Gastric cancer B lymphoproliferative disorder Hodgkin's lymphoma Stomach cancer	X-linked lymphoproliferative syndrome
Guillain-Barré syndrome, Type 1 diabetes	Mucoepidermoid carcinoma Prostate cancer Glioblastoma (90% association), skin cancer	Meningoencephalitis Pericarditis Myocarditis Thrombocytopenia Haemolytic anaemia Gastrointestinal ulceration
Multiple Sclerosis Hashimoto's thyroiditis	HHV-6 has been detected in lymphomas, leukemias, cervical cancers and brain tumours. Basal cell carcinoma. Glioma	Optic neuritis Temporal lobe epilepsy Liver failure
Graves' disease	Implicated in some of the same cancers as HHV 6	Drug-induced hypersensitivity syndrome Encephalopathy
	Kaposi's sarcoma Lymphoma Multicentric castleman disease (MCD) Primary effusion lymphoma (PEL)	

I suspect in CFS/ME the body is reacting against these microbes, with inflammation. That may cause both local inflammation wherever the virus hangs out, in addition to general inflammation. This is expensive in terms of energy and raw materials and has potential to kick an immunological hole in the energy bucket.

Martin Lerner, who died in October 2015 at the age of 86, had been working since 1993 on the idea that many cases of CFS/ME result from long-standing infection with herpes viruses. The most important of these is Epstein-Barr virus (glandular fever or 'mono', HHV 4), but he has also identified two other herpes viruses as a particular problem in CFS/ME sufferers, namely cytomegalovirus (HHV5) and human herpes virus 6 (HHV-6). He demonstrated that in CFS/ME sufferers there is what he called 'non-permissive replication' of the virus. By this he meant that there was sufficient viral replication going on in cells to disrupt cellular metabolism and cause cell death, but not sufficient to result in a positive DNA polymerase test, or antigenaemia with antibody response. This meant that such chronic infection would not be picked up by standard virology tests, including antibodies and polymerase chain reaction (PCR).

The grounds for starting treatments with antivirals

If tested, nearly all of us would show antibodies against one or more herpes viruses, showing we have been infected with such in the past. So whilst a positive antibody test is helpful, this should not be the only criterion for using antivirals. The criteria I would use are as follows:

1. A clear history of post-viral CFS.
2. All other interventions are already in place with respect to all that has gone before in this book. The 'battle' against any infection is not really a battle at all, but rather it's a war. Think of siege warfare – there are many different ways one can dislodge the enemy from its defensive position. Believe me, once these viruses are established in the body they are very well defended. We need a well-nourished, standing army with abundant energy and correct programming to fight infection efficiently. Attention to all these details should greatly improve the chances of a good response to antivirals. Importantly, these interventions greatly reduce the likelihood of drug resistance emerging – largely speaking, this is a problem of the immunosuppressed patient. People eating high-sugar, low-micronutrient, toxic Western diets are immunosuppressed.
3. A positive IgG antibody titre against herpes virus.

It may be that there are other bacterial co-infections. However, I think it is reasonable to start with antivirals and assess patient progress clinically. There are several reasons for this:

- First, one cannot know if a virus is clinically significant except by response to treatment. If the patient improves on antivirals then the virus is an important player.
- Second, antivirals do not upset the gut microbiome.
- Third, valacyclovir does seem to be a remarkably safe drug and well tolerated – if a patient worsens on this drug, one can assume this is a Herxheimer reaction (see Table 14.1, page 179) and that is good news.

Treatment regimes

- Valacyclovir 1 gram every six hours (that is, 4 grams per day). For larger patients, the dose is 1.5 grams every six hours and for small patients correspondingly less.
- Monitor creatinine at one, three and six months, then every three months. This can be done on a finger drop sample of blood – in other words, it can be done at home and sent direct to the laboratory.
- Drink at least 500 ml of water over and above normal requirements.

Initial response to treatment

- A Herxheimer response (see Table 14.1, page 179), with worsening of symptoms and a worsening 'energy score' continuing for two to six weeks after treatment begins, is a good prognostic omen because it indicates there is a viral infection present that is responding to treatment.
- Lerner found that increasing energy scores and decreasing symptoms were apparent at the fifth to sixth month of continuing valacyclovir.
- Lerner found that the above clinical improvements were accompanied by improvement in ECG (heart rhythm) monitoring.

Long-term maintenance

- As energy levels improve, the dose of valacyclovir can be reduced to, for example, one gram, two times a day.
- Continue treatment long term – this is different from one patient to another but the general rule of thumb is to take valacyclovir for two

months after symptoms have resolved. I do see this may be tricky to judge, but most people have a pretty good idea of what the antiviral is doing and at which point the response to such plateaus.
- Approximately 20 per cent of EBV CFS/ME patients require long-term maintenance of low-dose valacyclovir to prevent clinical relapse.

Dr Lerner went on to report on the outcomes of four studies using these regimes. These are detailed in Appendix 6 (see page 319).

CHAPTER 11 SUMMARY

The immunological hole in the energy bucket – Inflammation: chronic infections – Viral

- Life is an arms race between us and the microbes that would like to make their homes in our body.
- People eating high-sugar, low-micronutrient, toxic Western diets are immunosuppressed.
- There are three main areas of concern for CFS/ME sufferers:
    - The fermenting gut (see Chapter 7, page 107)
    - Chronic viral infection (this chapter)
    - Chronic bacterial infection (see Chapter 12, page 161)
- Herpes viruses (HHV1-8) are particularly implicated in CFS/ME:
    - Dr Martin Lerner reckons Epstein-Barr virus (EBV – HHV4) is causally involved in over 80 per cent of CFS/ME cases.
    - All these viruses infect the brain, peripheral nervous system and immune system – all areas affected by CFS/ME.
    - CFS/ME is often triggered by these infections, especially EBV (also known as glandular fever, mononucleosis, infectious mononucleosis, 'mono').
    - Neurological symptoms are common in CFS/ME and are known to be associated with herpes viruses.
    - Vitamin B12 by injection is often very helpful. Dr Patrick Kingsley, who treated over 5,000 patients with multiple sclerosis

(MS), used B12 injections routinely and to good effect – he too reckoned herpes viruses were causal in MS.

- Herpes viruses are associated with many cancers and autoimmune conditions – see Table 11.4 on page 154.
- Dr Martin Lerner worked in this area for over 30 years and there are many studies showing benefit to CFS/ME sufferers of treating active HHV viruses (see Appendix 6, page 319).
- There may be bacterial co-infections, but it is reasonable to tackle the viruses first with antivirals and assess patient progress clinically. There are several reasons for this:
  - First, one cannot know if a virus is clinically significant except by response to treatment. If the patient improves on antivirals then the virus is an important player.
  - Second, antivirals do not upset the gut microbiome.
  - Third, the drug valacyclovir does seem to be remarkably safe and well tolerated – if a patient worsens on this drug, one can assume this is a Herxheimer reaction (see Table 14.1, page 179) and that is good news.
- My criteria for treatment with antivirals are:
  - A clear history of post-viral CFS/ME.
  - All other interventions are already in place with respect to all that has gone before in this book.
  - A positive IgG antibody titre against herpes virus (the concetration as determined by titration).
- The antiviral treatment regime is:
  - Valacyclovir 1 gram every six hours (that is, 4 grams per day). For larger patients the dose should be 1.5 grams every six hours and for small patients correspondingly less.
  - Monitor creatinine at one, three and six months. This can be done on a finger drop sample of blood – that is, it can be done at home and sent direct to the laboratory.
  - Drink at least 500 ml of water over and above normal requirements.

- Initial response to treatment may be as follows:
  - A Herxsheimer response (Table 14.1, page 179), with worsening of symptoms and a worsening 'energy score' continuing for two to six weeks after treatment began, is a good prognostic omen.
  - Lerner found that increasing energy scores and decreasing symptoms were apparent at the fifth to sixth month of continuing valacyclovir.
  - Lerner found that the above clinical improvements were accompanied by improvement in ECG (heart rhythm) monitoring.
- Long-term maintenance may be as follow:
  - As energy levels improve, the dose of valacyclovir can be reduced to, for example, 1 gram two times a day.
  - Continue treatment long term – the general rule of thumb is to take valacyclovir for two months after symptoms have resolved.
  - Approximately 20 per cent of EBV CFS/ME patients require long-term maintenance with low-dose valacyclovir to prevent clinical relapse.

CHAPTER 12

The immunological hole in the energy bucket – Inflammation: chronic infections – Bacterial: Lyme and other co-infections

Chronic bacterial infections

It is well recognised that many chronic bacterial infections present with fatigue. Obvious examples include tuberculosis, bronchiectasis and syphilis. It astonishes me that the medical profession continues to ignore a range of more recently recognised chronic infections which also present with chronic, progressive symptoms. The most important of these is Lyme disease, but there are others.

These conditions again present with symptoms of CFS plus symptoms of inflammation – namely, myalgic encephalitis (ME). When I was at medical school, syphilis was dubbed the 'great mimic' because it could produce almost any pathology. Exactly the same could be said of Lyme disease. Interestingly, the infective organisms behind both Lyme and syphilis are spirochetes.

Lyme is now being implicated not just in CFS/ME but also in arthritis, dementia, heart disease and probably cancer. We are laying ourselves open to this, and other equally unpleasant infections, because of the immune-suppressing effects of Western diets and lifestyles. As I keep on saying, life is an arms race – deplete the defences and the microbes will prevail.

Biofilm – with chronic infection, the microbes throw up comfortable wrappings behind which they can hide

The production of biofilm is an intelligent response by microbes in their defence against attack. This is a further facet of the 'arms race'. Indeed, Dr Alan MacDonald has shown that in Lyme disease, borrelia conceal themselves in a substance called amyloid.[45] Amyloid has been known about for years and is associated with many chronic diseases but its reason for existing is unknown. However, if amyloid is indeed the shield behind which microbes hide, then this opens up very interesting avenues for treatment of any disease associated with amyloid – that is to say, it may be a marker for a chronic inflammation driven by infection. (Note the term 'amyloid' is a misnomer – the substance is not a starch but a tough protein with some sugars bound within.)

Examples of biofilm include dental plaque (*Streptococcus mutans*, the microbe responsible for dental decay, hides here), the coated tongue (microbes typically causing halitosis may hide here), gut mucopolysaccharide, fibrin clots, amyloid (plaques form in the brain and are associated with Alzheimer's) and other such possibilities.

Microbes may exist in more than one form to dodge the immune system's bullets

Microbes may exist in more than one form. Borrelia (the infective organism behind Lyme), for example, cycles from the cell-wall-deficient form known as the 'L-form' to the dormant or 'latent cyst' form. Encapsulating itself into the inactive cyst form enables the spirochete to hide undetected in the host for months, years or decades until some form of immune suppression initiates a signal that it is safe for the cysts to open and the spirochetes to come forth and multiply.

Chronic microbial infection exhausts the body's normal immune defences

One needs energy and raw materials to supply the immune system to allow it to fight infections effectively. It is a feature of the Armin tests (see page 163) for these chronic infections that, where such have been diagnosed, numbers of immune cells are almost invariably low. Dr Armin explains this in terms of a chronic immune exhaustion; that makes perfect sense to me. The immune system cannot keep up with demand – the microbes are winning the arms race. This is all the more reason to put in place all the other interventions I've described. Indeed, I have many CFS/ ME patients who recover substantially before we even get to the stage of testing for chronic infections. Simply on the law of averages, some must have been infected. But if one supports the immune system and stops feeding the little wretches (the bacteria, that is) with carbohydrates, then the body can do its own job of kicking arse!

Testing for Lyme and co-infections

There are many possible microbes which could be associated with ME (CFS plus inflammation). Ideally we would do all the tests for all patients, but if finances preclude then the list in Table 12.1 gives some guidance.

These tests (including the EliSpot and SerraSpot for Lyme) have 99 per cent sensitivity and 95 per cent specificity, which is good for any laboratory test.[46] If you wish to read more about how they work, see www.elispot.com. AONM are the UK distributors for Armin Labs (www.arminlabs.com/en) that carry them out.[47] The test requires special blood tubes which are easily posted, with results back five days after they have been received by the lab.

Treatment for chronic Lyme

Remember, as Pasteur famously said on his death bed: 'The microbe is nothing, the environment is everything.'

This is always difficult because by the time the patient has been diagnosed the organism has overcome the body's natural defences and made itself comfortably at home tucked into a warm and nutritious bed, wrapped up in biofilm.

Table 12.1. When to test for microbes associated with CFS/ME and how to treat them

Clinical picture	Test for	Treatment continued for two months after symptoms have settled
Post-viral ME	Epstein-Barr, HHV 3, HHV 5, HHV 6, HHV 8	Valacyclovir – see Chapter 11, page 151
Post-infectious ME with pneumonia or sexually transmitted chlamydia	Chlamydia pneumonia, Chlamydia trachomatis, Mycoplasma	Doxycycline 100 mg twice daily
Ticks Blood contamination No clear history	Anaplasma, Yersinia, Borrelia, Bartonella, Babesia – that is, Lyme disease	Anti-Lyme regime – see Table 12.2, page 165 Doxycycline 100 mg twice daily

It may be for some patients that improving energy delivery mechanisms together with the general approach to treating inflammation is sufficient to get rid of chronic Lyme. I say this because many of my patients recover well with these regimes and many must have had Lyme, since this disease appears to be such a common problem. However, some ME patients will *additionally* need the interventions I describe next.

Expose and weaken the microbes

First one has to expose the microbes to the antimicrobials by breaking down biofilms. If this additionally has to do with protective layers within the gut and mucus, then restoring normal gut function with respect to stomach acid, pancreatic enzymes, bile salts and so on may be very helpful – that is, all my usual package used to treat the upper fermenting gut (see Chapter 7, page 107). Enzymes, such as serrapeptidase 80,000 IU tablets (two capsules taken three times daily), are often used to break down biofilm and my guess is that the mechanism of action is to dissolve them.

Kill the microbes with antimicrobials

Having got all the above in place, one then has to consider antimicrobials to kill these co-infections. In dealing with them we have to take a 'tuberculosis-like' approach – that is, it is combinations of antibiotics that will get the result and these have to be taken over months, not weeks.

I have not been working with the above diseases for long enough to be expert. However, I can read the work of other doctors who are. The recommendations below are from these doctors. They sometimes use intravenous antibiotics – I have not included those regimes simply because they are almost impossible to put in place in the UK. I hope, and believe, that by first putting in the above regimes to improve the defences, this will make the oral regimes as effective as the intravenous ones.

Combinations of antibiotics are important to tackle the microbes in their various forms. It is important to combine antimicrobials for 'cell wall' and 'cystic' forms of Lyme together with those to get at intracellular microbes.

THE GROUNDS FOR STARTING TREATMENTS WITH ANTIBIOTICS

The criteria I would use are as follows:

- A history of post-infectious CFS/ME – sometimes there is additional clear clinical evidence of infection, such as tick bite, bull's-eye rash, erythema migrans or acute arthritis, but most often none such. (If one was lucky enough to be clinically diagnosed at this early stage then I would not even wait for positive test results but treat with doxycycline 100 mg twice daily for three weeks to nip this nasty infection in the bud.)

- Symptoms of inflammation (see Chapter 3, page 20).
- All other interventions described so far in this book are already in place. As detailed above, the battle against any infection is not a battle; it's a war.
- Positive tests showing evidence of immune activity against microbes. For some years I sat on the fence with respect to diagnosing Lyme and co-infections because I was not sure which tests I could trust. Simple antibody testing has a high incidence of false negative results; 'Western blot' testing seems to have a high incidence of false positive results. I now recommend EliSpot and SerraSpot testing, which, as I have said, are available through Armin Labs.

Treatment should be given for at least two months, and continued for two months after the patient is symptom free. This may be possible at a

Table 12.2. Antibiotic and herbal treatment regimes for chronic Lyme disease

Drug	Dose	Purpose	Alternative oral antibiotics
Doxycycline	100 mg twice daily	Tackle intracellular forms	
Metronidazole	400 mg three times daily	Tackle cystic forms	tinidazole 400 mg three times daily
Co-amoxyclav	500/125 mg two capsules taken three times daily*	Tackle 'cell wall' forms	cefuroxime 500 mg twice daily
Serrapeptidase (or other enzymes, such as pancreatic enzyme)	two 500 mg capsules three times daily	Break down biofilm	azithromycin 500 mg once daily, or ciproxin 500 mg twice daily
Possibly plaquenil	200 mg daily	Reduce unpleasant immune reactions – needs an eye check with optician once a month	
Herbal Treatments:			
Samento	500 mg three times daily		Samento often used with banderol
Possibly stevia	Ditto		
Banderol	Build up to 30 drops daily of the concentrate		

* A single Co-amoxyclav capsule contains 500 mg of amoxil and 125 mg of clavulanic acid. The dose is 2 of these capsules 3 times a day, making a daily dose of 6 capsules.

lower rate of dosing. Indeed, this is the general rule of thumb in treating any chronic infection.

RESPONSE TO TREATMENT

The response can be monitored clinically ('How do you feel?') and also with EliSpot blood tests to show (hopefully) that the white cells are reacting less against the microbes as the numbers (of microbes) come down.

I am on a very steep learning curve with respect to treating Lyme and co-infections. As I learn more I shall post information on my website.

Postscript

A recent study by Theophilus et al (2015) published in the *European Journal of Microbiology and Immunology* has shown that stevia had a significant effect in eliminating *Borrelia burgdorferi* spirochetes and persisters.[48] This is another avenue I am pursuing and no doubt more will open up as time goes by.

CHAPTER 12 SUMMARY

The immunological hole in the energy bucket – Inflammation: chronic infections – Bacterial: Lyme and other co-infections

- Lyme disease is the most important of the recently recognised chronic infections.
- Many doctors do not recognise Lyme as such.
- A key factor in treating Lyme disease is recognising the existence of biofilm – a comfortable wrapping, or shield, that is thrown up, and behind which the microbes can hide.
- Microbes can exist in many forms so as to dodge the immune system – *Borrelia* (the infective organism in Lyme), for example, cycles from the 'cell-wall-deficient' form, known as the' L-form' to the 'dormant' or 'latent cyst' form.
- Chronic microbial infection exhausts the body's normal immune defences – at this stage, the microbes are winning the arms race.
- Testing for Lyme disease and co-infections should be as shown in Table 12.2, page 165. (**NB:** Elispot and Serraspot testing are recommended for Lyme disease.)
- Treatment is two-fold:
    - One must expose the microbes and weaken them; this can be done using all my usual package of interventions for a fermenting gut (see Chapter 7, page 107) and also using substances such as serrapeptidase 80,000 IU tablets (two capsules three times daily), which break down biofilms.
    - Then one must kill the microbes with antimicrobials – see Table 12.2, page 165 for the criteria for treatment with antibiotics.
- Response to treatment should be monitored by use of the EliSpot tests and also by observing and recording clinical signs.
- Treatment should be given for at least two months, and continued for two months after the patient is symptom free. This may be possible at a lower rate of dosing. Indeed, this is the general rule of thumb in treating any chronic infection.

CHAPTER 13

Reprogramming the immune system

Like the brain, the immune system has memory. Largely speaking this is very helpful. But, as with the brain, if the wrong things are learned it is difficult to unlearn them. We cannot wind the clock back and start again.

Switching off allergy and autoimmunity by reprogramming the immune system

I recommend a two-pronged approach:

1. The general approach to treating any condition associated with inflammation (see Chapter 9, page 132)
2. The specific approaches for allergy and autoimmunity

My ideas for reprogramming the immune system come from the treatment of polymyalgia rheumatica (PMR) and temporal arteritis. These conditions are clearly pro-inflammatory and are highly damaging to the self. They are useless, self-destructive immune reactions and are both effectively treated with steroids – drugs which, in this context, have the effect of putting the immune system into a 'straitjacket'.* It is not allowed to react. However, what is interesting is

---

* **Historical note:** The straitjacket was invented in France in 1790 by an upholsterer named Guilleret, for Bicêtre Hospital and was first known as Camisole de Force. Some camisole!

that after several months of use, these drugs can slowly be tailed off and the patient is cured. So we must ask ourselves: what is the mechanism of this? How does this happen?

Things do not [just] happen.
Things are made to happen.

JOHN F KENNEDY
(29 May 1917 – 22 November 1963)

As detailed in Chapter 9 (specifically page 135), the immune system, I suspect, learns on the apprenticeship system. Put the mature cells in a straitjacket so that they do not react and the adolescents also learn that they too should not react. It seems to take several months of this straitjacket programming to see a clinical response. Since all the techniques detailed below also take some months to see a good clinical response, I suspect that the mechanism of action is similar – that is, immune tolerance is induced.

The five-pronged approach

In practice, we need to employ a five-pronged approach:

1. First, avoid all those factors, in as much as one can, which are switching the immune system on (see Chapter 9, page 132).
2. Second, put in place all possible interventions to make the immune system less twitchy and prone to inflammation (again, see Chapter 9, page 132).
3. Third, put the immune system into a drug-induced straitjacket and stop the inappropriate reactions of the mature white cells. Do this for several months, slowly reducing the dose at a rate at which symptoms do not flare.
4. Fourth, use antimicrobials to reduce the microbial load (see Chapters 11 [page 151] and 12 [page 161]). It may be that the above interventions will be *all* necessary to get a result.
5. Fifth, use proven methods to switch off the immune system. In order of practical application, I would do the following:

    1. oral immunotherapy (food drops – see page 171)
    2. enzyme potentiated desensitisation (EPD – see page 173)
    3. neutralisation (see page 173)

Put the immune system in a straitjacket

There are some clinical pictures which ME patients may suffer, in addition to severe fatigue, which may merit the use of the immune straitjacket. Examples of symptoms and appropriate straitjackets include (but are not limited to) immunosuppressives such as:

- Anti-inflammatory drugs such as NSAIDs
- Antihistamines for chronic urticaria (hives)
- Inhaled steroids for asthma
- Topical steroids for inflammatory skin conditions
- Steroids for autoimmune conditions such as rheumatoid arthritis or lupus
- Steroids for polymyalgia rheumatica and temporal arteritis (which I suspect result from allergy to gut microbes)
- Steroids for severe allergies, such as ulcerative colitis and Crohn's disease
- Rituximab for CFS and inflammatory arthritides – I do not recommend Rituximab for the treatment of CFS at this current time (one of the side-effects is death!) but one can infer the need for immune system re-programming from the results of its use
- Other immune-suppressive drugs, such as methotrexate, entanercept and gold injections, for rheumatoid arthritis, psoriatic arthritis, ankylosing spondylitis and juvenile idiopathic arthritis (all of which I suspect are driven by allergy to gut microbes)

It should be remembered that putting the immune system in a straitjacket is potentially dangerous – it may impair the normal, efficient response to infection as well as impairing normal cancer surveillance. Any such intervention should be done for as short a time as possible and treatment tailed off as soon as reasonably possible.

Putting the immune system into a straitjacket reduces symptoms in the short term – people feel better and that is highly desirable – but read my cautionary notes that follow.

Cautionary notes

It is tempting just to take the drugs alone and hope they will do the trick. This is a recipe for long-term drug dependency. Drugs should be withheld until all other interventions are in place – indeed, these other interventions (pacing, sleep, the ketogenic diet, the Basic Package of supplements, the mitochondrial package of supplements, the detox regimes, etc) alone stand a good chance of effecting a cure.

For the above to be effective the patient needs to be as free from inflammation symptoms as possible. They should return to just CFS symptoms, not inflammation symptoms (remember ME equals CFS plus inflammation). If patients are not free from inflammation symptoms, then the immune system is active and reacting and, therefore, not being educated 'the right way' – that is, towards being less prone to inflammation. If the patient is experiencing inflammation symptoms, then immune system education is all going in the wrong direction – it is *pro*-inflammatory. This means that the dose of any drug must be very carefully balanced. Too little and the education is incorrect or 'not enough'; too much and immune suppression occurs with all its risks of overwhelming infection, poor cancer surveillance and so on.

Too much of a good thing can be a bad thing

OLD ENGLISH SAYING (Deriving from *Proverbs* 25:16 – 'Hast thou found honey? Eat so much as is sufficient for thee, lest thou be filled therewith and vomit it.')

I think one has to be additionally cautious using symptom-suppressing medication – it is all too tempting to overdo things. Remember the cell damage from not pacing well (which may be a 'human' consequence of suppressing symptoms – that is, one feels better and so one feels one can do more) will also activate the immune system. It is only by a clear understanding of the above principles that the individual patient can balance up the treatments to maximise benefit with the lowest possible dose of drug in the shortest possible time (and the shortest time will be some months).

The above mechanisms may not be proven but this is a biologically plausible sequence of events which has clearly passed the clinical test of time. It may well be that there are some years before the science catches up but this is characteristic of the development of new ideas in a clinical setting.

Specific methods for switching off the immune system

1. Oral immunotherapy (food drops)

Incremental immunotherapy has long been recognised as being effective in inducing immune tolerance. The idea here is that one gradually increases the dose of antigen from a very low to a very high level over a period of time – typically two to three months – during which the immune system learns immune tolerance because the mature cells are not activated by a sudden hike in antigen. Indeed, incremental immunotherapy injections are still used to switch off hayfever and anaphylactic reactions to wasp and bee stings.

More recent studies show that immune tolerance can be induced with oral antigens. So, for example, we can turn off peanut anaphylaxis, birch-pollen-associated apple allergy and hayfever using oral immunotherapy. The idea is to take a tiny dose of the offending antigen under the tongue. The dose is so small that the immune system can ignore it. Importantly, the immune cells learn that this dose does not harm the body. Then one gradually increases the dose over several months so the adolescent immune cells learn that higher doses do not do harm and therefore these immune cells learn to tolerate a higher dose.

In their paper, 'Assessing the efficacy of oral immunotherapy for the desensitisation of peanut allergy in children (STOP II): a phase 2 randomised controlled trial', Anagnostou et al showed that over 80 per cent of the children in their study desensitised successfully over the six months of increasing doses of peanut.[49] In addition, Tang and colleagues carried out a study in 2015 that involved the use of a probiotic, *Lactobacillus rhamnosus*, alongside standard peanut oral immunotherapy. The inclusion of the probiotic seemed to make the therapy more effective.[50]

This potentially gives us an inexpensive technique for switching off our own food allergies. The idea is to list one's worst 10 food antigens, which must all be Paleo-ketogenic foods, and make up a soup which contains 10 grams of each food. This will produce a 100-gram soup (about a cupful). One can then dilute this down to 1/10, 1/100 and 1/1,000 strengths to provide:

White bottle – 1,000 mg (1 g) of total food per ml (i.e. the original soup)
Red bottle – 100 mg of total food per ml (i.e. diluted 10-fold)
Amber bottle – 10 mg of total food per ml (i.e. diluted 100-fold)
Green bottle – 1 mg of total food per ml (i.e. diluted 1,000-fold)

With the peanut anaphylaxis studies (as above), no child reacted to one drop of the 1 mg per ml peanut dilution. I have tried these drops for several patients and so far only one has experienced any sort of reaction to the green bottle drops. The idea is to very gradually increase the daily dose over several months until one can take the original soup on a daily basis. At this point one would expect to be able to tolerate those foods.

As I say, this is work in progress, but I have had some notable successes. This technique should not be tried with anybody who has suffered any anaphylactic reaction, or any reaction to antigens, which involves tissue swelling. While it is theoretically possible to have an anaphylactic reaction to this method, in practice this has never been observed, though one child did need an adrenaline injection on two occasions in the study by Anagnostou et al. (It was not full anaphylaxis and represents 0.01 per cent of the doses given in the study.)

Enzyme-potentiated desensitisation (EPD)

Enzyme-potentiated desensitisation (EPD) is a vaccine which can be used to desensitise patients to foods, inhalants and chemicals. It has some bacterial antigens. It was developed and refined by Dr Len McEwen over the past 30 years. It is supplied to the doctor who mixes the appropriate dose in a sterile environment, immediately prior to dosing. It is of proven benefit and works by manipulating the normal immune processes for creating and turning off allergies. Therefore success or failure depends largely on priming the patient in the best possible way. The beauty of it is that one injection can be used to desensitise to a great many allergens.

I learned this technique from Dr McEwen during the 1980s. Initially I used it in NHS general practice to treat a wide variety of allergic disorders, such as eczema, asthma, urticaria, irritable bowel syndrome and migraine, with excellent results. I also used it to treat patients with ME simply because at that stage of the game I did not know what else to try. I had a tool and I was going to use it! It surprised me how many patients did very well and indeed many ME patients I see now also do very well on EPD. That observation alone tells me allergy is a big player in ME.

Neutralisation

Neutralisation was the first technique I tried using during the 1980s to switch off allergies. It is of proven effectiveness. The idea of neutralisation is to inject a small dose of the allergen intra-dermally to raise a small weal. A positive reaction means allergy to that antigen, so one injects an even smaller dose. This should result in a lesser reaction, which may be positive. The first negative reaction switches off allergy to that antigen and this is called the 'neutralising dose' or 'endpoint'.

However, I found myself treating patients with multiple allergies. Since every allergen has to be dealt with individually as above, this quickly became a very time-consuming and expensive process. It could take me several hours to treat one patient. Furthermore, there was always potential for the endpoints (that is, the appropriate neutralising dose) to change – that meant the patient had to return for extensive retesting. In NHS general practice this quickly became impossible and therefore I moved on to using EPD. In private practice, neutralisation can escalate to become a very expensive intervention.

A list of practitioners using EPD and neutralisation can be found via the British Society for Ecological Medicine's website – please see www.bsem.org.uk.

CHAPTER 13 SUMMARY

Reprogramming the immune system

- In general, allergy and autoimmunity can be treated by a two-pronged approach:
    - First, the general approach to treating any condition associated with inflammation (see Chapter 9, page 132).
    - Second, the specific approaches for allergy (page 149) and autoimmunity (page 148).
- With regard to the specifics, we have five approaches:
    - First, avoid all those factors, in as much as one can, which are switching the immune system on (see Chapter 9, page 132).
    - Second, put in place all possible interventions to make the immune system less twitchy and prone to inflammation (again, see Chapter 9).
    - Third, induce immune tolerance by putting the immune system in a drug-induced straitjacket and stopping the inappropriate reactions of the mature white cells. Do this for several months, slowly reducing the dose at such a rate that symptoms do not flare (see page 170 for the specific drugs.)
    - Fourth, use antimicrobials to reduce the microbial load (see Chapters 11 [page 151] and 12 [page 161]). It may be that the above interventions will *all* be necessary to get a result.
    - Fifth, use proven methods to switch off the immune system. In order of practical application, I would do the following:
        - oral immunotherapy (food drops)
        - enzyme potentiated desensitisation (EPD)
        - neutralisation

PART III

Practical

The foundation stones of recovery – what everyone must do

CHAPTER 14

The path to recovery for those challenged by lack of energy or lack of time

. . . a journey of a thousand miles starts with a single step . . .

CHINESE PHILOSOPHER LAOZI (C 604 BC – C 531 BC)
in the *Tao Te Ching*, Chapter 64

And let's hope it's not quite a thousand miles . . .

CRAIG ROBINSON 2016

. . . it helps when you have someone holding your hand.

PENNY ROBINSON 2016

Recovering from this wretched illness requires time, energy and resources – the very things CFS/ME sufferers are lacking in. Theoretically one would put in place all possible interventions for recovery so that this can happen as quickly as possible. In practical reality, this is rarely possible and indeed is not desirable because it takes time for the body to adjust to the changes being made. The interventions I suggest are difficult – Rome was not built in a day! So we need to start with those interventions which provide the most 'bang for your buck'. This then gives one the energy to put in place the other interventions. In turn, this yields further improvements that can again be built upon – the virtuous circle.

It is always cheering to remember that the body wants to get well. If one only has 49 per cent of the package in place then one is still on the slippery slope downhill. If one gets 51 per cent in place then the body is in recovery. I do not mind how long it takes to recover so long as movement is in the right direction. Addressing all the underlying causes of CFS/ME also prevents other nasty diseases in the long term. So I can promise my patients that the years lost in early life will be made up for in later. (Greedy people like me want it all, so I do all the regimes now so I can function to my full potential in quality and quantity.)

> *Rivers know this: there is no hurry. We shall get there some day.*
>
> AA Milne in *Winnie-the-Pooh*

Of course, everyone is so very different and regimes always need tailoring. Below is a regime for an especially common problem – the severe CFS/ME sufferer who has little money and is housebound with little or no care package. In order of priority, take a leap of faith and do the following:

- See a doctor and get basic tests done to exclude obvious pathology. Everyone should have a basic package of tests which should include the following:
  - Haematology (anaemia)
  - Inflammatory markers (CRP, ESR, plasma viscosity)
  - Biochemistry (kidney function)
  - Measures of sugar metabolism and damage (total cholesterol, LDL cholesterol, glycosylated haemoglobin)
  - Liver function
  - Ferritin
  - Thyroid function (including free T4, free T3 and TSH)
  - Vitamin D
  - Sexually transmitted diseases (if relevant)
  - Autoantibody screen

- Sleep – ensure a good night's sleep; this may need medication to achieve. This then provides the energy to gradually put in place all the other elements of the package (see Chapter 16, page 196).
- Arrange food to be delivered weekly suitable for a no-cooking, no-food-preparation, Paleo-ketogenic diet. Ask a friend to help you set this up.

Table 14.1. Reasons why you may feel worse, initially, when adapting to a Paleo-ketogenic diet

The problem	The mechanism	The symptoms
Running out of fuel	Failure to keto-adapt*	Severe worsening of CFS symptoms
Hypoglycaemia	Adrenaline symptoms	Fatigue and foggy brain Irritable, palpitations, tremor
Addiction withdrawal symptoms (sugar, caffeine)	Lack of endogenous opiates	Fatigue and foggy brain Headache, irritability, cravings
Food allergy withdrawal	Allergy and addiction are two sides of the same coin – see row above	Ditto
Detoxification reactions	Acute poisoning as toxins are mobilised	Fatigue and foggy brain Feel poisoned, malaise, rashes, return of old symptoms
Herxheimer reactions	Allergic reactions to dead microbes as they are 'seen' by the immune system	Fatigue and foggy brain Fever, malaise

* The ketogenic diet is helpful for many reasons, but it takes time to keto-adapt. Often people start this diet by reducing carbohydrates. However, even a small amount of carbohydrate will spike blood sugar and therefore insulin. High insulin prevents fat-burning. When the sugar 'hit' runs out, the body has no sugar left to burn and cannot access the stores of fat to get energy that way so there will be a window of time where there is no fuel from sugar and no fuel from fat. This causes acute fatigue. The temptation is to consume more carbohydrate or sugar in order to 'feel better' but this only worsens the situation and causes cycles of severe fatigue. It is important to know this so that one can guard against it and recognise when it is happening.

- Read the pacing chapter (Chapter 15, page 183) every day (or as often as you can manage) until you've really 'got' it.
- Take the Basic Package of nutritional supplements (see Chapter 18, page 220).
- Take the Basic Package of mitochondrial supplements (see Chapter 18, page 222).
- Get hold of vitamin B12 injections and self-inject 0.5 mg daily in the morning.
- Think about the environment in which you live – is it toxic with people, emotion, atmosphere, chemicals, electromagnetic radiation, mould, dust, noise or air pollution? (See Chapter 20 [page 233] and Appendix 5 [page 315].)
- Are you financially secure? Ask for help with benefits (see Appendix 9, page 329).
- It is common for CFS/ME sufferers initially to worsen after dietary changes and introducing nutritional supplements. This may give clues as to mechanisms but the commonest problems are shown in Table 14.1.

Time

See how far this gets you. It may take six months to see the full benefits from dietary changes and supplements. The above interventions are a blueprint for good health for life for everyone.

Where you go from here depends on your clinical picture and possible past exposures to infection or toxins, but a further comprehensive set of tests, all available through the Natural Health Worldwide website (www.naturalhealthworldwide.com), would include:

- Tests of organ function
  - Comprehensive digestive stool analysis with parasites – being a stool test, this can be done at home by the patient.
  - Mitochondrial function – contained within this profile are many helpful nutritional tests.
  - Adrenal stress profile – this is a saliva test and so can be done at home by the patient.

- Toxicity tests. The following tests can both be done at home with urine samples and sent through the post:
  - Toxic metals in urine after taking a chelating agent (DMSA – see page 355) – this test gives some additional helpful information on friendly minerals.
  - Toxic organic chemical exposure.

- Test for chronic bacterial infection with organisms such as borrelia, bartonella, babesia, anaplasma, chlamydia, mycoplasma, toxoplasma, yersinia and rickettsia from Armin Labs.
- Test for chronic viral presence such as Epstein-Barr virus ('mono'), cytomegalovirus, varicella zoster, HHV6, coxsackie virus, HHV9 – note these tests concentrate on herpes viruses which appear to be the biggest problem in ME. Again, these tests can be ordered directly through the Natural Health Worldwide website (page 385).

If you are still stuck at this stage then you need professional help, again available from Natural Health Worldwide. Indeed, the interpretation of tests is as important as the test results and again professional help may be essential.

You can't stay in your corner of the Forest waiting for others to come to you. You have to go to them sometimes.

AA MILNE in *Winnie-the-Pooh*

CHAPTER 14 SUMMARY

The path to recovery for those challenged by lack of energy or lack of time

- When you have not much money, very little energy and a poor or non-existent care package, it is difficult to know where to start.
- Take a leap of faith and do these things:
    - See a doctor and get basic tests done to exclude obvious pathology – see tests listed on page 178.
    - Read Chapter 16, page 196, to ensure a good night's sleep becomes the norm.
    - Arrange food to be delivered weekly suitable for a no-cooking, no-food-preparation, Paleo-ketogenic diet. Ask a friend to help you set this up.
    - Read the pacing chapter (Chapter 15, page 183) every day (or as often as you can manage) until you've really 'got' it.
    - Take the Basic Package of nutritional supplements – see Chapter 18, page 220.
    - Take the Basic Package of mitochondrial supplements – see Chapter 18, page 222.
    - Get hold of vitamin B12 injections and self-inject 0.5 mg daily in the morning.
    - Think about the environment in which you live – is it toxic with people, emotion, atmosphere, chemicals, electromagnetic radiation, mould, dust, noise or air pollution? (See Chapter 20 [page 233] and Appendix 5 [page 315].)
- Expect to see an initial worsening of symptoms for the reasons described in Table 14.1, page 179.
- It may take six months to see clinical improvements after putting in place the above interventions.

- Depending on your clinical picture and possible past exposures to infection or toxins and further tests, decide where to go next.
- The following tests (from www.naturalhealthworldwide.com) will give direction to your path:
    - Tests of organ function
        - Comprehensive digestive stool analysis with parasites – being a stool test, this can be done at home by you, the patient.
        - Mitochondrial function – contained within this profile are many helpful nutritional tests.
        - Adrenal stress profile – this is a saliva test and so can be done at home by you, the patient.
    - Toxicity tests
        - Toxic metals in urine following a chelating agent, DMSA – this test gives some additional helpful information about friendly minerals. As this is a urine test, this can be done by you, the patient, at home.
        - Toxic organic chemical exposure – again, as this is a urine test, this can be done by you, the patient, at home.
    - Test for chronic bacterial infection
        - Bacteria such as borrelia, bartonella, babesia, anaplasma, chlamydia, mycoplasma, toxoplasma, yersinia and rickettsia from Armin laboratories.
    - Tests for chronic viral presence
        - Such viral presence as Epstein-Barr virus, cytomegalovirus, varicella zoster, HHV6, coxsackie virus, HHV9 – note these concentrate on herpes viruses which appear to be the biggest problem in ME.
- All these tests can be accessed through Natural Health Worldwide (www.naturalhealthworldwide.com). You can also access practitioners through this website who can help you with the interpretation of these tests and advice as to where to go next.

CHAPTER 15

Pacing

Much old wisdom about resting and pacing has been lost in the hubbub of modern life:

A good rest is half the work.

YUGOSLAVIAN PROVERB

How beautiful it is to do nothing and then rest afterwards.

SPANISH PROVERB

Moreover, in the context of this book, rest and pacing are the most important factors in allowing CFS/ME sufferers to get better. Not to do so results in much worse fatigue, pain and a postponement of recovery.

Pacing is a part of normal life

We all have to pace activity – increasingly so with age. Indeed, the failure of 'normal', healthy people to pace well puts them at great risk of CFS/ME. In those with CFS/ME, it is often the case that years of stress and pushing themselves to accomplish their goals in life will pre-date the onset of their condition. CFS sufferers are often the sort of people who get things done at the expense of sleep, holidays and diet, and consequently they end up feeling very fatigued. As a result, they invariably also suffer from the progressive cell damage that goes with such severe and unremitting levels of fatigue. Then a toxic stress, which may be infectious, poisonous, financial or emotional, becomes the last straw which finally pushes them over the edge – more of this in Craig's Catastrophe Theory chapter (page 271).

Exercise makes things worse

An invariable feature of the CFS/ME sufferer's history is that exercise (either mental, physical or emotional) makes the symptoms worse. Indeed, this very fact distinguishes CFS/ME from depression – exercise tends to improve the symptoms of people who are 'simply' depressed. In CFS/ME, the desire is there but the performance lacking. Indeed, the very personality that often gets people into CFS/ME stops them from getting out of it. All CFS/ME sufferers tend to push themselves to their particular energy limit every day, and sometimes even beyond that limit, and this tendency actively prevents recovery. This means CFS/ME sufferers have one day doing as much as symptoms permit, overdo things and then need three days to recover. Whilst on this rollercoaster ride of activity and dives, one cannot hope to improve overall. It is akin to an economic 'boom-and-bust' cycle – money is borrowed to fuel economic activity but then at some point the level of borrowing becomes unsustainable and a downturn, or even a recession, inevitably follows. (Perhaps you can tell why I decided upon a career in medicine rather than economics!) But the point is clear – CFS/ME sufferers engage in cycles of activity, unsupported by their 'real' energy levels, followed by periods of forced inactivity, where the body 'recovers' from such unsupported activity. Many people find it helpful to use the analogy of energy as 'money', because this is something which is much more familiar to everyday lives.

The starting place for recovery is to reduce your energy expenditure to the point at which you feel absolutely fine doing absolutely nothing. To achieve this you will have to put in place many other interventions in addition to pacing, as described elsewhere in this book.

Pacing

The symptoms of pain and fatigue arise when energy demand exceeds energy delivery. These are essential symptoms which protect us from ourselves; without such we would carry on functioning all day and all night and drop dead within a few days. At risk of repetition, I shall again quote the Mr Micawber equation from Charles Dickens's *David Copperfield*:

> *Annual income twenty pounds, annual expenditure nineteen pounds nineteen and six, result happiness. Annual income twenty pounds, annual expenditure twenty pounds nought and six, result misery.*

. . . and so it is with energy. Indeed, the financial analogy is very helpful in understanding the need to pace activity. I always think that energy is very much like money – it is hard work earning it and great fun spending it!

We run into serious financial (whoops, I mean 'energy') problems when demand exceeds delivery. In this event we can 'borrow' energy with the biochemical tricks as detailed below (page 186). However, this comes at a terrible price, first because we then have the pain of lactic acid and, second, because we rapidly build up an energy debt. This energy debt has to paid back with interest – to be precise, the interest rate is 300 per cent. This is akin to running one's life borrowing energy (money) from a loan shark – all one's energy (money) is spent on catch-up (paying the interest) and there is never enough left over for recovery.

Pacing is what you have to do to stay in energy credit. If you do not pace properly and slip into energy debit, then you get stuck in an energy poverty trap created by this loan shark. His name is anaerobic metabolism and his method is the Cori cycle (page 187).

Neither a borrower nor a lender be.

POLONIUS IN *HAMLET*, Act I Scene 3
(William Shakespeare)

What happens when energy demand exceeds energy delivery

The most efficient way to make energy is to burn the fuel acetate in mitochondria with oxygen. Acetate ideally comes from ketones, but glucose will do. This is called aerobic metabolism and is very efficient. One molecule of acetate produces 32–36 molecules of our universal energy currency ATP (depending on how efficient the system is).

Should energy demand exceed delivery, there are at least two ways by which ATP can be made ('borrowed'), but they are both horribly inefficient, as I have said, and take hours, possibly days, for normal aerobic metabolism to be restored. This catch-up involves pain (lactic acid burn) and greatly increased energy demands because one has to repay not just the debt but additional cripplingly high interest rates.

The biochemical explanation for this that comes next is for those with time, energy and a biochemical bent.

The biochemical mechanisms for borrowing energy and repaying the energy debt

Essentially there are two mechanisms for borrowing energy and repaying the debt. Both are greatly demanding of raw materials, time and energy. These are:

1. The adenylate kinase reaction
2. Anaerobic metabolism

1. The adenylate kinase reaction

When ATP ('TP' stands for 'tri-phosphate', which is three phosphates) releases energy it is converted into ADP ('di-phosphate', or two phosphates) and this ADP is normally then passed into mitochondria, courtesy of translocator protein, where it is recycled back to ATP. However, if ATP is being used up faster than it can be made, then:

> Two molecules of ADP can combine to make one molecule of ATP and one of AMP (one phosphate).

$$2\ \text{ADP} \rightarrow \text{ATP} + \text{AMP} + \text{energy}$$

or

> ADP can be converted to AMP directly with the production of energy from breaking a high-energy phosphate bond.

$$\text{ADP} \rightarrow \text{AMP} + \text{energy}$$

The problem is that both the above mechanisms result in the production of AMP and this is poorly recycled. The effect is to drain mitochondria of recyclable ADP. The body then has to make brand new, *de novo* ATP and this takes time, energy and raw materials.

Anaerobic metabolism

In this event, ATP is made in the absence of oxygen and without mitochondria. It is hopelessly inefficient since one fuel molecule of acetate makes just two molecules of ATP together with lactic acid. It is the acid that causes such pain. The business of returning lactic acid to our acetate fuel is called the Cori cycle and takes place in the liver. However, this job requires six molecules of ATP to

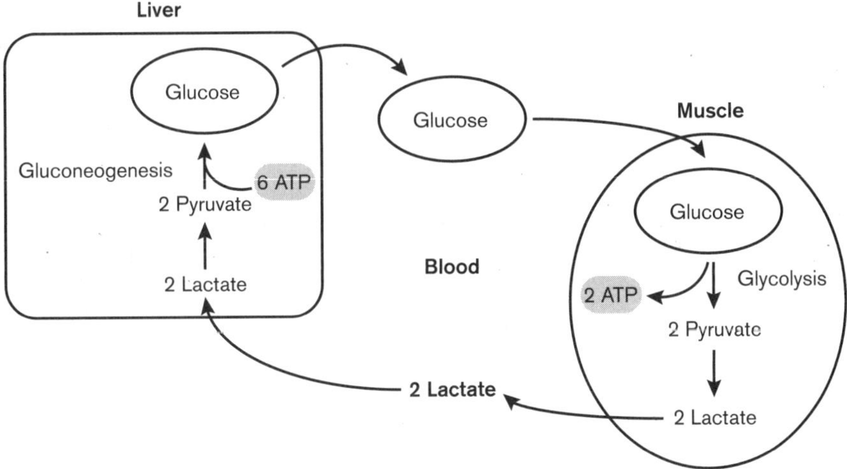

Figure 15.1. The Cori cycle – look at how much ATP is needed to recycle lactate! Three times as much!

achieve. This is why I can be so precise about the interest rate – borrowing two molecules of ATP costs six molecules of ATP for payback.

Borrowing short-term energy results in long-term problems

Borrowing short-term energy results in long-term problems as follows:

1. The production of lactic acid, as in anaerobic metabolism, causes symptoms:
   a) In skeletal muscles – athletes call this 'lactic acid burn' (muscles feel heavy); the burn is severe – as I have said already, it prevents athletes winning gold medals. CFS/ME sufferers describe the feeling as 'walking through treacle'. It is part of the explanation for fibromyalgia.
   b) In the heart, lactic acid burn results in pain which is called angina. Remember, the heart is a muscle and so suffers in the same way as all muscles.
   c) In the brain, lactic acid, I suspect, causes headache (there are several different types of headache in CFS/ME).
   d) In mitochondria, acidity (from lactic acid) inhibits mitochondrial function further; this contributes to the spiralling down of all energy delivery mechanisms resulting in the CFS/ME sufferer 'suddenly hitting a brick wall' – they become pole-axed and paralysed. It is another one of those vicious cycles in CFS/ME.

2. To restore normal energy delivery is demanding of raw materials. We can make brand new ATP through a bit of biochemistry called the 'pentose phosphate shunt' (page 71), but this is greedy of raw materials. We can help the body by supplying it with D-ribose, the immediate raw material for making *de novo* ATP. This is an excellent rescue remedy when one has really overdone things. Interestingly, caffeine helps the body scavenge AMP, and so small amounts of green tea, coffee or dark chocolate can be helpful. These may additionally help to restore the normal circadian rhythm. Some CFS/ME sufferers find that D-ribose taken in green tea or black coffee is a perfect pick-me-up.
3. To restore normal energy delivery mechanism takes time. This is for at least two reasons – (1) it takes time to generate enough ATP to recycle lactic acid and (2) it takes time to make *de novo* ATP. I believe this explains the pathological delayed fatigue that we see in CFS. The body is having to recycle lactic acid and make new ATP. Indeed, although the chest pain in CFS is angina it is not diagnosed as such because, by contrast with the angina that doctors normally see and which results from poor blood supply, the angina in CFS patients is caused by lactic acid burn and is very prolonged. So doctors don't 'recognise' it as angina, because of its prolonged nature, and CFS sufferers get diagnosed with 'atypical chest pain' – which is no diagnosis at all! Terms such as 'atypical' are doctors' ways of saying 'I don't know what this is or why it is happening'!

'Rabbit's clever,' said Pooh thoughtfully.
'Yes,' said Piglet, 'Rabbit's clever.'
'And he has Brain.'
'Yes,' said Piglet, 'Rabbit has Brain.'
There was a long silence.
'I suppose,' said Pooh, 'that that's why he never understands anything.'

AA Milne in *Winnie-the-Pooh*

This symptom of delayed fatigue is what differentiates the pathological fatigue of CFS/ME from the normal person with fatigue at the end of the day – the normal person recovers after a good night's sleep; the CFS/ME sufferer does not.

I hope the above demonstrates the intellectual imperative to pace – without understanding the biochemical essentials of pacing, the determination to do such cannot follow.

Ipsa scientia potestas est – *Knowledge itself is power.*
Sir Francis Bacon in *Meditationes Sacrae* (1597)

The practical rules for pacing

Imagine that a normal healthy person has £1,000 worth of energy to spend in a day. The CFS/ME sufferer only has £100. What is more, this has to be spread out throughout the day in such a way that there is £20 'change' at the end. This allows energy for healing and repair. You initially have to do less in the short term in order to achieve more in the long term.

A fatigue-ometer would be a very useful gadget to make people pace. Until that arises one has to listen to one's body!

In Craig's case, he literally does 'listen' to his body – his tinnitus. He suffers from this constantly and has done so for the last 20 years. The higher the pitch, the greater the urgency there is for him to take a rest. About a year ago, for a period of about two weeks of proper rest, Craig had no tinnitus.

Rest and pace throughout the day

- By rest, I mean complete mental, physical and emotional rest from exercise, visitors, telephone calls, reading, computers, talking, child minding, noise and TV. All the above count as activities which have to be carefully rationed through the day. When you rest, lie horizontal because this reduces the work of the heart. (It is much harder work pushing blood round a vertical body, uphill and down dale, than when horizontal, with everything on the flat.)
- You should have a proper rest, perhaps when you actually go to bed, regularly in the day, even on days when you feel well. Ideally sleep. *Homo sapiens* evolved in hot climates where it is normal to have a siesta in the afternoon. Most people experience an energy dip after lunch. Young babies and older people return to this more normal sleep pattern and ill people should do the same. An afternoon sleep is normal. I do it! It is called power-napping.
- Do things in short bursts. You will be more efficient if you do things for 10–40 minutes (whatever your window of time is), then rest for the same length of time. I had one patient who could only walk 30 metres, but by walking 15 metres and resting, then going on again, she got up to walking a mile a day without delayed fatigue.
- Vary your activity. This applies to the brain as well as the body – for example, listening to the radio or music uses a different part of the brain to watching TV. Washing up (sitting on a high stool, please) uses different muscles to walking.

- Do things by the clock. We are creatures of habit and the physical body likes things to happen on a regular basis; ask any farmer who keeps animals – they thrive on routine. Sleep and eat at regular times and pace activities so you do about the same every day and during the same time slots. I know that life has a habit of getting in the way of this ideal, but as a general principle, stick to it.
- Do not overdo things on a day when you feel well. Short-term symptoms mislead.
- Be careful with adrenaline – this temporarily masks the symptoms of overdoing it and can lead one astray.
- Do not live life on the edge – a useful analogy is that CFS/ME sufferers often live life on the edge of a cliff. A minor stress will tip them off the edge and down to the beach below; it is a hard climb back. We should walk back from the edge onto the grassy slope. If we fall on this grassy slope, then we do not hurt ourselves and it is a small business to pick ourselves up and go on again. Again, see Craig's Catastrophe Theory, Chapter 24, page 271.

Prioritise, get organised and accept help – reduce energy expenditure on the routine

- Apply for benefits.
- List the 10 most important things in your life. Then scrub out and cancel the bottom half.
- Do not be house-proud. Get a cleaner and dishwasher. Give up ironing – a nonsensical, energy-sapping waste of time and effort; ironing came into fashion to kill nits and fleas in the seams of clothes and had a purpose once. I don't iron.
- Accept offers of 'meals on wheels' from others.
- Shop online so food is delivered.

In a nutshell – The 10 commandments for reducing energy expenditure

(Credit for this wonderful list goes to my patient Sylvia Waites)

Thou shalt not be perfect nor try to be.
Thou shalt not try to be all things to all people.

Thou shalt leave things undone that ought to be done.
Thou shalt not spread thyself too thin.
Thou shalt learn to say 'No'.
Thou shalt schedule time for thyself, and for thy supporting network.
Thou shalt switch off and do nothing regularly.
Thou shalt be boring, untidy, inelegant and unattractive at times.
Thou shalt not even feel guilty.
Thou shalt not be thine own worst enemy, but thine own best friend.

Pattern of recovery

The first stage – windows of improvement – is when the sufferer starts to see windows of time when he/she feels better (but cannot do more). These may just be a few hours initially or a day or two. At this stage do not be tempted to do more activity – that will just postpone your recovery and complicate things. As I have said before, the trouble is the very personality that often gets people into CFS/ME does not help them to get out of it. Many CFS/ME sufferers have a little devil on their shoulder that beats them up every time they try to rest.

The second stage – feel fine doing nothing – is when the sufferer must feel completely well whilst doing absolutely nothing. The reason why it is so important to get to this stage is because that is the best test of how the body is functioning. The blood test for cell-free DNA is a measure of tissue damage (page 66), and this tissue damage potentially is a disease-amplifying process. The reason for this is that when there is lots of cellular debris swilling around the body, the immune system makes antibodies against it and this has the potential to set up either allergies or possibly autoimmunity. When there is lots of immune activity there is excessive production of free radicals and this puts an extra stress on the antioxidant system. The bottom line is that feeling ill puts a great stress on the body, energy is expended uselessly in coping with this stress and the whole business of recovery is further delayed.

The third stage – feel fine doing nothing every day – is when the sufferer feels absolutely fine doing absolutely nothing (and of course this never really happens in true life because life has a habit of getting in the way) *and* this level of wellness is maintained for some days or, even better, weeks. That is to say one's level of wellbeing becomes established, more robust and less susceptible to the fluctuations of everyday life. Suddenly one starts to have a future and one's horizons pick up. Then one can move into . . .

The fourth stage – activity programme. IT IS ABSOLUTELY ESSENTIAL THAT THE THIRD STAGE HAS BEEN REACHED BEFORE ATTEMPTING

THIS. Carefully start a very gradual, graded activity programme. The deal is that you are allowed to increase your activity, which may be mental or physical, on the grounds that you feel fine the next day. I do not mind people feeling tired at the end of the day – that is physiological and helps you to have a good night's sleep. However, if the fatigue is delayed and so you wake up the next morning feeling exhausted as a result of the previous day's exertions then you have overdone things and must pull back. IT IS ESSENTIAL THAT YOU *LISTEN* and DO PULL BACK – OTHERWISE YOU RISK A RELAPSE AND RETURNING TO AN EARLIER STAGE OF THE PROCESS. This explains why there is no standard activity programme to follow because however much you can or cannot do depends entirely on how you feel. I suppose one way around this would be to do daily blood tests for cell-free DNA, but this would be rather impractical!

So long as you continue to feel well and do not get delayed fatigue then the graded activity programme can be continued. But, always go very gradually so as not to risk the gains that have been made. However, during all this time it is very important to hold the whole regime of diet, sleep, supplements, pacing and detoxing in place.

The fifth stage – additional exercises to restore numbers of mitochondria – is when you get to a stage where you feel well all the time and activity levels are acceptable; then you can start to do exercises to increase the numbers of mitochondria and so improve cardiovascular fitness. AGAIN, DO NOT ATTEMPT THIS UNTIL STAGE FOUR HAS BEEN WELL ESTABLISHED; OTHERWISE, A RELAPSE MAY BE A RISK. And again IT IS ESSENTIAL THAT YOU *LISTEN* and DO PULL BACK if necessary. (See Appendix 2, page 301, for the details of how to progress with exercise and the actual types of exercise that are recommended.)

The sixth stage – balance up the regime with lifestyle. Only now dare we relax the regime. Actually, as we age we all get a measure of chronic fatigue syndrome. It is pretty obvious why this is the case – energy levels are dictated by mitochondrial performance and the ageing process is dictated by mitochondrial performance. The very interventions I recommend to treat CFS/ME all slow the normal ageing process. So, as we age we can stay just as fit and just as well, but we have to work much harder at it. So the level of supplementation and lifestyle changes one ends up doing depend very much on the individual. Magnesium injections are a real nuisance, but once mitochondrial function is restored, usually they are no longer necessary. Simply taking magnesium by mouth, in the bath, or whatever, is sufficient to do the job.

Again, once antioxidant status has been restored, then the need for B12 injections is very much reduced. But there is also no doubt that some people feel a lot better for the odd B12 jab, it has no known toxicity and I am happy for people to continue with these in the long term. Indeed, because as we age our ability to absorb micronutrients, particularly B12, declines, whilst at the same time we become less efficient biochemically, our requirement for these micronutrients increases, and so you could argue that everybody over the age of, say 60, would benefit from regular B12 injections. You might think that this is evolutionary nonsense since primitive man did not need B12 injections, but then on the other hand, by the age of 60, most of us are on the evolutionary scrap heap and so evolutionary rules do not apply!

Long term – Not only do the lifestyle changes, nutritional supplements, sleep, detox regimes and so on help to get rid of CFS, but these are all the interventions I use in the prevention and treatment of cancer, heart disease and other degenerative conditions such as Alzheimer's, arthritis, organ failures, etc. Therefore, I can say with confidence to my CFS/ME patients that once they get on the regimes, not only should they improve but their best years could be ahead of them and their risk of developing these diseases, associated with the ageing process, is substantially reduced. I am greedy – I want the best quality of life for as long as possible, so I too observe all the regimes I impose on my CFS/ME patients; this also helps me to understand how difficult they are.

CHAPTER 15 SUMMARY

Pacing

- Pacing should be a part of everyone's plan for a healthy life.
- Pacing and rest are absolutely vital in CFS/ME to start the process of recovery and ensure the continuation of such a recovery.
- CFS/ME sufferers often have a history of pushing themselves to their limits and have a tendency to continue with these patterns even after they have fallen ill.
- This tendency of CFS/ME sufferers to 'push' leads to a vicious cycle of 'boom-and-bust', whereby they overspend their energy on 'good days' and then spend days recovering.

- There are good, substantiated biochemical reasons as to why this 'boom and bust' happens in CFS/ME patients – these reasons involve the ways in which the body can 'borrow' energy to keep going when it really should be resting. Understanding these biochemical mechanisms gives the intellectual imperative to understand why pacing and resting are so vital to recovery from CFS/ME. (See pages 186 to 189.)
- CFS/ME sufferers must always pace and rest so that they have energy left at the end of the day – this energy is their recovery energy.
- Thinking of energy as money is a very useful analogy – CFS/ME sufferers should always aim to have some money (energy) left at the end of the day so that their bodies can spend this money (energy) on recovery.
- CFS/ME sufferers should not engage in 'borrowing' energy (money) by the biochemical mechanisms as mentioned above because the interest rates on these energy debts are exorbitant and drain further energy (money) from their energy (money) bank in the paying back of that interest.
- The practical rules for pacing include:
    - Understanding that rest means *complete rest* from *all* activities – for example, listening to the radio while lying on your bed is *not* resting.
    - Doing things in short bursts – 20–40 minutes or whatever suits the individual sufferer.
    - Having a sleep during the day – that is, an afternoon siesta.
    - Varying activities regularly – this is less tiring for the body than continuing with the same activity.
    - Having a strict daily routine.
    - Never overdoing things on days when you feel 'better'.
    - Organising your life and home as best as you can to reduce energy spent on these things.
    - Giving yourself a break! See the 10 commandments on page 190.
- Be aware of the stages of a typical pattern of recovery and only start gentle exercise regimes when all previous 'stages' of the recovery process have been consolidated – see pages 190 to 193 and Appendix 2 (page 301).

POSTSCRIPT

Crucial to good pacing is good record keeping. There are many ways to achieve this, especially with new technology and apps. In Appendix 3 (page 308), Craig Robinson has included the methods that he uses, which are low tech and rely on pencil, paper, highlighters and a physical diary. There are two elements to his record keeping:

- Weekly activity sheet for pacing
- Page-to-a-day diary record of activities, protocol compliance, diet and symptoms.

CHAPTER 16

Sleep

Without a good night's sleep on a regular basis all other interventions are to no avail. In the short term, I often advise whatever is necessary, possibly prescription drugs (see page 210), to ensure sleep. However, the goal must be to find out why sleep is poor and address those underlying causes. All living creatures require a regular 'sleep' (or period of quiescence) during which time healing and repair take place. You must put as much work into your sleep as your diet. Without a good night's sleep on a regular basis, all other interventions are undermined.

We are all born as babies with the gift of sleep and somewhere down the line that ability may be lost. Retracing those footsteps can be helpful diagnostically. So let's start with babies.

Poor fuel delivery mechanisms

When babies are born they are fully keto-adapted – that is to say, they run their entire metabolism on fats and ketones. During the first weeks of life, the baby's brain uses an astonishing 60 per cent of all energy consumption in the body – another beautiful example of how the brain loves to run on fats and ketones. Unfortunately, we turn babies into carbohydrate addicts at a young age. Many babies are reared on bottled milk which has a high proportion of sugars and carbohydrates, and this is bad news for the developing brain and baby. Even those babies who are breast-fed may suffer – breast milk reflects what is going into the mother's bloodstream and if she is a sugar and carbohydrate addict, then her baby will also become such. Indeed, we are currently seeing epidemics of oral thrush in babies – usually dismissed by nurses and health visitors as a minor annoyance, but symptomatic of the fact that already a baby is overwhelmed by sugar so that yeasts can comfortably make themselves at home. In the mouth this presents with a white coating of the tongue; in the scalp as cradle cap. Some baby girls even develop perineal thrush and the little boys get balanitis.

So this brings us to, I suspect, the commonest cause of insomnia – namely, nocturnal hypoglycaemia. Blood sugar levels fluctuate rapidly and as they fall there is an outpouring of adrenaline that wakes us up. This out-pouring of adrenaline is, I suspect, partly responsible for the nightmares and vivid dreams often experienced by CFS / ME sufferers. What makes this problem even worse in CFS / ME sufferers is alcohol – this has disastrous effects on blood sugar because it stimulates insulin production and inhibits the production of glucagon (the hormone that increases blood sugar), causing even wider fluctuations in blood sugar levels. Alcohol may come from the diet or the fermenting gut. The keto-adapted infant can happily burn fat and this fuels him through the night. The keto-adapted adult can do the same.

The treatment of nocturnal hypoglycaemia is clearly the ketogenic diet.

Allergy

At this point many parents will be saying, 'Oh, but my baby never slept!' A common cause of this is allergy and I suspect this starts with the hyperactive baby in the womb. Allergy and addiction are two sides of the same coin – we become addicted to our allergens and allergic to our addictions! Short-term small doses of that allergen, therefore, give relief, but one then gets rebound worsening a few hours later. This may explain why many allergic conditions, such as asthma, migraine, headaches, arthritis, mood changes or irritable bladders, cause most problems in the middle of the night or early morning. The Paleo-ketogenic diet is the starting point for treating allergy.

A common problem in babies is colic and the commonest cause of that is allergy to dairy products. Cows' milk protein is a tough antigen. Dairy products eaten by Mum easily pass into breast milk to cause allergic reactions in her baby. I know. Both my daughters suffered from such and this was the start of my personal journey into understanding and treating allergy (see Chapter 10, page 143).

Sleep apnoea: obstructive

Sleep apnoea is a major disturber of sleep. It simply means that breathing ceases for windows of time during sleep. There are two reasons for this – namely, obstructive and central.

In obstructive sleep apnoea, the airways are narrowed and collapse in on themselves and clinically this presents with noisy breathing or snoring. If the collapse is complete, no air may pass through for some time and there is complete obstruction of the airways. Oxygen levels in the blood rapidly fall, the brain detects this, and there is an immediate stress response and partial waking – clearly very disruptive to sleep.

Obstructive sleep apnoea occurs when the tissues lining the airways become swollen, or 'oedematous', and there are four reasons for that:

1. **Allergy:** The commonest cause of airway narrowing and snoring I suspect is allergy to dairy products, but it may be to other foods as well.
2. **Hypothyroidism (underactive thyroid):** Another name for hypothyroidism is myxoedema and that reflects the fluid retention we see in tissues. This may present with a change in voice, such as hoarseness or loss of singing ability. Dr Kenneth Blanchard estimates that at least 20 per cent of Western women are hypothyroid.[51]
3. **Metabolic syndrome:** Aside from being overweight, metabolic syndrome also results in fluid retention and this too may be sufficient to partially obstruct the airways.
4. **Pickwickian syndrome*:** This is an extreme version of metabolic syndrome in which the sufferer is grossly overweight. I am not sure if the obstruction is due to fat deposits in the tissue or fluid retention, but the result is the same. I have to say it was my experience when I was a young mother in Nottinghamshire that the health visitors did not seem satisfied

---

* **Historical Note:** Dickens showed his full range of observational and descriptive powers when introducing to the reader the 'fat boy', Joe, who displays all the signs and symptoms of sleep apnoea.

> *'Sleep!' said the old gentleman, 'he's always asleep. Goes on errands fast asleep, and snores as he waits at table.'*

More recently, in 1956, a poker-playing businessman developed similar symptoms to those of Joe in *The Pickwick Papers*. However, it took financial loss for him to seek hospital care. The patient played poker once a week and on this particular occasion he had been dealt a hand of three aces and two kings – a full house. However, because he had dropped off to sleep he failed to take advantage of this opportunity. A few days later he checked himself into hospital!

with the weight gain of infants until the babies' cheeks met in front of their noses! It seemed then that the only definition of baby health was obesity.

Sleep apnoea: central

In central sleep apnoea there is no obstruction, but breathing ceases because the brain forgets to initiate breathing – the respiratory sensor itself seems to have gone to sleep. I was involved in a legal group action for farmers all of whom had been seriously poisoned by organophosphates. Central sleep apnoea was common amongst them. This told me that organophosphates, potent inhibitors of brain neurotransmitters, have the potential to switch off the respiratory centre. This squared very nicely with the work of Barry Richardson whose theories on cot death received wide acceptance at the time.[52] His ideas were scientifically based and biologically plausible. His hypothesis beautifully and elegantly explained the statistics of the cot death epidemic. In a nutshell he identified fire retardants in cot mattresses to be the root cause. These fire retardants included arsenic compounds, phosphorus compounds and antimony compounds, which, when fermented by microbes which thrive on babies' mucus – namely, *Scopulariopsis brevicaulis* – were broken down into toxic gases – namely, arsine, phosphine and stibine, respectively. These toxic gases work very much like organophosphates – they are cholinesterase inhibitors. Essentially they switched off the babies' respiratory centre and stopped them breathing. We also know these organophosphate-like chemicals have the potential to cause cardiac dysrhythmias. This theory beautifully explained the clinical evidence of the cot death poison gas theory as listed in Table 16.1.

The point I am making here is that I suspect central sleep apnoea is a symptom of toxicity.

Diagnosis of sleep apnoea

Ideally diagnosis takes place in a sleep laboratory, but this is expensive and rather artificial – sleep is always impaired in a strange environment. The diagnosis of sleep apnoea may simply come from a sleeping partner who notices either obstructed breathing or cessation of breathing. A pulse oximeter, which records blood oxygen levels during the night, may show dips in blood oxygen levels. Some of my patients have set up a camera to video them whilst asleep. It makes for dull viewing but can result in a diagnosis. There is also an app for your smartphone that can record your whole night's sleep and play back to you the 'noisy bits'.

Table 16.1. Explaining cot death

Fact:	**Explanation: because . . .**
Cot death occurs more often during a mild illness when a baby has a temperature	An increase in a baby's body temperature from the normal 37°C (98.6°F) to 42°C (107.6°F) causes a 20-fold increase in poison gas production
Cot death is more common in boys than girls	Boys run a basal metabolic rate which is 15 per cent higher than girls, so they are hotter and evaporate more toxic gases from the mattresses
It occurs more in winter when parents overwrap their babies and turn the central heating on	An increase in a baby's body temperature from 37°C (98.6°F) to 42°C (107.6°F) causes a 20-fold increase in poison gas production
Many deaths occur in the early morning when the central heating turns on automatically. Indeed, the incidence of cot deaths exactly parallels heating bills	Ditto
More common in babies that were over-wrapped or who had caps on their heads	Ditto
Cot death peaks at age 2–5 months	It takes a couple of months for the mattress to become impregnated with *Scopulariopsis brevicaulis*. At six months the baby has the strength to lift his/her head away from the toxic gases
Cot death is more common in low birthweight or otherwise disadvantaged babies	Low birthweight babies are not as physically strong as healthy babies so cannot move their heads away from the poisoning Possibly they are also more susceptible to toxic stress
Cot death babies often have been irritable	Toxic gases cause headache
Cot death is rarer with brand new mattresses	It takes time for the mattress to become impregnated with *Scopulariopsis brevicaulis*
Cot death is more common in babies lying on their fronts or side	They cannot escape inhaling the toxic gases
Cot death is more common in babies on secondhand mattresses – i.e. hand-me-downs such as occurs with a second child or army babies	The mattress is pre-inoculated with *Scopulariopsis brevicaulis* by the previous babies
Success of the 'back to sleep' campaign	Babies lying on their backs breathe fresher air, or rather the poison gases are somewhat diluted
Absence of abnormal post-mortem findings	This is an acute poisoning. The poison gases rapidly evaporate off
One study showed that babies dying of cot death have abnormally high levels of antimony in their blood (from stibine gas)	Antimony is fermented into stibine, one of the suspect poisonous gases

Fact:	Explanation: because . . .
High instance in aboriginal babies	Aboriginal babies are traditionally placed on sheep fleeces which may come from sheep dipped in organophosphates or it may be that the fleeces had a naturally high arsenic content because Australian soils are high in arsenic
Absence of cot death in Japan	Where boron is used as a fire retardant.

Treatment of sleep apnoea

Treatment of sleep apnoea depends on the cause as shown in Table 16.2.

The conventional treatment of obstructive sleep apnoea involves a CPAP (continuous positive airways pressure) machine. This works by increasing the pressure in the airways to blow them, and keep them, open. This is effective but cumbersome and often poorly tolerated. Much more logical and satisfying is to identify the underlying cause.

Hypervigilance

From an evolutionary perspective, hypervigilance for tribal survival would have been very helpful. These people would have made the sentries at the opening of our caves. They would have been so anxious that they would have heard a sabre-toothed tiger break wind a mile away. These constitutionally hard-wired worriers would have kept the tribe safe during the dark hours. The laid-back, unconcerned warriors and hunters would have slept soundly through the night. By day, warriors and hunter–gatherers would have been out

Table 16.2. Sleep apnoea – causes and treatments

Clinical picture	Cause	Treatment
Obstructive sleep apnoea	Allergy	Paleo diet*
	Metabolic syndrome	Ketogenic diet*
	Pickwickian syndrome	Ketogenic diet plus 5:2 diet*
	Hypothyroidism	See Chapter 5 (page 81) for treatment of hypothyroidism
		Consider surgical excision of the uvula
Central sleep apnoea	Toxic stress Head injury – see page 202 Infection – see page 204	See Chapter 20 on detoxification (page 233)

* Please see my books *Prevent and Cure Diabetes* and *The Paleo-Ketogenic Cookbook.*

there hunting food for the tribes while the hypervigilant fretters would have had a chance to rest.

Some people are born hypervigilant. Some acquire hypervigilance through childhood experience – bullying, sexual abuse, insecurity, being unloved, unresolved concerns, all have the ability to hard-wire a child for sleeplessness for life. I remember one patient who told me that as a boy his father suffered from severe asthma and was not expected to live. The boy tried to stay awake at night to make sure his father was still breathing to reassure himself he was still alive. That boy carried that hypervigilance into adult life and CFS/ME.

As a child I shared a bedroom with my sister and a bed with my soft toy of a seal. Of course, my seal was imparted with magical qualities which kept me safe through the night – I could not go off to sleep without hugging my best friend. Later on, the sentry in my bedroom became my pet dog Nancy who now snuggles up to me at night. She has become my sentry at the gate and this supplies my primitive emotional brain with a sense of security that helps sleep. I know I do not sleep so well when I am away from home and she is not with me. I am quite sure Craig would not sleep half so well without Penny to snuggle up to!*

Treatment: Many people prevented from sleeping by hypervigilance benefit from psychological techniques to help them deal with past traumas – these are beyond the scope of this book. However, hypervigilance is the commonest reason for me to prescribe medication. For many it is long-term medication (see page 210).

Neurological damage

After the First World War a strain of Spanish 'flu swept through Europe, killing 50 million people worldwide. Some people sustained neurological damage and for some this virus wiped out their sleep centre in the brain. This meant they were unable to sleep at all. All these poor people were dead within two weeks; this was the first solid scientific evidence that sleep is more essential for life than food and water. These conclusions were supported when, in the 1980s, a University of Chicago researcher, Allan Rechtschaffen, performed a

---

* **Editor's note:** Very true! And before Penny, there was 'LitTed', my little blue teddy bear bought for me by my father's squadron – I still have him – he is three months older than me and looks a lot better on it!

series of sleep deprivation experiments on rats. After 32 days of total sleep deprivation, all the rats were dead. This was further confirmed by a follow-up study in 2002.[53]

It may well be that there are other viruses which damage the sleep centre to a lesser degree – but this lesser damage will also have a negative impact on sleep.

I also have patients who have sustained a head injury and been unable to sleep properly since. I suspect that these people require mild hypnotics for life in order to sleep and function normally. The same is true for patients poisoned by organophosphates and toxic metals (especially mercury).

Sleep disturbed by heat

A falling body temperature is a trigger for sleep. A rising body temperature in the morning (driven by thyroid and adrenal hormones) wakes us up.

Being hot at night is a major sleep disrupter as any woman with post-menopausal flushes will testify to. Interestingly, it seems that one mechanism by which alcohol is so damaging to the liver is that it encourages the wrong gut microbes and increases their movement through the gut wall (bacterial translocation) so that they have to be dealt with by the liver. The liver uses a great deal of energy to cope with this and some is wasted as heat. Indeed, running a fever is a major defence against bacteria. I suspect this is one mechanism by which the upper fermenting gut disturbs sleep. This is because alcohol is a product of a fermenting gut and so the mechanism as described above will occur in the presence of a fermenting gut. The treatment of this is found in Chapter 7 (see page 107).

For menopausal hot flushes I have no perfect answer. I find it astonishing that despite the high prevalence of symptoms in menopausal women there is remarkably little research on the mechanisms by which hot flushes occur. In my webpage on menopause, too long to include here, I argue that symptoms result from the out-pouring of hormones from the pituitary (which is trying to stimulate the ovaries to produce eggs but they have of course run out of these). This is made much worse by metabolic syndrome. These hormones are either hormone mimics or thermogenic in their own right. For example, LH (luteinising hormond) and FSH (follicle stimulating hormone) mimic hormones such as bradykinin and vasopressin, both of which cause hot flushes. We can reduce the out-pouring of these hormones with a ketogenic diet and reducing food intake in the evening – I will keep repeating it: we should breakfast like an emperor, lunch like a king, sup like a pauper. We can further mitigate flushes with pregnenolone (50 mg daily). Clonidine (a bradykinin inhibitor) in tiny doses (25–50 mg) at night is often helpful.

In the event of a hot flush at night, get as cool as possible as quickly as possible. If you can, sleep under an open window. Drink ice cold water – I suggest leaving a half-full ½ litre water bottle in the deep freeze during the day. Top up with water and keep next to the bed – the ice keeps all the water ice-cold over night. Drinking ice cold water brings the body temperature down faster than anything else.

Chronic infection may present with insomnia. Part of the mechanism may well be due to heat – running a fever is how the body naturally deals with infection. Furthermore, the two groups of microbes most commonly associated with CFS/ME are the herpes viruses (Epstein-Barr or 'mono', shingles/chicken pox) together with Lyme disease and co-infections. We also know that many cases of dementia are caused by the same. Tackling the chronic infections of CFS/ME may be a vital part of dealing with sleep (see Chapters 11 [page 151] and 12 [page 161]).

Sleep disturbed by the need to pee

One should be perfectly able to go through the night without needing to pee. Indeed, to pee in the night would put one in terrible danger during our evolutionary past – imagine having to creep out of the cave with a T-rex lurking. (I know they weren't around at the same time as our human ancestors, but you know what I mean!)

We have a hormone – namely, anti-diuretic hormone (ADH) – which shuts down the kidneys during the night and prevents them making urine. The need to pee is driven either by a full bladder or an irritable one.

Full bladder. In CFS/ME I can see two possible mechanisms which may stop this working as it should:

(i) The first is that there is a general suppression of the HPA (hypothalamus-pituitary-adrenal) axis in CFS/ME, and ADH secretion may be impaired. This should improve as energy delivery mechanisms are improved.

(ii) The second has to do with poor cardiac output in CFS/ME – people with severe CFS/ME are in borderline heart failure. During the day there may not be sufficient cardiac output for the kidneys to work normally. As detailed in Chapter 4, page 51, it is much easier to pump blood on the flat, so the kidneys are better perfused when lying down. Suddenly the bladder fills at night and one needs a pee. Again, this symptom will improve as energy delivery mechanisms are improved.

Irritable bladder. The bladder can react allergically just like any other part of the body. It reacts to antigens in urine. Perhaps the commonest is yeast from the fermenting gut. The idea here is that microbes in the fermenting gut are miniscule compared with human cells and spill over into the bloodstream. (This is called 'translocation'.) Again, because they are tiny they pass through the kidney into urine. A urine infection is defined as more than 10,000 microbes per millilitre (ml). However, the bladder may sensitise to much less. This explains why women suffer recurrent cystitis and men recurrent prostatitis, which respond to antibiotics even though the urine cultures are negative. The treatment is as for the fermenting gut (see Chapter 7, page 107). However, there are other possible allergens – I have one patient whose severe interstitial cystitis was triggered through working with photographic chemicals in a dark room which had no ventilation – she now finds any chemical will irritate her bladder. For others, foods are a problem – especially citrus fruits.

Hypothyroidism and hypoadrenalism

In Nature, levels of thyroid-stimulating hormone spike at midnight, levels of T4 (thyroxin) at 4 am and T3 at 5 am. The rising level of T3 wakes the adrenal gland up and we then see a spike of adrenal hormones including DHEA and cortisol. Correction of thyroid function and adrenal function often results in improved sleep (see Chapter 5, page 81).

Light and melatonin and sleep waves

The timing of sleep is ultimately controlled by light. It is light landing on the skin that switches off melatonin production. Melatonin is the sleep hormone without which we cannot sleep – in the Richardson ground squirrel (*Spermophilus richardsonii*), night time levels may be 20–40 times higher than day time. Melatonin is produced in the brain by the pineal gland and I suspect its production too is impaired in CFS/ME. Indeed, I suspect melatonin dysfunction is another 'acquired metabolic dyslexia' – as we age we all get less good at producing it.

The first step is to switch off production during the day. It is light which does this; again this makes perfect evolutionary sense – we do not want to fall asleep whilst running around naked in the African sunshine! Switching off melatonin is best achieved with full spectrum sunlight. I suspect this is part of the mechanism by which so many people have now become 'owls' – we spend too much time indoors and do not get the necessary full spectrum light exposure. I love to work in my conservatory surrounded by natural light. Living and working next to large windows improves energy levels and productivity as demonstrated by a myriad of studies. For example, a recent study showed that office workers with windows received 173 per cent more white light exposure during work hours, and slept an average of 46 minutes more per night. Workers without windows reported poorer scores than their counterparts on quality of life measures related to physical problems and vitality, as well as poorer outcomes on measures of overall sleep quality, sleep efficiency, sleep disturbances and daytime dysfunction.[54]

By contrast, we need a pitch-black room to sleep in – it may be necessary to use black-out curtains. Many people comment that their sleep is worse when the moon is full; the valley I look out on appears floodlit when the moon is full and bright – it certainly wakes me up. Wolves are more active with the full moon perhaps because their sleep too is disrupted.

Melatonin 1–9 mg at night is often helpful for sleep. The dose is remarkably variable. It is not common, but some people get depressed with melatonin, so be aware. This is possibly a seasonal affective disorder (SAD) -like effect – melatonin levels are higher in hibernation and this is associated with low mood.

We are told that melatonin should be avoided in autoimmunity, but I can see no biologically plausible mechanism for this. Indeed, melatonin is a useful antioxidant and therefore – quite the other way – I would think it is indicated in autoimmunity. In UK NHS paediatric practice, melatonin is a first-line treatment for children with sleep disorders.

Finally, sleep does not gradually creep up on us during the evening – it comes in waves. There is a sleep wave about every 90 minutes and you will get to sleep most efficiently if you learn to recognise and ride the sleep wave. Often there is a lesser one earlier in the evening, which is when people drop off to sleep in front of the telly, or they jump and make a cup of tea to wake themselves up because 'they are not ready to go to bed' – actually they are. My sleep wave comes at 9.20 pm and I like to be in bed reading well before this – it is immediately recognisable now and I have learnt to expect it.

The general principles of treating insomnia

The general principles of treating insomnia are:

1. Identify possible causes as above and treat.
2. Get the physical essentials for a good night's sleep organised.

We are all creatures of habit and the first step is to get the physical essentials in place:

- A dark room – the slightest chink of light landing on your skin will disturb your own production of melatonin (the body's natural sleep hormone). Have thick curtains or blackouts to keep the bedroom dark; this is particularly important for children. If you should wake up, do not switch the lights on and do not keep on looking at your watch!
- A source of fresh, if possible cool, air.
- A warm comfortable bed – we have been brainwashed into believing a hard bed is good for us and so many people end up with sleepless nights on an uncomfortable bed. It is the shape of the bed that is important. It should be shaped to fit you approximately and then very soft to distribute your weight evenly and avoid pressure points. Tempur mattresses can be helpful (if expensive), as are water beds.
- Do not allow a bed fellow who snores – you need different rooms!
- Until you become keto-adapted, a high-fat, low-carbohydrate snack just before bedtime (e.g. nuts, seeds) helps prevent nocturnal hypoglycaemia. Once keto-adapted, sleep is improved by eating early in the evening and not snacking later. Many people observe that, once keto-adapted, fasting improves sleep quality.
- Perhaps restrict fluids in the evening if your night is disturbed by a full bladder (but see above and address the underlying issues, page 204).
- No stimulants, such as caffeine or adrenaline-inducing TV, arguments, phone calls, family matters or whatever before bedtime! Caffeine has a long half life – none after 4 pm.
- Learn to recognise the sleep wave – as I said, one comes every 90 minutes. A regular pre-bedtime routine is really helpful – your 'alarm' should go off at 9 pm, at which point you drop all activity and move into your bedtime routine.

Busy brain – learn a 'sleep dream'

Getting the physical things in place is the easy bit. The hard bit is getting your brain off to sleep. An astonishing statistic is that throughout life, the brain makes a million new connections every second. This means that it has a fantastic ability to learn new things, so it must be perfectly possible to teach your brain to go off to sleep – it is simply a case of pressing the right buttons.

Getting off to sleep is all about developing a conditioned reflex. The first historical example of this is Pavlov's dogs. Pavlov was a Russian physiologist who showed that when dogs ate food, they salivated. He then 'conditioned' them by ringing a bell whilst they ate food. After two weeks of conditioning, he could make them salivate simply by ringing a bell. This of course is a completely useless conditioned response, but it shows us that the brain can be trained to do anything.

Let's apply this to the busy brain. First, you must get into a mind-set which does not involve the immediate past or immediate future. That is to say, if you are thinking about reality then there is no chance of getting off to sleep – more of this in a moment. Then use a hypnotic (see pages 210–11) which will help induce sleep. Apply the two together for a period of 'conditioning'. This may be for a few days or a few weeks. The brain then learns that when it gets into that particular mind-set, it will go off to sleep. Then the drug becomes increasingly irrelevant. However, things can break down during times of stress and a few days of drug may be required to reinforce the conditioned response. But it is vital to use the correct 'mind-set' every time the drug is used, or the conditioning will weaken.

I do not pretend this is easy, but to allow one's mind to wander into reality when one is trying to sleep must be considered a complete self-indulgence. Treat your brain like a naughty child – it must simply not be allowed to free-wheel.

Find a sleep dream that suits you

Everyone has to work out their best mind-set. It could be a childhood dream, or recalling details of a journey or walk, or whatever. It is actually a sort of self-hypnosis. What you are trying to do is to 'talk' to your subconscious. This can only be done with the imagination, not with spoken language. I dream that I am a hibernating bear, snuggled down in my comfortable den with one daughter in one arm and the other in the other. Outside the wind is howling and the snow coming down and I am sinking deeper and deeper down . . . cripes! I am going now!

As I have said, this is a form of self-hypnosis. We know that the hypnotic state is characterised by extreme responsiveness to suggestion. You can use this information for conditioning yourself in self-hypnosis. Here is a standard procedure to follow. Lie down in bed, ready for sleep, initially with your eyes open. (The room needs to be dark.) Mentally give yourself the suggestion that your eyes are becoming heavy and tired – that as you count to 10, your eyes will become very heavy and watery and that you will find it impossible to keep your eyelids open by the time you reach 10. If you find that you cannot keep them open and have to close them, then you are probably under self-hypnosis. At this point deepen the state by again slowly counting to 10. Between each count, mentally give yourself suggestions that you are falling into a deep hypnotic state. Try to reach a state where you feel you are about to fall asleep. Give yourself the suggestion that you are falling more deeply down into sleep. Some people may get a very light feeling throughout the body; others may get a heavy feeling.

Let us assume that your eyes did not become heavy. Then repeat the procedure. You can count to 100 if you need this period of time to assure eye closure. The closing of the eyes is the first sign you are in a receptive frame of mind. Let us assume that you get the eye closure. Take a longer count to get yourself in the very relaxed state. Once you achieve this, you should be able to respond properly. The difficult bit is not allowing your brain to wander off into other areas. You must work hard at concentrating on the counting and the responses that achieves.

If you respond properly, give yourself the 'post-hypnotic suggestion' that you will be able to put yourself under later by counting to three, or using any specific phrase you desire. Continue using it every day and give yourself the post-hypnotic suggestion every time you work with it, so that at each succeeding session you will fall into a deeper state and the suggestions will work more forcefully with each repetition.

Each time that you work towards acquiring the self-hypnotic state, regardless of the depth that you have achieved and whether or not you have responded to any of the tests, give yourself the following suggestions: 'The next time I hypnotise myself, I shall fall into a deeper and sounder state.' You should also give yourself whatever suggestions you desire as though you were in a very deep state of hypnosis. You may ask, 'If I'm not under hypnosis, why give myself the suggestions?' You do this so that you will begin to form the conditioned reflex pattern. Keep at it. One of the times that you work at achieving self-hypnosis the conditioned response will take hold . . . you will achieve self-hypnosis from that time on. It is like learning to drive a car with a clutch. At first you must consciously go through the process of putting your foot on the clutch and shifting gears. Usually there is a grinding of the gears and you feel quite conspicuous about this, but gradually you learn to do this almost automatically and you gain confidence in your driving ability. The same is true of hypnosis. As you work at your task, you gradually get the feel of it and you achieve proficiency in it.

What to do should you wake in the night

If you do wake in the night, do not switch the light on, do not get up and potter round the house, or you will have no chance of dropping off to sleep again. Relieve any discomfort, such as the need to pee, getting too hot or cold, etc, then use your sleep dream again.

Natural preparations to help sleep

These all work differently and so I like to use low-dose combinations until you find something that suits. Choose from the following, and start with:

- Melatonin 3 mg (per tablet) 1–3 tablets at night. This may work better if used sublingually (under the tongue).
- Valerian root 400 mg (per capsule) 1–4 capsules at night. This is a herbal preparation which is shorter acting and can be taken in the middle of the night.
- Nytol (diphenhydramine) 50 mg, Piriton (chlorphenamine) 4 mg or doxylamine 25 mg. These are sedating antihistamines available over the counter. The dose is 1–2 tablets at night. Try them one type at a time to see what suits you best. They are longer acting – don't take them in the middle of the night or you may wake up feeling hungover.
- Kava kava 60–120 mg. At one stage this was banned in the UK (and still is in the Republic of Ireland) because of potential liver toxicity. However, that results if the liver is deficient in micronutrients or over-loaded by toxic stress. Attention to these issues minimises and probably negates any theoretical toxicity.

Do not use alcohol for sleep. Yes, it gets you off to sleep, but it is disruptive subsequently because it induces hypoglycaemia. In addition, it requires a huge amount of raw materials and energy from the liver to detox it, opening up a large hole in the energy bucket.

Prescription drugs for sleep

Those CFS/ME sufferers who are hard-wired for hypervigilance or have neurological damage (traumatic, toxic or viral) may need prescription hypnotics long term. It is vital that any such use is combined with all the above interventions, and especially the sleep dream (page 208). This helps to prevent the problem of 'tachyphylaxis' – that is, habituating to a drug so that the dose has to be increased. The deal is always, 'I will prescribe but you must sleep dream.' The sleep dream is hard work and requires discipline and mental energy – it is all too easy to let the brain wander and expect the drug to do its work – but that is short-term gain and long-term pain.

Prescription drugs in the order of what I would try first are:

- Amitriptyline 5–25 mg. I would start with 5 mg initially. Most CFS/ME patients are made worse and feel hungover with 'normal' doses
- Short-acting zaleplon (Sonata 10 mg), if the problem is dropping off to sleep.
- Medium-acting zopiclone (Zimovane 3.75–7.5 mg).
- Long-acting clonazepam 0.5–2 mg, or possibly more. This may be doubly helpful because it is anti-inflammatory (it damps down the NMDA receptor).
- Diazepam 2.5 mg is helpful if sleep is disturbed by muscle spasms. (It is a good muscle relaxant.) Possibly up to 10 mg for short periods.

Different people will respond to different combinations of hypnotics. For example, one person may take a melatonin and two valerian capsules at night, plus a zaleplon when they wake at 3.00 am. Somebody else may be best suited by 10 mg amitriptyline at night with a Nytol. Don't be afraid to try combinations – there are no serious side effects that I am aware of with any of these used in combination. However, don't change more than one thing at any time, otherwise you will get confused and won't know what has worked best for you. Furthermore, the dose may vary from day to day and week to week – many people have a good idea of how much they need according to the stress of the day.

Addiction and dependence

Understandably people worry about being addicted to sleep medications. However, I do not think of this as addiction so much as dependence. In this respect I am dependent on a good night's sleep so that I can function the next day. For the CFS/ME sufferer, a poor night's sleep results in a poor day and so recovery is postponed by 24 hours. When I was being hounded by the General Medical Council I became a complete insomniac. Without Nytol, melatonin and valerian I would not have slept at all and my defence would have been seriously compromised as a result.

People then point out that sleeping pills, and anticholinergics (including sedating antihistamines), are associated with cognitive dysfunction and dementia. I suspect that the real issue is not the pills but the insomnia. We know lack of sleep is a major risk factor for dementia (and, indeed, cancer and heart disease). For example, a study by Shastri et al (2016) concluded, 'There is a clear relationship between obstructive sleep apnoea, cognitive decline and dementia.'[55]

I suspect it is the underlying causes of insomnia (as detailed above) that are the risk factors for the three deadly killers – heart disease, cancer and dementia. Address those causes properly and the impact of sleep pills fades into insignificance by comparison. They may also, of course, become redundant.

CHAPTER 16 SUMMARY

Sleep

- Good sleep is absolutely *essential* to recovery from CFS/ME and for continuing good health.
- There are many reasons why modern Westerners do not manage good restorative sleep – these are listed below, with the action required to correct them:
  - Nocturnal hypoglycaemia: waking up because of blood sugar swings – treat with ketogenic diet.
  - Allergies – treat with Paleo-ketogenic diet, cutting out the common food allergens, such as dairy, wheat. Further interventions for more stubborn allergies may be needed (see Chapter 10 on allergy, page 143).
  - Sleep apnoea: obstructive – this could be caused by allergy (treat as above), hypothyroidism (see Chapter 5, page 81, for treatment), metabolic syndrome (treat with ketogenic diet) or Pickwickian syndrome (lose weight via Paleo-ketogenic diet)
  - Sleep apnoea: central – most likely a symptom of toxicity (see Chapter 20 [page 233] on how to detox).
  - Hypervigilance: perhaps you are naturally hypervigilant or perhaps a past trauma has made you so – treatment is psychological therapy or use of prescription drugs as below.

- Sleep disturbed by heat – if caused by menopause, treatment is ketogenic diet and reducing food intake at night, along with possibly pregnenolone 25–50 mg daily. If caused by chronic infection, then see Chapters 11 (page 151) and 12 (page 161) on chronic infections.
- Sleep disturbed by the need to pee – if there is a full bladder then improving energy delivery systems as recommended elsewhere in this book will help. If there is an irritable bladder, then the treatment is as for fermenting gut – see Chapter 7, page 107.
- Hypothyroidism or hypoadrenalism – treat as in Chapter 5, page 81.

- We must also get the conditions for sleep right by:
    - Sleeping in a pitch-black room
    - Having a source of fresh cool air
    - Having a warm, comfortable bed – not a hard bed but one that moulds to your body shape
    - Until you become keto-adapted, eating a high-fat, low-carbohydrate snack just before bedtime, such as nuts or seeds
    - Restricting fluids in the evening if your night is disturbed by a full bladder
    - Avoiding stimulants, such as caffeine or adrenaline-inducing TV, arguments, phone calls, family matters or whatever, before bedtime
    - Learning to recognise the sleep wave and to use the techniques of a sleep dream and self-hypnosis – see page 208 for more detail.
- Even with all these treatments and interventions, some CFS/ME sufferers still have difficulty sleeping. In this event, do not shy away from natural or even prescription hypnotics to help establish a good sleep regime. More often than not, these drugs can be removed once sleep patterns have been restored.
- Naturals sleep-inducers include:
    - Melatonin 1–3 × 3 mg tablets at night
    - Valerian root 1–4 × 400 mg capsules at night

- Nytol (diphenhydramine) 50 mg, Piriton (chlorphenamine) 4 mg, doxylamine 25 mg – these are sedating antihistamines available over the counter
- Kava kava 60–120 mg.

- Prescription hypnotics include:

  - Amitriptyline 10–25 mg
  - Short-acting zaleplon (Sonata 10 mg) – if the problem is dropping off to sleep
  - Medium-acting zopiclone (Zimovane 3.75–7.5 mg)
  - Long-acting clonazepam 0.5–2 mg, or possibly more
  - Diazepam 2–5 mg, possibly up to 10 mg for short periods of time – helpful if sleep is disturbed by muscle spasms.

CHAPTER 17

The Paleo-ketogenic diet

The diet I advocate may seem boring but my job is to get you well, not to entertain you. Take a leap of faith and just do it! So what follows are the simple Rules of the Game followed by a suggested daily menu.

Rules of the diet game

Table 17.1, page 216, sets out the rules in order of priority. It is a reminder of what was in Chapter 6, page 101, or will be news to you if you have skipped to the practical details.

Example daily menu

In the plan set out in Table 17.2, page 218, I am using net carbs (sugars and starches, with fibre excluded) on the grounds that soluble fibre is fermented into short-chain fatty acids. Linseed is a good example – it is said to have virtually zero carbs because although 100 grams contains 29 grams of total carb, 27 grams consist of fibre and so just 2 grams of starch and sugar.

The idea of this approach is to get into ketosis. Check that you are by testing your urine with ketostix.

Wait until you are keto-adapted before trying D-ribose. This is because it may lower blood sugar by stimulating insulin release – this is not a problem once you are running your body on ketones, and indeed lowering insulin levels further helps the body switch into fat burning.

Table 17.1. Dietary rules in order of priority

Rules	Why you need to observe them
No alcohol – 90 per cent of CFS/ME sufferers are alcohol intolerant	Directly toxic to brain and liver. Suppresses the immune system, increasing the risk of infection and cancer.
	Stimulates insulin and inhibits glucagon, worsening metabolic syndrome. Switches on other cravings – e.g. sugar and snacks.
	Uses up micronutrients and causes deficiencies.
Greatly increase intake of fat and fibre – if you get hungry, eat more fat	The body should be powered by fat and fibre, not starch and sugar. Switching to such is called keto-adapting; it may take two to three weeks to switch into fat-burning mode.
	Please note our epidemics of cancer, heart disease and dementia are driven by starch- and sugar-based diets. Fat is protective. Fibre is fermented by friendly microbes to produce short-chain fatty acids – a useful fuel. Much more detail in *Prevent and Cure Diabetes.*
No sugar No fruit sugar – fructose is even more pernicious than the white stuff No honey Nothing ending in '-ose'	Triggers wobbly blood sugar levels and metabolic syndrome. Directly toxic to brain and liver. Fruit sugar inhibits the enzyme glycogen phosphorylase and this worsens the problems of low blood sugar. Sugars suppress the immune system, increasing the risk of infection and cancer.
	Sugars are easily fermented in the upper gut to produce alcohols, including D-lactate. Sugar feeds unfriendly gut microbes, including yeast. (See Chapter 7 for fermenting gut, page 107.) Stevia and xylitol, though less problematic, keep the sugar craving going. There is evidence to suggest they stimulate insulin release which would reduce blood sugar, increase carbohydrate craving and switch off fat burning – all undesirable metabolic effects.
No artificial sweeteners	Aspartame and other such are toxic to the liver. Artificial sweeteners keep alive the psychological craving for sugar.
Low starch diet (care with all grains, root vegetables and pulses)	Starches may be rapidly digested and spike blood sugars, further driving metabolic syndrome. Starches may be fermented by unfriendly gut microbes (see Chapter 7 for fermenting gut, page 107).
Starches to be eaten just once a day and then in very modest amounts	Reverse metabolic syndrome. Squeeze the liver glycogen sponge dry. Too much starch and sugar spikes insulin and this switches off fat burning.
No snacking	Reverse metabolic syndrome. Squeeze the liver glycogen sponge dry.

Rules	Why you need to observe them
All foods to be eaten within a 10-hour window of time – e.g. breakfast at 8 am, supper finished by 6 pm	A 14-hour window of time for fasting reverses metabolic syndrome and encourages fat burning. Squeeze the liver glycogen sponge dry. Encourage the body to be fuelled by fat.
Cut out all foods containing gluten, dairy and yeast	These are major allergens – allergy kicks a hole in the energy bucket. If you suffer headaches, bowel symptoms, joint and muscle pain, asthma or upper respiratory tract symptoms, then this is a priority.
No milk protein either	Milk protein is also a growth promoter and a risk factor for cancer.
No hydrogenated fats – i.e. margarine and 'spreads' Do not use nut, seed, fish or vegetable oils for cooking – make sure cold-pressed oils really are cold-pressed	Heating and hydrogenation of long-chain cis (left-handed) oils flips them into toxic, trans (right-handed) oils. Cook with medium-chain fats such as lard (from beef, pig, lamb, poultry) or coconut oil. Goose fat is gorgeous! These tough saturated fats are not denatured by heat.
Avoid added chemicals	One can be allergic to anything, including chemical additives. Many people require detoxification in the liver and so add to its burden.
Caffeine	If tolerated, then use at breakfast and lunch. Avoid after 2 pm or you risk disturbing sleep.
Chocolate	Most people are addicted to the sugar and the milk of a chocolate bar. If you can enjoy a square of 70 per cent and not scoff the whole bar then you are not addicted.
Other addictions – nicotine, cannabis, social highs, etc	You can't have an upper without a downer. One addiction leads to another. To recover you must give them all up. (Ouch!) But I did, so you can too.
Eating organic	This of course is highly desirable, but for many, unaffordable and impossible. Do your best.

Weekly shopping-list based on seven days of the example daily menu

- 7 pots Coyo yoghurt, 125 grams size
- 70 grams linseed
- 14 eggs
- 1.75 litres Grace coconut milk (or soya milk) to make kefir
- Kefir sachet or grains
- 6 bars 90 per cent dark chocolate
- One pot peanut butter
- One pot tahini
- 7 tins of fish or meat, 120 grams size

- 7 avocados
- 1.75 litres Grace coconut milk – to use with berries
- 700 grams berries
- 7 chops or pieces of fish
- 560 grams green vegetables
- One lettuce
- 300 grams tomatoes
- One large cucumber
- One pot of 'Not Really Dairy' mayo

Table 17.2. A daily plan for getting into ketosis

When	To eat	Calories (kilo-calories)	Carbs (grams)	To drink
On rising				Spring or bottled water, still or fizzy, 500 ml Herbal tea
Breakfast	Large pot Coyo yoghurt, 125 grams	229	0.6	Bottled water, still or fizzy, 500 ml
	Stir in whatever amount of linseed you need to deal with constipation – say 10 grams	53	0.2	Small coffee with 1 tspn D-ribose (Do not use D-ribose until you are keto-adapted – that takes two weeks)
	2 boiled eggs	150	1.2	
	250 ml of kefir (assuming coconut milk)	50	1.0	
Mid morning	4 squares 90 per cent dark chocolate	237	0.6	Bottled water, still or fizzy, 500 ml
	Dessertspoonful of peanut butter	63	2.1	Herbal tea
Lunch	Tin of sardines in sunflower oil – 120 grams	92	0.1	Bottled water, still or fizzy, 500 ml
	1 avocado – say 100 grams	160	2.0	Small coffee with 1 tspn D-ribose (Do not use D-ribose until you are keto-adapted – that takes two weeks)
	125 ml of Grace coconut milk	138	3.8	
	with 50 grams of berries – say blueberries	23	5.8	
Mid afternoon	4 squares 90 per cent dark chocolate	237	0.5	Bottled water, still or fizzy, 500 ml
	Dessertspoon of tahini	60	1.3	Herbal tea
Supper	Meat or fish – say 125-gram pork chop	290	nil	Bottled water, still or fizzy, 500 ml
	Green vegetables – say 80 grams	35	4.4	Herbal tea
	Large salad (lettuce, tomatoes, cucumbers) with dollop, say tablespoon, of 'Really Not Dairy Mayo'	80	0.2	
	125 ml of Grace coconut milk with	138	3.8	
	50 grams of berries	23	5.8	
Total		2058	33.4	

CHAPTER 17 SUMMARY

The Paleo-ketogenic diet

- I am not here to entertain you . . .
- Take a leap of faith and follow the guidelines as above.
- Just do it! *
- There is more guidance on my website at: www.doctormyhill.co.uk/wiki/Ketogenic_diet_-_the_practical_details. There is also more in my book *Prevent and Cure Diabetes* and in the recipe book that is in development.

* **Historical note:** Nike's iconic 'Just Do It' slogan has been described as one of the best taglines of the twentieth century. The slogan was pitched by advertising executive Dan Wieden, nearly 30 years ago. In a recent interview Wieden admitted that it was inspired by Utah killer Gary Gilmore, who was sentenced to death in 1977 for robbing and murdering two men. Gilmore reportedly said 'Let's do this' as he waited to be shot by a firing squad (Sharkey L, 2015).[56]

CHAPTER 18

The nutritional supplements you need to recover

So often I hear, perhaps most surprisingly from doctors, that all one needs is 'a balanced diet' (oh dear, what is that?!) and that nutritional supplements are unnecessary. These people are like those who used to say that the Earth was flat. Indeed, I call them nutritional flat Earthers.

I used to do nutritional tests routinely. Now I no longer bother because I know what the results will be. Everyone is deficient because of Western diets and lifestyles. We must give our bodies the nutrients that they need in order that they can function as intended.

> *Give us the tools, and we will finish the job.*
>
> WINSTON CHURCHILL
> (30 November 1874 – 24 January 1965)
> 'Give Us the Tools' speech, 9 February 1941

There is much more detail on the 'whys' in my book *Sustainable Medicine*. However, we should all be taking a Basic Package of nutritional supplements, with bolt-on extras should problems arise. Those packages are as follows:

1. The Basic Package

The Basic Package is what we should all be taking as supplements even if nothing is wrong. The doses would be reduced slightly for children depending on their size, but remember children have a greater requirement for nutritional supplements than adults because they are developing and growing. Requirements for supplements also increase in pregnancy for obvious reasons. The supplement one has to be careful with during pregnancy is vitamin A – not more than 10,000 IU daily.

The Basic Package is:

Multivitamins: B1 – 25 mg, B2 – 25 mg, B3 – 50 mg, B5 – 100 mg, B6 as its active form pyridoxal-5-phosphate – 25 mg, B12 – 30 mcg, inositol – 12 mg, PABA – 10 mg, folic acid – 400 mcg, vitamin A – 2,000 IU, vitamin E – 50 mg.

Multi-minerals (including extra vitamin D and B12): Because I could not find a good preparation on the market containing all essential minerals I have a company that makes one up for me which contains the following per ONE gram of 'multi-mineral mix' (MMM):

- Calcium (as calcium chloride) – 60 mg
- Magnesium (as magnesium chloride) – 70 mg
- Potassium (as potassium chloride) – 40 mg
- Zinc (as zinc chloride) – 6 mg
- Iron (as ferric ammonium chloride) – 3 mg
- Boron (as sodium borate) – 2 mg
- Iodine (as potassium iodate) – 0.3 mg
- Copper (as copper sulphate) – 0.2 mg
- Manganese (as manganese chloride) – 0.2 mg
- Molybdenum (as sodium molybdate) – 40 mcg
- Selenium (as sodium selenate) – 40 mcg
- Chromium (as chromium chloride) – 40 mcg
- Vitamin B12 (as methylcobalamin) – 1,000 mcg
- Vitamin D (as cholecalciferol) – 1,000 IU.

Dosage of MMM: The daily dose is 1 gram (one blue scoop) per 2 stone of body weight (12.5 kg or 28 lb) to a maximum of 5 grams (five scoops) per day. The daily dose should be dissolved in cold water – ½ pint of water per 1 gram of the mix (the maximum dose made up in 3 pints of water) and taken throughout the day. **Start off with just ½ pint of mix daily and build up slowly to allow your stomach to adjust to the changes; otherwise it may cause nausea and loose bowel movements.** You can use with ascorbic acid to optimise absorption – with fresh lemon juice this is palatable. It also makes one drink water; this is something many people forget to do! MMM is suitable for all age groups, including babies and pregnant women. The dose is not critical as there is a very wide margin of safety for all essential minerals. (The above doses assume one gets nothing from diet. As diet and gut function improve the dose may be reduced. Most people end up taking 2–3 grams daily.)

Essential fatty acids: Ideally these omega-6 and omega-3 fatty acids should be taken in the ratio 4:1. This ratio is present in hemp oil, so use this as a dressing, or simply take a dessert spoonful daily. In CFS/ME sufferers the enzyme delta-6-desaturase needed to break down linolenic acid (the form of omega-3 in linseed) may not be working so I additionally recommend VegEPA (see page 386), 3 capsules daily to ensure good levels of downstream essential fatty acids.

Vitamin C: At least 2 grams; ascorbic acid is the least expensive and best form of vitamin C. However, it may not be tolerated, in which case I recommend magnesium ascorbate. This should be taken last thing at night on an empty stomach. Vitamin C is poorly absorbed; most remains in the gut, and this protects us against infection and fermentation.

Vitamin D: No toxicity has ever been seen in doses up to 10,000 IU daily. This is roughly equivalent to an hour of Mediterranean sunshine. It is highly protective against infection and osteoporosis.

Salt (sodium chloride): This too is an essential mineral. Western diets are high in salt and people eating such are often overdosing with salt. The Paleo diet is low in salt; furthermore, the ketogenic diet increases salt requirement. Once established on these diets you need to add 5 grams (1 teaspoon) daily of salt, ideally unrefined sea salt, to the diet.

2. The Bolt-on Extras for fatigue and to slow the ageing process (the 'mitochondrial support' package)

In addition to the Basic Package, the following should be added daily:

- Coenzyme Q10 as ubiquinol, 200 mg
- Vitamin B3 as niacinamide, 500–1,500 mg – slow release
- Acetyl-L-carnitine, 1 gram
- D-ribose, 10–15 grams (2–3 teaspoonfuls)
- Vitamin B12, either 5 mg sublingually or, ideally, 0.5 mg by injection (self-inject) in the morning

3. The Bolt-on Extras for healing and repair

In addition to the Basic Package, the following should be added daily:

- Glucosamine, 250 mg
- Organic silica and boron (e.g. silboron)

4. The Bolt-on Extras for detoxing

In addition to the Basic Package, plus mitochondrial support, plus healing and repair, because detoxing also places demands on these mechanisms, the following should be added:

- Iodine (iodoral), 14 mg daily
- Glutathione, 250 mg daily
- Extra zinc, 30 mg and selenium, 500 mcg at night
- Epsom salt baths or sauna-ing (at least weekly, more often if possible – see Chapter 20, page 233)
- Detox clays weekly such as zeolite, 10 grams – see Chapter 20, page 233
- The methylation package – high dose B12; vitamin B6 as piridoxal-5-phosphate, 100 mg; and folic acid as methyltetrahydrofolate, 800 mcg daily – see Chapter 20, page 233.

5. The anti-infection Bolt-on Extras

The following should be taken if exposed to infection or at the first symptoms of such:

- Vitamin C to bowel tolerance (I take 8 grams in one dose, then a further 8 grams two hours later. Vitamin C kills viruses directly and the ensuing diarrhoea washes the rest away.)
- Zinc and vitamin C lozenges – zinc and vitamin C are directly toxic to microbes in the mouth and pharynx

CHAPTER 18 SUMMARY

The nutritional supplements you need to recover

- Western diets and lifestyles lead to deficiencies in nutrition – much more about this in my book *Sustainable Medicine*.
- Everyone, whether ill or not, should take the Basic Package of nutritional supplements.
- The Basic Package consists of:
    - Vitamins
    - Essential fatty acids
    - Extra vitamin D
    - Minerals
    - Extra vitamin C
    - Salt
- The Bolt-on Extras for fatigue and anti-ageing, in addition to the Basic Package, are:
    - Coenzyme Q10 as ubiquinol, 200 mg
    - Vitamin B3 as niacinamide, 500–1,500 mg – slow release
    - Acetyl-L-carnitine, 1g
    - D-ribose, 10–15 g (2–3 tsp)
    - Vitamin B12, 5 mg sublingually or ideally B12 by injection – self-inject 0.5 mg daily in the morning
- The Bolt-on Extras for healing and repair, in addition to the Basic Package, are:
    - Glucosamine, 250 mg daily
    - Organic silica and boron (Silboron contains 1.5 mg silicon and 3.8 mg boron)
- The Bolt-on Extras for detoxing, in addition to all the above, are:
    - Iodine (iodoral), 14 mg daily
    - Glutathione, 250 mg daily
    - Extra zinc, 30 mg and selenium, 500 mcg at night

- Epsom salt baths or sauna-ing (at least weekly, more often if possible – see Chapter 20, page 233)
- Detox clays weekly such as zeolite, 10 g weekly
- The methylation package – high dose B12; vitamin B6 as piridoxal-5-phosphate, 100 mg; and folic acid as methyltetrahydrofolate, 800 mcg daily

• The anti-infection Bolt-on-Extras, taken in addition to the Basic Package are:

- Vitamin C to bowel tolerance (I take 8 g in one dose, then a further 8 g two hours later.)
- Zinc and vitamin C lozenges (zinc, 2 mg and silicon, 1.5 mg every hour)

CHAPTER 19

Avoiding, treating and preventing infections

As I have said in several earlier chapters, life is an arms race – and you and I are a potential free lunch for microbes. As Pasteur famously said on his death bed, 'The microbe is nothing; the environment is everything.'

So, we concentrate on avoidance, then on the environment – that is, our bodies – making things as inhospitable as possible for the microbe; then, if that fails, we attack the said microbe without mercy! Infections are a major trigger for CFS/ME initially as well as triggering relapses. This makes dealing with them effectively all the more important in order to maintain the momentum of a recovery.

Avoid exposure to microbes (do your reasonable best)

Make sensible lifestyle choices such as:

- Choose your foreign holidays with care – avoid those which require vaccination and those which require major dietary changes.
- Be mindful that hospitals, GP surgeries, airports, schools and other such accumulate viruses and antibiotic resistant bacteria.
- Choose your sexual partners with care – This is difficult because sex hormones induce symptoms of recklessness and madness! Oxytocin is the 'love' hormone – it must have been what Puck gave Titania so she fell in love with Bottom in *A Midsummer Night's Dream*. Sexually transmitted diseases are a real danger and need to be guarded against; I don't mean

to hand down 'Commandments' about lust, but I am reminded of that wonderful quote by Field Marshal Bernard Law Montgomery, 1st Viscount Montgomery of Alamein, KG, GCB, DSO, PC (17 November 1887 – 24 March 1976), who said:

> *As God once said, and I think rightly . . .**

Treat at the first sign of infection

- Take vitamin C to bowel tolerance – that is, a sufficient dose to cause diarrhoea. Not only does this kill microbes directly, but it reduces the toxic load from the gut so that more energy can be divested to the immune system.
- Stick with your low-carb ketogenic diet – sugar and fruit sugar feed infection. The worst thing one can give a sick patient is fruit, yet hospital wards are stuffed with these poisonous items! No wonder we are seeing epidemics of antibiotic resistant infections – we are feeding the little wretches too well.

> *Feed a cold; starve a fever*
>
> AN OLD WIVES' TALE which dates back to 1574 from the original 'Fasting is a great remedie of feuer' (sic)

- Take zinc lozenges or zinc drops, 10 mg, four times daily – suck these in the mouth as this is directly toxic to microbes.
- Allow inflammation to develop. The body reacts against viruses with inflammation and the result of inflammation is either directly toxic to the virus or helps to physically expel viruses from the body. For example, viruses are very temperature sensitive – for the body to run a fever is a good thing

---

* **Explanation** – Monty was implying, by his use of words, that he was able to make judgements as to which of God's pronouncements had been made 'rightly'! I make no such claims about my ability to make judgements about the 'rightness' of the Seventh Commandment (Exodus 20:14) concerning adultery but I simply make the point that sexually transmitted diseases are dangerous and efforts should be made to avoid them, as with all infections.

as fever kills viruses (and bacteria). A good snotty nose helps to wash out viruses from the nose and a hacking cough blasts the bugs from the lungs. Symptoms may be uncomfortable but should be welcomed as an appropriate way to get rid of virus. This is why I hate to see symptom-suppressing cold remedies such as paracetamol, antihistamines, alcohol, decongestants and cough mixtures which interfere with the body's natural mechanisms of killing and expelling virus. SO DO NOT SUPPRESS SYMPTOMS – THEY ARE NATURE'S WAY OF EXPELLING INFECTIONS. We suffer symptoms for very good reasons – they protect us from ourselves. We need to suffer pain, fever, chills, malaise and loss of appetite to make us rest and recuperate. I suspect many disease processes are switched on when the immune system is inappropriately switched off by a symptom-suppressing medication. Shockingly, doctors routinely recommend anti-inflammatories, painkillers, antihistamines, antipyretics and stimulants for infectious diseases – I believe this is contributing to our current epidemics of post-infectious fatigue and hospital-acquired, antibiotic-resistant bacteria.

- Sunshine includes ultraviolet rays which kill many microbes. Long-wave ultraviolet light penetrates skin and irradiates the blood. In the pre-antibiotic era this was perhaps the most effective treatment for tuberculosis. If you can sunbathe, then do so.
- Be nice to yourself – Always do this. You don't need to be ill to be nice to yourself!
- Do not be afraid to use antimicrobial medicines if needed. I have a low threshold for using antibiotics, antivirals or antifungals which may be prescription or herbal. It is much better to use these antimicrobials early on, otherwise one risks chronic infection or even chronic allergy to microbes. I would have no qualms about using antivirals such as valacyclovir early on to treat any herpes infection from chickenpox to glandular fever. We know that the early use of antivirals in shingles greatly reduces the risk of post-herpetic neuralgia – a nasty pain which may persist for months following infection. I suspect the mechanism of this is allergy to virus in those nerves sensitised by infection – see 'Allergic Muscles' in Chapter 23, page 263. Similarly, people who have tendencies to infection such as bronchitis, cystitis or sinusitis should have a ready supply of antibiotics so that any such infection can be nipped in the bud.
- Keep warm, overwrap, maybe induce a fever – Do this because all microbes are killed by heat. Heat helps inflammation and whilst the symptoms of inflammation are uncomfortable, this is desirable with acute infection. Indeed, cytokines produced as part of the inflammatory

response induce fatigue and illness behaviour. There is no doubt that people who tend to run cold all the time are more prone to picking up infections and, indeed, this is the basis of the age-old adage to wrap up well in cold weather or you will catch a chill. It would be interesting to measure your basal temperature. Low temperature can be indicative of borderline hypothyroidism and this can certainly present with recurrent infections. Children are very good at running a temperature at the first sign of viral infection, but adults are less good. At one stage Boots used to market a product called rhinotherm which blasted hot air into the nose – the idea was that you inhaled this at the first sign of a cold and for some people it got rid of the virus. I know some patients can get rid of a virus by giving themselves a temperature – that is, using a hot bath to get themselves as hot as possible and then wrapping up in blankets with a hot water bottle to make themselves 'sweat it out'. I know some athletes deliberately go running in order to induce a temperature and sweat out a virus, but I have to say this is extremely risky and not something I would recommend as it could trigger a flare of CFS.

- The only exception to using paracetamol for fevers is in some children who tend to get fits if their temperature goes up too high. In this event paracetamol and tepid (have you ever had a fever and cold water splashed on you?) sponging should be used to prevent this happening. It is therefore doubly important in these children that micronutrients are used to improve the immune response.

Remember, feeling ill is Nature's way of making you rest. This allows the body to spend energy on immune function. So often CFS/ME sufferers are tipped into their illness by a viral infection plus stress which they then try to address with dwindling energy. Good nursing care is needed – rest, warmth, good food and love. I have seen several athletes who thought they could get rid of their infection through exercise; sometimes that works because the heat generated kills virus, but exercise takes energy away from the immune system and, indeed, intensive exercise is a recognised immunosuppressant.

Prevent infection by making your body inhospitable to microbes

Many CFS/ME sufferers either had their illness triggered by infection or they suffer regular infections that seem to drag them down. Typically they present with symptoms of inflammation such as malaise, sore throat, swollen lymph nodes, catarrh, fever and feeling 'flu like. In order of frequency Table 19.1 lists factors that increase susceptibility to infection.

Table 19.1. Factors that increase susceptibility to infection

Problem	Why	Treatment
High-carbohydrate, high-sugar diets	Carbohydrates nourish microbes and encourage them to flourish.	See my book *Prevent and Cure Diabetes.* Treat with ketogenic diet – see Chapters 6 (page 101) and 17 (page 215).
Allergy	Dairy allergy often presents with recurrent sore throats, tonsillitis, croup and catarrh.	Treat with Paleo-ketogenic diet – see Chapters 6 (page 101) and 17 (page 215).
Hypochlorhydria (low stomach acid)	The overwhelming majority of infections come in through the mouth. Even those microbes that are inhaled get stuck onto sticky mucus from the nose or bronchi, which is coughed up and swallowed. They should find themselves in an acid bath in the stomach which kills them.	The fermenting gut often starts and continues with hypochlorhydria. See Chapter 7 on the fermenting gut (page 107).
Poor immune function	Deficiencies of zinc, vitamin C, vitamin D and selenium. Western diets, micronutrient deficiencies and toxic stress are immunosuppressive.	Take the Basic Package of supplements including at least 5,000 IU of vitamin D daily – see Chapter 18 (page 220).
Hypothyroidism		See Chapter 5 (page 81).
Poor quality gut flora	Allow unfriendly bacteria to flourish.	Probiotics are of proven benefit in protecting against infection. Eat prebiotics such as vegetable fibre to feed friendly bacteria.
Being cold	The lower the temperature, the lower the innate immune response to viruses.	Wrap up and keep warm. Fever kills microbes.
Vitamin D deficiency	We see more infection during the winter months partly because of the cold but largely because vitamin D deficiency is so common.	High dose vitamin D possibly 10,000 IU daily – no toxicity has been seen at this dose.
Chemical poisoning	Chemicals can have immuno-suppressive effects.	For detox see Chapter 20 (page 233).

CHAPTER 19 SUMMARY

Avoiding, treating and preventing infections

- There is a three-pronged approach:
  - Avoid infections as much as possible.
  - Attack microbes aggressively.
  - Make the environment (of your body) as inhospitable as possible for microbes.
- Avoid infections as much as possible:
  - Choose your foreign holidays with care – avoid those which require vaccination and those which require major dietary changes.
  - Be mindful that hospitals, GP surgeries, airports, schools and other such accumulate viruses and antibiotic-resistant bacteria.
  - Choose your sexual partners with care – though this is difficult because sex hormones induce symptoms of recklessness and madness!
- Treat aggressively:
  - Take vitamin C to bowel tolerance.
  - Follow a low-carb, ketogenic diet.
  - Take zinc drops – 10 mg four times daily.
  - Allow inflammation.
  - Grab what sunshine you can.
  - Be nice to yourself – rest, warmth and love!
  - Do not be afraid to use (prescription or herbal) antimicrobials if needed.
  - Keep warm, overwrap, maybe induce a fever.
  - Do not use symptom-suppressing medication.
- Prevent infection by making your body inhospitable to microbes:
  - Paleo-ketogenic diet – this deprives the microbes of food (see Chapters 6, page 101, and 17, page 215)
  - Treat any fermenting gut issues (see Chapter 7, page 107)

- Take the Basic Package of micronutrients (see Chapter 18, page 220).
- Take probiotics (see Chapter 7, page 107, and Appendix 8, page 327).
- Treat hypothyroidism (see Chapter 5, page 81).
- Take vitamin D – 10,000 IU daily.
- Consider detox regimes (see Chapter 20, next).

CHAPTER 20

Detoxing

. . . let us cleanse ourselves from everything that contaminates body and spirit . . .

2, CORINTHIANS 7:1

We live in an increasingly polluted world and whether we like it or not we are all toxic. We should all be doing detox regimes to keep the body burden as low as possible.

There are two major sources of toxin: toxins from within the body (endogenous) and toxins from outside (exogenous). The reason why we have evolved a detox system is to deal with the toxins that normally arise from within the body. However, modern diets have increased this burden from within the body and this burden has been further increased by toxins from outside the body.

Toxins coming from within the body

There are three major sources of endogenous toxins – normal metabolism, plant foods and, in recent times, the fermenting gut:

Free radicals: One cannot burn fuel in the presence of oxygen to produce energy without producing some 'exhaust fumes'. These exhaust fumes are free radicals – for the biochemists they are molecules with an unpaired electron; highly reactive and very damaging. These are mopped up by our antioxidant system, which includes frontline enzymes such as super-oxide dismutase (it needs zinc, copper and manganese), glutathione peroxidase (it needs selenium and glutathione) and coenzyme Q10 (co-Q10). These antioxidants pick up the unpaired electrons and pass them down the line through other antioxidants, such as vitamins A and E, before they are dumped in the ultimate electron acceptor, vitamin C.

Toxic substances from normal metabolism, such as bilirubin, porphyrins, uric acid, neurotransmitters and other such.

Toxins from plants: Plants contain a variety of substances: some good, some bad. Yes, some plants contain an energy source that we can use together with substances good for our health, such as antioxidants, polyphenols, resveratrols, vitamins, fibre and other such. However, they also contain natural toxins which protect them from being eaten by animals – these include lectins, cyanides, glycoalkaloids and so on. This makes perfect biological sense – if you look at life from the point of view of a plant it does not want to be eaten. It makes itself as toxic as possible. By contrast, prey animals do not generally need to make themselves toxic – their defence is to run away. This means that animal foods are intrinsically less toxic than plant foods.

Fermenting gut: Modern, Western human beings power their bodies with sugars and starches. There is potential for those foods to ferment in the upper gut and that produces toxins such as alcohol, D-lactate, hydrogen sulphide and many other such, all of which have to be detoxified in the liver. Thankfully the liver is usually well able to do this. However, if it is overwhelmed by other dietary toxins, such as alcohol, caffeine, chemical additives, pesticide residues and so on, then there is a risk of overwhelming the liver and running into problems of toxicity.

Toxins coming from outside the body

An increasing source of toxic exposure comes from the outside world. These toxins include:

- **Social toxins and food additives:** Many have to be detoxified in the liver and include caffeine, nicotine, alcohol, food additives, flavourings and colourings, and artificial sweeteners. For example, aspartame, a particular hate of mine, is broken down to produce the more toxic metabolite and pesticide formaldehyde.
- **Cosmetics:** These include makeup, perfumes, hair dyes, deodorants, toothpastes, piercings.
- **Prescription drugs:** These greatly increase the burden on the liver.
- **Pollution:** Those we acquire through pollution of food, water and air – pesticides, volatile organic compounds (VOCs), noxious gases and toxic

metals. So, for example, when I do fat biopsies in patients I invariably find toxic chemicals such as organochlorines, polybrominated biphenyls (fire retardants), benzene compounds and other such. When I look for toxic metals in the urine using DMSA (see page 238), again, almost invariably, I find significant levels of lead, mercury, nickel, aluminium, arsenic and other such toxic metals.

Treatment of toxicity

Of course, the treatment of the toxic patient depends very much on the cause of that toxicity and also avoiding the toxin wherever possible. To get rid of endogenous toxins (those originating from within the body) the liver requires the raw materials to do so (micronutrient supplements) together with the energy to detox. An astonishing statistic is that at rest the liver uses 27 per cent of all the energy generated in the body – this is more than the heart and brain combined. It may be that my CFS/ME patients are particularly susceptible to poisonings because they do not have the energy to detox. Much of the energy spent in the liver goes towards the business of detoxing.

The mechanisms for getting rid of endogenous toxins are also effective for getting rid of some (but not all) exogenous toxins (those originating from outside the body) – so for example, there are mechanisms for detoxifying alcohols produced from the fermenting gut, but these can be up-graded to deal with alcohol in beers, wines and spirits. Similar mechanisms detoxify prescription drugs and food additives, such as preservatives, sweeteners, E-numbers, colourings, flavourings and so on. No wonder the liver is overwhelmed and needs help.

1. First steps that we should all take to detox and keep the load as low as possible

We should all put in place as many interventions as we can to reduce our toxic load – the necessity for this is evident from the above lists. The interventions we can put in place both help the liver directly and also provide alternative routes of detoxing, thereby reducing the load that falls to the liver itself:

- The most obvious is a Paleo-ketogenic diet. This partly reduces our burden of many plant toxins (from grains, pulses and root vegetables) and also substantially reduces the burden of fermenting sugars and starches. So, by concentrating on a high-fat, low-carbohydrate and low-sugar diet, we necessarily consume fewer plant toxins and also we deprive the microbes that cause the fermenting gut of their food – namely, sugar. We should also be aware that many toxic metals bio-accumulate where there is upper fermenting gut.

We acquire a toxic load of metals in two steps. First we are exposed to them – the two commonest examples are mercury from dental amalgam and lead from drinking water. Then we absorb them. However, the absorption of both of these common toxic metals, for example, is greatly enhanced by the fermenting gut. One of the products of a fermenting gut is hydrogen sulphide and this sulphide converts poorly absorbed inorganic metals into well-absorbed organic metals with the potential to bio-accumulate. In this way, we can see how the fermenting gut 'helps' the absorption of toxic inorganic metals. These toxins then bio-accumulate in the heart, brain, bone marrow and kidneys – places where the liver cannot get at them.

This bio-accumulation is worse when the body is deficient in friendly trace elements – if it cannot, for example, access zinc for enzyme systems then the body will grab something which 'looks' similar, such as arsenic or nickel. If it cannot access selenium then it will grab something which 'looks' similar, such as lead or mercury. This means that the synthesis of super-oxide dismutase, dependent on zinc, or glutathione peroxidase, dependent on selenium, will both be less efficient. This in turn means that the body will be able to call on fewer of these powerful antioxidants, thereby weakening its own detox systems. This has the potential to develop into a particularly vicious cycle. But this is a cycle that we can break. In fact, this gives us the basis for the next interventions . . .

- Take multivitamins, multiminerals and essential fatty acids – many are used in the liver for detoxing and to improve antioxidant status.
- Eat protein – this is broken down into amino acids (such as methionine) and short-chain polypeptides (such as glutathione) which are important co-factors for excreting toxins.
- Vitamin C increases excretion of toxic metals in urine. I suggest 2–3 grams at night because this is additionally helpful in treating the upper fermenting gut – vitamin C is directly toxic to the harmful microbes.
- Prevent constipation – foods should spend 60–90 minutes in the stomach, 6 hours in the small intestine and 24 hours in the large intestine for efficient digestion and absorption. Longer than this increases any problems of fermentation and absorption of toxins.
- Iodine – deficiency is pandemic! Iodine displaces toxic 'halides', such as fluoride and bromide. It also binds to toxic metals and increases their excretion in urine. I suggest at least 1 mg (1,000 mcg) daily.

- Take additional micronutrients to improve antioxidant status, viz:
  - Superoxide dismutase – copper 1 mg, manganese 3 mg and zinc 30 mg;
  - Glutathione peroxidase – selenium at least 200 mcg and, if deficient, up to 500 mcg at night and glutathione 250 mg – as above, many micronutrients, like glutathione, multitask
  - Coenzyme Q10 as ubiquinol – 100 mg daily
  - Vitamin B12 is an excellent antioxidant and if I have a patient obviously deficient or poisoned, then vitamin B12 by injection provides instant antioxidant cover and protection whilst all else is being corrected. I suggest 1 mg (1,000 mcg) by daily injection. If injections are not possible, then nasal B12 drops do spike blood levels more effectively than oral B12. I suggest 5,000 mcg intra-nasally daily.

- Provide raw materials for the methylation cycle – again, another essential detox tool. This includes vitamin B12 as above, methyltetrahydrofolic acid (the active form of folate/B9) 800 mcg, vitamin B6 as pyridoxal-5-phosphate 50 mg and glutathione 250 mg. (This could be in addition to the glutathione taken to improve antioxidant status as above – a daily dose of 250–500 mg is recommended.)
- Quench thirst with water – The kidneys clearly require water to flush out toxins, but essentially the kidneys are simply a passive filtering system followed by an active scavenging system to recover nutrients such as sodium and glucose. They are passively, not actively, involved in detoxification. The liver is much more important and its size reflects this.

2. Avoid toxins from the outside world and possibly test for them

Test for:

Pesticides and volatile organic compounds: There is no single test which screens for all toxic organic chemicals, but Great Plains Laboratory offers a useful test which can be easily done on a urine sample – namely, Toxic Organic Chemical Profile.

Toxic metals: Measure toxic metals in urine after taking a chelating agent. Measuring toxic metals in urine, blood and hair is unreliable because heavy metals are very poorly excreted. These tests often produce false negative results – that is, the result looks normal when the body's burden is actually high. Toxic metals bio-concentrate in organs such as the heart, brain, bone marrow and kidneys and so are not available to measure. The answer is to use a chelating agents, such as DMSA; this is well absorbed from the gut, grabs toxic and friendly minerals alike, and pulls them out through the urine. It is excellent for diagnosing toxicity of heavy metals such as mercury, lead, arsenic, aluminium, cadmium, nickel and probably others. DMSA can be used to pull these metals out of the body through the urine.

THE 'TOXIC ELEMENTS IN URINE' TEST

This test is available from Biolab (page 384). Biolab cannot supply DMSA but it can be purchased online.

TEST PROCEDURE

Consume no fish or seafood for three days beforehand. On waking, empty the bladder. Take DMSA in one dose at a dosage of 15 mg/kg. (DMSA is remarkably safe stuff and the dose is not critical.) Most people need 750–1,250 mg of DMSA (50 kg to 83 kg body weight). Collect all the urine you pee for the next six hours. Measure the total volume. Then send 20 ml of that sample to Biolab.

INTERPRETATION OF THE TEST

- If the toxic elements are high then you are partly poisoned by such. Remember the 'normal' range for mercury, lead, nickel and arsenic should be zero.
- Expect to see high levels of copper as DMSA is a good chelator of copper – this does not mean copper toxicity.
- Expect to see high-normal or high levels of manganese, zinc, chromium and selenium. If these are within reference ranges then you may be deficient.

How to get rid of toxic metals

1. Try to identify and get rid of the source of contamination

Sometimes the source remains a mystery. The fermenting gut enhances the absorption of toxic minerals and so deal with any fermenting gut issues first (see below.) As previously mentioned, a possible mechanism for this relates to hydrogen sulphide, which is produced with fermentation. If present it will stick to metals in the gut and convert them from poorly absorbed inorganic metals to well-absorbed organic metals.

2. *Interventions to increase the excretion of toxic metals from the body*

- Take high-dose trace minerals, such as zinc 30 mg or selenium 500 mcg to displace minerals from binding sites within the body, then combine this with glutathione 250–500 mg or methionine 250–500 mg which grab the toxic mineral and allow it to be excreted. The toxicity of paracetamol can be largely mitigated by methionine – indeed, there was once a move to combine all paracetamol tablets with methionine; this would hugely reduce the death rates from over-dosing, but since this would increase the cost of paracetamol by several pence the initiative was abandoned. In the battle between pennies and dead patients, the pennies always win. For all patients with Gilbert's syndrome (where the liver cannot detox via glucuronidation [see page 357]), providing extra glutathione is very helpful.
- Clays in the gut. Many toxins are excreted in bile, which is a fatty liquid. However, these are reabsorbed in the gut in the so-called entero-hepatic circulation. To counter this, clays help to grab these toxic metals and hold them in faeces so preventing their reabsorption. This is a benign way to enhance faecal excretion. However, clays should not be used continuously since they also chelate the friendly minerals. I recommend using them once a week; good examples are zeolite, bentonite or kaolin (say 10 grams as a single oral dose).
- High-dose fats and oils. Dr Patricia Kane (patriciakane.net) has shown that intravenous phospholipids are effective in mobilising chemicals from the body. Oral lipids probably work as well but take longer. I suggest high-fat diets using the cleanest organic oils you can get hold of. Organic hemp oil is ideal since it has the perfect proportion of omega-6:3 oils – namely, 4:1.[57]
- Use a chelating agent such as DMSA, as already mentioned. The word 'chelation' comes from the Greek χηλή, 'chela', or a 'crab's claw'. DMSA literally grabs toxic metals so that they can be excreted in urine. Indeed, this is the basis of the test for toxic minerals described in the 'The "Toxic Elements in Urine" Test' sidebar. The DMSA will have 'grabbed' the toxic minerals and these can then be measured. If there is a toxic load then DMSA can also be used to detoxify these toxins because of its ability to grab and dispose of them. Because DMSA also chelates friendly minerals, it (the DMSA) should be taken only once a week. One should take no

supplements of friendly minerals on one's 'DMSA day', but then take good doses of minerals to rescue the situation for the other six days of the week. My experience is that most poisoned patients need at least two to four months of weekly DMSA after which the test can be repeated. This gives us two points on the graph and an idea of how much more, if any, chelation is required to reduce the body load to an acceptable level. Note, one can never get the body load to zero – all one can do is establish a reasonable equilibrium with the external environment.

- High-dose vitamin C. If tolerated, take 4 grams at night (too much may cause diarrhoea).
- High-dose iodine, such as Lugols iodine 12 per cent solution – one drop contains about 5 mg of elemental iodine; take one to two drops daily. Iodine is also well absorbed through the skin.

How to get rid of toxic organic compounds (pesticides and VOCs)

We then come to the problem of VOCs and pesticides which have been dumped in fat and fatty organs (brain and immune system, viz bone marrow and lymph nodes).

Test for toxic organic chemical exposure

As I mentioned before, the Great Plains Laboratory has recently launched a new test – namely, Toxic Organic Chemical Exposure. This is a urine test, available from Biolab. I do not have enough experience of this test to know how reliable it is, but watch this space. A normal result should be zero because the chemicals looked for are man-made. The trouble is we live in such a toxic world that we all carry a chemical burden. The best we can do is keep that burden as low as possible through a combination of avoidance and improved excretion.

How to get rid of toxic organic compounds

As with toxic metals, the liver cannot get at these chemicals because they are stuck elsewhere in the body's tissues. This is where heating regimes are so helpful because they mobilise chemicals from these tissues.

Many of the pesticides and VOCs are in adipose tissue, which is just under the skin. The idea of heating regimes is to heat up this subcutaneous fat and literally boil off these toxins. They migrate through the skin onto the surface where they dissolve in the fatty lipid layer that covers the skin. Once there they can then be washed off with soap and water in a shower.

In the early days I used far-infrared (FIR) sauna-ing exclusively, simply because my severely ill CFS/ME patients do not tolerate heat at all well. Five to 10 minutes of FIR sauna-ing would warm up the skin and subcutaneous layer without making the patient intolerably hot. However, it is my view that all the heating regimes should work just as well as FIR sauna-ing because the principles of detoxing – that is, mobilising chemicals on to the surface of the skin and washing them off – are the same.

I have now collected figures from over 30 patients who have undergone heating regimes to get rid of toxic compounds. These have been assessed by specialised Acumen tests before and after. The tests have been chosen for particular situations but include fat biopsies, translocator protein studies and DNA adducts. The tests prove to my satisfaction that heating regimes are effective. These heating regimes include sauna: traditional and FIR; and Epsom salt hot baths. I would expect sun-bathing and exercise to be just as effective but my CFS/ME patients do not tolerate or have access to either. For CFS/ME sufferers, the best tolerated remains FIR sauna because they are so heat intolerant – one can get FIR sleeping bags so the patient does not even need to sit up. As I have said, just five to 10 minutes at a time can be effective.

It is not essential to sweat for these regimes to be effective – the idea is to 'boil off' toxins in the subcutaneous layer onto the lipid layer on the surface of the skin from where they can be washed off. The washing off is as important as the heat, or toxins will simply be reabsorbed.

My experience, roughly speaking, is that 50 episodes will halve the body load. One would expect chemicals to come out exponentially, so one never gets to zero but ends up in some sort of equilibrium with the environment which is as low as reasonably possible. Indeed, because we live in such a toxic world I think we should all be doing some sort of heating regime at least once a week. I am lucky enough to be able to exercise – I deliberately overdress to make sure I get hot and sweaty, then shower off subsequently – what a treat that is!

The results that I have collected are currently being analysed by Dr Norman Booth, a doctor of physics at Mansfield College, Oxford, with a view to their being published. However, simply looking at the raw data tells me that these regimes are effective.

Indeed, it is my view that because we live in such a toxic world we should not wait until we become ill with some nasty illness, such as CFS or cancer; we should be using detox regimes on a regular basis and those regimes, in my opinion, should include heating regimes.

Conclusion – the benefits of regular detox

Take advantage of what is available locally to detox your system on a weekly basis. For those people lucky enough to live in a hot climate, an hour of sunbathing followed by a dip in the sea is ideal. We English seem to relish hot baths and the effect of detoxification is further enhanced by adding Epsom salts into the bath. The idea here is that not only are the toxins pulled out by the heat but magnesium and sulphate pass through the skin into the body – both magnesium and sulphate are essential co-factors to allow detoxification. This was established in a lovely study by Dr Rosemary Waring at Birmingham who showed that both magnesium and sulphate levels in the blood increased markedly following such hot baths, as did the excretion of magnesium sulphate in the urine.[58] Her formula was for 500 grams of Epsom salts in 15 gallons of water. We English also love to mix our metric and imperial measurements! (OK, OK . . . 15 gallons is 68 litres.)

For countries with a tradition of such, sauna-ing is an excellent method of detoxifying through the skin. Indeed, I recall a case of one family who were all poisoned by organophosphate and had high levels in their fat biopsies. They decided to take themselves off for a three-week holiday in Eastern Europe at a lovely hotel which offered regular massage, sauna-ing, hot springs and mineral bath treatments. They all cycled from one treatment to the next. The results were little short of astonishing – after three weeks of treatment their toxic load of organophosphates had reduced substantially, almost to background levels.

Indeed, similar research was conducted by Dr William Rea in the United States and he used similar regimes of massage, gentle exercise, sauna-ing and showering to achieve very similar biochemical results.

It is also my clinical experience, and I know that is a very subjective measure, that the reduction of toxic load is also paralleled by clinical improvement and wellbeing. It may well be that part of the reason we feel so well after the traditional sun, sand and sea holiday is because we substantially reduce our toxic load.

So, in conclusion, we have a system of detoxification that is biologically plausible, within the scope of the vast majority of people, and of proven effectiveness. I recommend sauna-ing to you all!

CHAPTER 20 SUMMARY

Detoxing

- We live in an increasingly toxic world and we are all toxic.
- Being toxic puts a strain on our body's systems and can also cause illness in its own right.
- There are two categories of toxin:
    - Toxins from within the body
    - Toxins from the outside world
- Sources of toxins from within the body include:
    - The natural production of free radicals as a result of how our metabolism works
    - Toxic substances from normal metabolism, such as bilirubin, porphyrins, uric acid
    - Toxins from the plants that we eat
    - Toxins such as alcohol, D-lactate and hydrogen sulphide that result from a fermenting gut, which is as a result of modern carbohydrate diets
- Sources of toxins from the outside world include:
    - Food additives
    - Cosmetics, perfumes, hair dyes, deodorants, toothpastes, piercings
    - Prescription drugs
    - Those we acquire through pollution of food, water and air – pesticides, volatile organic compounds, noxious gases and toxic metals
- Detox treatments (page 235) include:
    - Paleo-ketogenic diet
    - Multivitamins, multiminerals and essential fatty acids
    - Eating protein
    - Vitamin C which increases excretion of toxic metals in urine – take 2–3 grams at night
    - Iodine – 1 mg (1,000 mcg) daily

    - Quench thirst with water

- Additional micronutrients to improve antioxidant and methylation status (page 237) include:

    - Superoxide dismutase – copper 1 mg, manganese 3 mg and zinc 30 mg
    - Glutathione peroxidase – selenium (at least 200 mcg and, if deficient, up to 500 mcg at night) and glutathione (250 mg)
    - Coenzyme Q10 as ubiquinol – 100 mg daily
    - Vitamin B12 is an excellent antioxidant. I suggest 0.5 mg (500 mcg) daily by injection. If injections are not possible, then 5 mg (5,000 mcg) sublingually daily.
    - Provide raw materials for the methylation cycle. This includes vitamin B12 as above, methyltetrahydrofolic acid 800 mcg, vitamin B6 as pyridoxal-5-phosphate 50 mg and glutathione 250 mg.

- Also, identify which external toxins you have and then directly get rid of them.
- Test for these external toxins with Toxic Organic Chemical Profile from Great Plains Laboratories or other tests for toxic metals.
- Get rid of these external toxins by:

    - High-dose trace minerals such as zinc 30 mg or selenium 500 mcg
    - Clays such as zeolite 10 g weekly, bentonite or kaolin.
    - High-dose fats and oils – organic hemp oil is ideal since it has the perfect proportion of omega-6 to omega-3 oils – namely, 4:1.
    - Use a chelating agent such as DMSA.
    - Heating regimes, especially sauna-ing (see page 240).

CHAPTER 21

The emotional hole in the energy bucket

Human behaviour flows from three main sources: desire, emotion, and knowledge.

PLATO (428/427 or 424/423 BC – 348/347 BC [age c. 80])

You should have the knowledge by now, and I know you will have the desire to get better. So, what about the emotions?

Background

The brain is hugely demanding of energy. At rest it consumes 20 per cent of the total energy production of the body. This is because the business of generating electrical impulses and neurotransmitters requires large amounts of energy. Optimising expenditure of brain energy is a vital part of recovery. All CFS/ME sufferers have an emotional hole in the energy bucket because the brain is understandably overactive with stress, worry and anxiety, all caused by the situation that their CFS/ME has put them in.

We have a major problem here with respect to the medical profession because this is the only 'cause' of CFS/ME which they consider. We know this because it is reflected by the standard treatments – antidepressants, cognitive behaviour therapy and graded exercise. The latter treatment is guaranteed to make CFS worse – if it does not then the patient does not have CFS! By definition, exercise worsens CFS. (In fact, this emotional hole is often a *consequence* of CFS, and only rarely the single *cause*. But we still have to plug it if we want to get better as quickly as possible.)

Worse, if a patient refuses to comply with psychiatric treatments, then either they are ignored and denied state or other benefits, or they risk a more serious psychiatric diagnosis which may give the psychiatrist powers to take them into a psychiatric unit, against their wishes, under psychiatric section. This seems to be a very particular problem with children and there are many horror stories involving them. I recommend the document written by Jane Colby FRSA, Executive Director of The Tymes Trust, *False Allegations of Child Abuse in Childhood Cases of Myalgic Encephalitis (ME)*,[59] dated July 2014 that can be found via my website. Jane Colby states that:

> *There is no cure for ME (Myalgic Encephalitis). In its absence, management regimes are prescribed, typically based on cognitive behavioural therapy (CBT) and graded exercise therapy (GET). In the case of children, this may involve the application of Child Protection powers to enforce treatment. NICE [National Institute for Health and Care Excellence] confirms that patients may withdraw from treatment without effects on future care, but parents who decline, or withdraw children from, management regimes, which may have worsened their illness, can find themselves facing investigation for child abuse or neglect, or have their child forcibly confined to a psychiatric unit. Tymes Trust has advised 121 families facing suspicion/investigation. To date, none of these families has been found to be at fault.*

These cases are very delicate and I am therefore wary of making things worse for the parents and children by disclosing details in this book but one case has garnered so much publicity that I really cannot make things worse by repeating the facts here.

Karina Hansen – Denmark

Karina had been struggling with ME since the age of 16. In Denmark, CFS/ME sufferers are deemed to be suffering from a 'functional disorder' and the recommended treatments are GET, CBT and antidepressants. A Danish psychiatrist, Per Fink, considered it to be in Karina's best interests to be taken into his Hammel Neurocenter psychiatric clinic. Karina and her parents hired a lawyer to fight this and were granted a power of attorney over Karina and managed to win a reprieve against Per Fink. However, Fink then wrote to the Danish Ministry of Health asking for the power to remove Karina's parents' legal rights over her. On 12 February 2013, five policemen, two doctors, two social workers and a locksmith forcibly removed the bedbound Karina, whilst she pleaded with them to allow her to remain at home with her family. Karina's mother was physically restrained. Since that time, Karina's parents' rights of power of attorney have been disregarded and Fink has installed, as legal guardian, a retired policeman named Kaj Stendorf. Fink has refused all requests from Karina's family to visit her, including birthdays and Christmas.[60] (Update: On 17 October 2016, after three and a half years of incarceration, Karina finally returned home. The arrangement was on a trial basis but it is hoped will become permanent.)

Not only do the powers-that-be within the psychiatric lobby line up against parents and their children with CFS/ME but also other areas of speciality too. Again, the following case has been widely publicised.

Mary Kidson's daughter – UK

Mary Kidson's 16-year-old daughter, who suffers with CFS, was forcibly removed from her mother by Herefordshire Social Services on 5 March 2013. This poor girl was not permitted to see, speak to or take part in social events and activities with close maternal family members or her own friends, or even do simple things like see and cuddle her much-loved dog. Her education was completely disrupted. Mary Kidson was taken to court for 'attempting to poison' her daughter with thyroid extract and oestrogen tablets. Fortunately, she was cleared by a jury after a three-week trial at Worcester Crown Court.[61] The 55-year-old was accused of three counts of unlawfully and maliciously administering drugs, endangering life or inflicting grievous bodily harm, with all the offences alleged to have happened between 2010 and March 2013. Dr Neil Fraser, a specialist in hormonal medicine in children, and Dr Sally Stucke, a consultant paediatrician, both gave evidence against Mary Kidson. It has been difficult to obtain up-to-date information on this case, as is usual in these matters, but about a year ago, this was posted on a petition website, signed by in excess of 39,000 people:

> *We have some wonderful news to share with you. Mary now has unsupervised contact with her daughter and Herefordshire Social Services have produced an exit plan which has been formally agreed. An education plan is in place and plans for her daughter to be in touch with her friends soon are also agreed.*

Psychiatrists come up with diagnoses which are not diagnoses at all but simply clinical pictures. These include 'somatisation', 'chronic pain syndrome', 'conversion disorder' (hysteria), 'Munchausen's syndrome' or, in the case of children, 'Munchausen's syndrome by proxy'. I do recommend reading Dr James Davies's book *Cracked*. This is a marvellous critique of Western psychiatric practice, which simply funnels patients into drug treatment categories.[62] These categories are laid down by *The Diagnostic and Statistical Manual of Mental Disorders* (DSM-5), compiled and published by the American Psychiatric Association.[63] A lovely analogy Davies draws is with the night sky – psychiatrists are still drawing lines between stars and diagnosing 'Gemini', 'Taurus' and 'Aries'. They are diagnostic flat-Earthers who ignore modern science. We need astronomers, not astrologists, to diagnose and treat CFS/ME.

We have not moved far since Nicholas Culpepper, a medical herbalist (1616–1654), stated:

> *Three kinds of people mainly disease the people – priests, physicians and lawyers – priests disease matters belonging to their souls, physicians disease matters belonging to their bodies, and lawyers disease matters belonging to their estate.*

Indeed, much of my job I see as protecting CFS/ME patients from the psychiatric profession by establishing the underlying physical and pathological causal mechanisms which manifest clinically with CFS/ME.

By relying on symptom-supressing drugs to treat CFS/ME, care and compassion have gone out of the window. Psychiatrists are dangerous, as evidenced by the recent Mazars report into deaths at Southern Health NHS Foundation Trust. In the Mental Health section during a four year period between 2011 and 2015 there were 1,454 unexpected deaths of which 857 underwent no investigation to determine why.[64] Just imagine this happening in any other walk of life?

How does one know there is an emotional hole in the energy bucket?

We know because we have symptoms of such:

Feeling stressed. Stress is the symptom we experience when we have to gear up energy delivery to cope with demands. That stress may be good for us, or bad for us, depending on the energy equation. So, for example, if we have plenty of energy then we can enjoy the normal stressful challenges of life. If we do not have the energy to deal with such challenges we suffer the deeply unpleasant mental and physical symptoms of stress – for example, we may experience the consequences of constant demands being made on the adrenal glands. Problems arise when the stress is unremitting because eventually the output of the adrenal gland will fall so we cannot 'gear up' energy delivery mechanisms to allow us to deal with stress (see Chapter 5, page 81).

Worrying. Worry is additionally exhausting and wasteful of energy. This is not only a risk factor for CFS/ME but makes symptoms worse because of the massive energy drain that it can cause. I believe the symptom of worry is caused when we think (know) that we do not have the necessary energy delivery to cope with the upcoming energy demands. CFS/ME sufferers face situations like this many times a day.

Anxiety or obsessional thinking. This includes such things as: the brain being wired; being unable to let go of worries; having the same thoughts going round and round in the brain; feeling disempowered. All of these activities spend emotional energy. Anxiety may be entirely appropriate to the situation faced. However, some people are constitutionally hard-wired for anxiety – it runs in some families. Others acquire an anxious tendency because of life's experience. One such example would be an unhappy, insecure childhood with bullying and physical, psychological or sexual abuse – indeed, we know this is a risk factor for some cases of CFS/ME. All mothers are evolutionarily programmed for worry – this improves the chances of their children surviving. I suspect it partly explains why we see much more CFS/ME in women than men, along with the hormonal factors previously discussed (see page 41).

Weepiness or extremes of emotion. This is often accompanied by feelings of an inability to 'cope' with minor irritations. These feelings also sometimes 'annoy' CFS/ME sufferers who know that they would otherwise be able to cope very well – this annoyance can set up an emotional vicious cycle.

The emotional vicious cycle can be very destructive. It can go something like this:

A. Inability to cope with situations that previously the CFS/ME sufferer would have sailed through
B. Loss of self-esteem and self-worth, accompanied by feelings of inadequacy

C. Further inability to cope with situations because of reduced emotional resilience as a consequence of reduced self-esteem and self-worth
D. Further loss of self-esteem and self-worth, accompanied by feelings of inadequacy . . . etc . . .

Sometimes CFS/ME sufferers attempt to break out of this vicious cycle by trying to 'do things' to 'prove' to themselves that they are still capable. So, they try to return to work, or go on a bike ride, or whatever, if they are able. This may give a (very) temporary boost to self-esteem but will be followed by a 'crash' if they are not physically ready for this type of activity.

The key is to treat the emotional hole, alongside all the other physiological problems, and move forward like this 'in tandem'. It is a very fine balancing act of keeping the spirits up whilst not using too much precious energy in so doing. It is about forgoing a little of 'today' for much more of 'tomorrow'. However, CFS/ME sufferers must 'allow' themselves to spend some energy on things that they enjoy. This is one way of plugging the emotional hole; others are discussed below. Additionally, please see Appendix 3 (page 308), where methods of dealing with these emotions are discussed with respect to record keeping.

The treatment of stress, anxiety and worry – plugging the emotional hole in the energy bucket

The principles of treatment are always to identify and address the underlying causes.

1. Reduce demands on the system

- Reread Chapter 15 on pacing (see page 183). Energy borrowed has to be paid back at 300 per cent interest – avoid the loan shark.
- Lifestyle interventions – reduce the load. List 10 ways in which you spend energy. Put them in order of importance. Stop doing the bottom 50 per cent.
- Be ruthless about getting rid of emotional baggage. That may include ignoring unsupportive or draining family members. Indeed, to recover, you must be emotionally ruthless and selfish – often this is the very opposite of the personality which gets people into CFS/ME in the first place.
- Surround yourself with 'energy-givers' rather than 'energy-vampires'.

- Do not be too proud to ask for help. Money is very helpful in reducing stress. Getting the financial benefits that you may be entitled to is an essential part of recovery.

2. Improve energy delivery mechanisms

- Read the rest of this book. We need energy to deal with stress.
- Recognise when you are using addictions to cope with stress – they may bring short-term gain but there will be long-term pain because addictions mask the symptoms and allow CFS/ME sufferers to slip into energy deficit.
- Reread Chapter 16 on sleep (see page 196) – I can cope with anything in the day, given a good night's sleep, but not otherwise. I suspect the benefit of many psychiatric prescriptions derives from better quality sleep.

There is a time for many words, and there is also a time for sleep.

HOMER, *The Odyssey*

3. Psychological techniques

There are many psychological techniques, such as meditation, relaxation techniques, mindfulness and counselling, for helping people to cope with worries. It is beyond the scope of this book to detail these. However, improving energy delivery mechanisms gives one the energy to adopt and put in place these interventions. The starting point is to recognise you have a problem, swallow your 'pride' and ask for help.

4. Medication to reduce anxiety

There is an obvious vicious cycle detailed above since we need energy to cope with the stress and stress wastes energy. What may be helpful to break this cycle is prescription medication. We have to be careful with this because many prescription medications inhibit mitochondria directly – that may be part of the process by which many CFS/ME sufferers become intolerant of drugs. Those drugs which I find most helpful clinically are as follows:

- Medications to improve sleep – see page 210
- Herbal teas, rescue remedy, valerian

- Diazepam 2 to 5 mg for occasional use in stressful situations. Often just the knowledge that the drug is available is all that is needed – this is a useful 'get out of jail free' card.

People naturally have concerns about using drugs to treat anxiety because of the potential for addiction. However, in the absence of prescription medication, people turn to other addictions. Benzodiazepines, correctly used are, in my view, safer than sugar, alcohol, cigarette smoking and cannabis. It may be that nicotine is less dangerous – vaping is preferable to cigarette smoking. The key to using these drugs is to 'buy' a window of time to give one the energy to put in place the necessary physical interventions to improve energy delivery mechanisms so that in the long term these drugs are not required.

I never initiate the prescribing of SSRIs such as Prozac – there is a risk of suicidal ideation. Suicide is common in CFS/ME. SSRIs are addictive drugs and many struggle to stop them. Similarly, I try to avoid beta blockers in CFS/ME because they are good inhibitors of mitochondria.

Addiction and dependency

The key to avoiding addiction and dependency is to have windows of time drug-free. It is diazepam taken on a regular basis – that is, before the effects of the previous dose have worn off – which results in dependency.

With respect to sleep, we must clarify terms. I am dependent on a good night's sleep to be well – without that I develop unpleasant symptoms very quickly. Prescription drugs to help sleep may make one dependent on them but this is not addiction. Addiction is a condition of taking a drug excessively and being unable to cease doing so without other adverse effects. Stopping your hypnotic may result in a poor night's sleep but no more than that. This is not addiction but dependence. The key is to use drugs to help sleep in conjunction with psychological techniques to avoid dependency (see page 210). Once good sleep is established, then the drug can be slowly withdrawn.

The same principles apply to anxiety-blocking drugs – they must be used in parallel with interventions to reduce and deal with stress.

5. Obtain the state and other benefits to which you are entitled

Much of my time is spent in helping CFS/ME patients gain appropriate state and other benefits. This is also an essential part of managing their medical condition since financial security is essential for good emotional health.

6. Connect with others

CFS/ME can be very isolating and these feelings of isolation can set up more vicious cycles that only worsen the situation. Connecting with others for housebound or bedridden CFS/ME sufferers used to be well nigh impossible before the advent of the internet and social media. There has been a lot of misinformation written about the negative impact of support groups upon illness outcomes, with some psychiatrists stating that such support groups reinforce 'illness beliefs' and prolong disability. This is not so. Linking with other sufferers can provide a life-line to many people, where not only support and understanding can be found, but sometimes deep friendships develop. One caveat is that time spent on social media can 'fly by' and one can end up using energy that one does not really have. So, as with all things, be careful to pace your time on social media and do factor it into your energy equation. Appendix 9 (page 329) lists many support groups, both online and also 'physical'.

Love, caring and carers

This is not meant to be a cheesy homily on care and love – others are much better at that than me.*

However, I must include a few home truths . . .

It is essential and fundamental to a happy life that we all care for and are cared for by someone. Now my daughters have left home I am lucky to have my Patterdale terrier Nancy – my fun is watching her enjoy herself chasing rats and rabbits. After dark we go out round the barns ratting. Wednesday afternoons is Terrierorist Club – out on rabbiting walkies. Our pets are more emotionally intelligent than humans and Nancy picks up on my every mood. Many a cat or dog has transformed the life of a CFS/ME sufferer.

She clawed her way into my heart and wouldn't let go.

MISSY ALTIJD

It is important to recognise that the business of caring requires huge amounts of energy – physical, mental and emotional. The carers need care

---

* **Editor's note:** Sarah is better at this than she thinks – actions speak louder than words.

too. Indeed, caring for someone with CFS/ME is so damaging to relationships because energy has to be a two-way thing, and the CFS/ME sufferer cannot reciprocate in full. This must be recognised and acknowledged with politeness which, at least, is not energy sapping. A 'please' and 'thank you' go a long way. A caring soulmate is an essential part of recovery.

If you live to be a hundred, I want to live to be a hundred minus one day, so I would never have to live without you.

AA MILNE in *Winnie-the-Pooh*

Personal Comment by Craig

I have read *The Great Gatsby* more times than is good for one's health. I am often heard quoting from it:

I wish I had done everything on Earth with you.

(from the screenplay, not the book!)

Do not be like this!
Do not try to 'catch up' for 'lost years'.
Do not mourn the loss of things not done.
Do not try to do everything with anyone!

Instead, celebrate each milestone, and like Gatsby 'believe in the green light', but believe in it not as some unobtainable, unrequited lost love or experience but rather as an horizon, something always to aim for and always to look forward to. Be resolute in all the physiological interventions. Keep going and never ever give up!

Never give in – never, never, never, never, in nothing great or small, large or petty, never give in except to convictions of honour and good sense. Never yield to force; never yield to the apparently overwhelming might of the enemy.

WINSTON CHURCHILL
(10 November 1871 – 12 March 1947)
in a speech given to Harrow School, 29 October 1941

CHAPTER 21 SUMMARY

The emotional hole in the energy bucket

- The brain is hugely demanding of energy. At rest it consumes 20 per cent of the total energy production of the body and so this is an area of energy expenditure which must be fully addressed.
- Emotional holes do exist in CFS/ME but there is a major problem here with respect to the medical profession because this is the only 'cause' of CFS/ME which they consider.
- This means that treatments such as antidepressants, cognitive behaviour therapy and graded exercise are often prescribed. This is not helpful, with the latter guaranteed to make CFS/ME worse.
- This leads to serious mistreatment of some CFS/ME patients.
- Symptoms of a significant emotional hole include:
  - Feeling stressed
  - Worrying
  - Anxiety or obsessional thinking
  - Weepiness or extremes of emotion
- This can lead to an 'emotional hole vicious cycle' whereby CFS/ME patients lose self-esteem as a result of an inability to 'cope' with things that would have been 'child's play' beforehand, and this loss of self-esteem leads to a further widening of the emotional hole, resulting in a lessening of the ability to 'cope' and so on . . .
- Treatments for the emotional hole include:
  - Reduce demands on the system – pacing, reduce the load, get rid of emotional baggage, surround yourself with energy givers not energy vampires – ask for help
  - Improve energy delivery systems – see the rest of this book
  - Try psychological interventions – meditation, mindfulness, counselling, relaxation techniques
  - Try medication to break the cycle of worry – herbal teas, rescue remedy, valerian, diazepam
  - Try medications to improve sleep – see page 210
  - Obtain all state and other benefits to which you are entitled
  - Connect with others
- Understand the need to care and be cared for.

CHAPTER 22

Reprogramming the brain: brain perception of imbalances in the energy equation

Brain perception of energy

What goes on in the body is monitored and perceived by the brain. This includes fatigue. So how does the brain know when there is an imbalance? More importantly, in terms of illness management, what if its perception of such an imbalance is wrong? Such a misperception by the brain could help to explain why some CFS/ME sufferers do not improve despite having worked hard and corrected all those elements of energy delivery and energy demand that have been highlighted so far as needing to be corrected. The brain may not realise that, with all these interventions in place, it is now 'safe' to spend energy. It is stuck in 'energy conservation/survival mode', or 'safe mode'. As detailed in Craig's chapter on Catastrophe Theory (Chapter 24, page 271) this is a little like the phenomenon of having a phantom limb:

> *. . . we should first consider a different example, that of the 'phantom limb'. The brain has an internal map of the body and also of what is going on in the body, and this internal map may not always reflect reality. So, a limbless person may still feel as though he has a (painful) limb because of this 'incorrect' internal body map that his brain is still relying on. In effect, the brain has not 'updated' its internal map of the body in the light of new information. In a similar way, it is possible that the immune system has*

> *such an internal map of what is going on within itself and this map will reflect the situation as it has subsisted for some time, rather than the situation as it actually is now. So, just as the brain 'registers' a limb, or limb pain, because that is the situation which has subsisted for some time, even though this is no longer the reality, so does the immune system 'register' CFS because that is the situation that has subsisted for some time, even though the reality is now that the patient is in a non-CFS state.*

Kick-starting the brain

So, how can we kick-start the brain out of 'safe mode' into 'normal functioning mode'?

Let's look at addiction. We use addictions to cope with the uncomfortable feelings of stress which arise, I believe, when the energy equation is compromised, by which I mean when energy demand exceeds available energy delivery. We use some addictions to 'plug' the emotional hole, or other holes, in our energy buckets – the common ones are sugar and carbohydrates, nicotine, alcohol and cannabis.

Prescription drugs that are used to plug emotional holes include benzodiazepines, SSRIs (yes – they are addictive), antidepressants and antipsychotics. We use these addictions when, through force of circumstance, we do not have enough love, laughter, sunshine, exercise, sleep, games, music and security (of relationships, finance, future, etc).

We use other addictions to kick our mitochondria into life. Caffeine is an adrenaline-like drug which stimulates mitochondria to increase output. However, this is not sustainable in the long term – you can't have an upper without a downer. I suspect addictions to substances like amphetamine, cocaine and ecstasy work by fooling the brain into thinking that it has a bottomless supply of energy.

> *If your day is gone, and you want to ride on, cocaine.*
>
> ERIC CLAPTON (30 March 1945 – lyrics to "Cocaine")

These drugs allow addicts to dance all night and be mentally sharp and outrageously funny. However, it's a dangerous ploy – if energy demand exceeds energy delivery, dramatically and suddenly, then we risk death, and of course we all know that this is possible with these drugs.

However, it may be possible to use stimulant drugs judiciously, in combination with all the other treatments in this book for CFS/ME, to facilitate an otherwise delayed or 'not happening' recovery. This is not to say that there is a psychological block to 'recovery' at all. Rather it is the case that there is an 'unconscious unwillingness' of the brain to move out of 'safe mode'. This is not 'psychological sickness behaviour' but rather a physiological response which requires a physiological 'kick'.

Dr Jon Kaiser (see next section) puts it this way:

> *I believe it is reasonable to imagine very sick mitochondria as being stuck in a dysfunctional mode similar to a heart muscle that is 'fibrillating'. In ventricular fibrillation, if all you do is inject supportive drugs (i.e. lidocaine), nothing happens. It is only upon 'kick starting' the heart with a jolt of energy that a normal heart rhythm once again occurs.*

In this sense, also, I can't emphasise enough the importance of doing 'all the other treatments'. If the underlying physical problems have not been fully addressed, then it is dangerous medicine to use stimulants to kick the brain into ignoring the energy equation. To emphasise this point – one should only consider this use of stimulants if one is sure that all that can be done to address the various components of energy delivery and energy demand has, in fact, been done. One does not want the brain ignoring a 'valid energy equation' but rather one wants to 'kick-start' the brain out of a 'safe mode' of operating that is no longer relevant to the individual's current, and improved, circumstances. It is a fine line, both to identify and to walk, and needs professional oversight and monitoring by an experienced CFS/ME specialist.

The Synergy Trial

For some time I have been following the work of Dr Jon Kaiser who has been treating CFS/ME with a combination of supplements to support mitochondria, together with low doses of methylphenidate (Ritalin) – he calls this combination KPAX 002 ('KPAX').[65]

Dr Kaiser set up the Synergy Trial where he looked at reduction of symptoms in patients taking KPAX versus placebo. Altogether 36 per cent of KPAX patients improved by more than 20 per cent over four weeks (fatigue, motivation, concentration and activity) – interestingly the sickest patients improved most. Please see this ClinicalTrials.gov webpage for full details of this study – clinicaltrials.gov/ct2/show/study/NCT01966276.

This trial does not separate out the effects of mitochondrial support and methylphenidate. It would make more sense to me to compare patients taking mitochondrial support with patients taking mitochondrial support *and* methylphenidate. However, this trial does raise the possibility that some patients could be kick-started into recovery by using methylphenidate. It may be that we are already doing this with the active thyroid hormone T3 – that too is a neurotransmitter and I already have many patients whose recovery has been kick-started by this drug. Many of them, once they have achieved functioning at a high level, have found that they can reduce T3 to physiological doses without a worsening of their symptoms.

Implications for management

I think it is reasonable to trial these interventions when all other treatments are in place – there is a checklist of such other treatments in Appendix 7 (page 325). The drug options would be:

- Methylphenidate (Ritalin 10–20 mg daily – in regular use to treat narcolepsy and ADHD in children)
- Modafinil (Provigil 100–200 mg daily – in regular use for narcolepsy, sleep apnoea, appetite suppression)
- Tertroxin (pure T3, 20–60 mcg, possibly more) or Armour thyroid (T4 + T3, 1–3 grains, possibly more – needs regular monitoring with thyroid function tests).

All the above also require:

- Regular home checks of pulse and blood pressure
- GP to be informed and ideally oversee the regime

My guess is that it would take 6 to 12 months for the brain to 'relearn' the new energy equation. I do not foresee dependence on these drugs for life (but I may be wrong).

CHAPTER 22 SUMMARY

Reprogramming the brain: brain perception of imbalances in the energy equation

- Some CFS/ME sufferers do not improve despite having worked hard and corrected all those elements of energy delivery and energy demand that have been highlighted as needing to be corrected.
- It may be that the brain is stuck in 'energy conservation/survival mode', or 'safe mode'.
- This is most definitely not 'psychological sickness behaviour' but rather a physiological response which may be helped by a physiological 'kick'.
- It may be possible to use stimulant drugs judiciously, in combination with all the other treatments in this book for CFS/ME, to facilitate an otherwise delayed or 'not happening' recovery.
- It is essential that *all* other treatment possibilities are in place before this is attempted (see Appendix 7, page 325)
- There is evidence for this possible treatment option – Dr Kaiser set up the Synergy Trial where he looked at reduction of symptoms in patients taking KPAX (a combination of mitochondrial supplements and Ritalin) versus placebo. Altogether 36 per cent of KPAX patients improved by more than 20 per cent over four weeks.
- The implications for management are that, as long as *all* other treatments options are in place, there is room for a trial of one of these drugs:
    - Methylphenidate (Ritalin 10–20 mg daily – in regular use to treat narcolepsy and ADHD in children)
    - Modafinil (Provigil 100–200 mg daily – in regular use for narcolepsy, sleep apnoea and appetite suppression)
    - Tertroxin (pure T3, 20–60 mcg, possibly more) or Armour thyroid (T4 + T3, 1–3 grains, possibly more) – needs regular monitoring with thyroid function tests.
- All the above also require:
    - Regular home checks of pulse and blood pressure
    - GP to be informed and ideally oversee the regime

CHAPTER 23

Common associated problems:

fibromyalgia, osteoporosis, female sex hormone imbalances

When sorrows come, they come not single spies
But in battalions.

CLAUDIUS IN *HAMLET*
(William Shakespeare, April 1564 – 3 May 1616)

Fibromyalgia

Fibromyalgia 'simply' means pain in the muscles and connective tissue. Doctors can be very naughty and pass this off as a diagnosis. They may prescribe painkilling or anti-inflammatory drugs which may provide short-term relief. However, in suppressing symptoms, one ignores the underlying cause and that has the potential to worsen the condition by accelerating the underlying pathology. Please see my book *Sustainable Medicine* for more on the importance of understanding symptoms and addressing root causes of illness.

Often by the time patients come to see me they are taking a cocktail of toxic drugs, often including opiates. This makes it particularly difficult to unravel the original underlying causes.

Just like 'CFS/ME', 'fibromyalgia' is not a diagnosis but a symptom and again one must ask the question 'What is the cause?' In order of likelihood the possible causes are as follows.

Overtraining

All athletes suffer mild muscle and connective tissue pain if they have overdone things – this results from mild tissue damage which then takes a few days to heal and repair. During this time of healing and repair, rest and pacing are essential. All my CFS/ME patients constantly push themselves to their (very restricted) limit because it takes so little before they reach their 'limitations' – for example, walking to the toilet from the bedroom could well be 'overdoing things' for many CFS/ME sufferers. Consequently, they pay for this with muscle pain.

Poor energy delivery mechanisms

Poor energy delivery results in an early switch into anaerobic metabolism with the production of lactic acid. That is painful – it is what produces a 'stitch' when running. Please see Chapter 4 (page 51) for more detail on this.

Magnesium deficiency

Calcium is required for muscles to contract, but magnesium is needed for relaxation. Indeed, magnesium has been dubbed nature's tranquilliser. I have many patients who find that muscle pain is relieved by magnesium – the following are especially helpful:

Transdermal magnesium. When this idea was first mooted I was deeply cynical. I could not believe that such a tiny dose of magnesium could be helpful. However, my clinical experience has been that this is often extremely helpful. Importantly, this is cheap, easy to apply and convenient. Epsom salt baths are particularly helpful. We know magnesium is well absorbed through the skin and has additional benefits with respect to detoxing.

Magnesium by injection. I often use this treatment for improving mitochondrial function, but also often for muscle pain. The major drawback is that the injections can themselves be painful. This is simply because they are hypertonic (the solution has less solute and more water than the body fluid into which it is being injected) – giving the injection very slowly, to allow the magnesium to disperse, gets round this problem. Also, some of my patients add 0.05 ml of lignocaine (a local anaesthetic) to the 0.5 ml dose of magnesium sulphate. This makes the injection painless at the point of the injection site.

Allergic muscles

Allergy never ceases to surprise and amaze me for the multiplicity of symptoms that it can cause. It is now clear to me that any part of the body can react allergically. Irritable bowel syndrome is partly due to allergy in the gut, migraine is allergy in the brain, asthma is allergy in the lungs, so why not allergic muscles? The more I look for this condition the more I find it, and it is obvious when you look for it!

How do allergic muscles start? What seems to happen is that muscles get sensitised as a result of mechanical damage. Tearing or bruising the muscle means that it comes in direct contact with blood, which may be carrying food antigens or I suspect microbial antigens from the gut. I suspect the allergy is switched on at that time and the pain which follows the muscle damage and which persists long term is mis-attributed to damage, when actually it is sensitisation. So a torn muscle in the back from, say, lifting a heavy load, could sensitise to, say, dairy products, and it is the consumption of dairy subsequently which keeps the problem on the boil. I suspect that polymyalgia rheumatica is muscles becoming allergic to gut microbes.

The diagnosis is made more difficult because we often see delayed reactions, which start 24 or 48 hours after allergen exposure and last for several days. Muscles can only react in one way, which is with contraction, and this can vary from low grade cramp and muscle tics or jumping, to acute lancinating pain. I suspect the type of reaction depends on how much of the food is being consumed – regular consumption results in chronic low grade spasm and cramp, but the odd inadvertent exposure in somebody who is normally avoiding that food can cause acute lancinating pain so severe that the sufferer literally collapses. Typically this just lasts a few seconds. Pain is triggered by stretching the affected muscle. Initially any stretch will cause it; then, as things settle down, only a sudden stretch will do that. The sufferer protects him/herself from the pain by moving slowly. Other muscles in the vicinity of the allergic muscles may also go into spasm to protect against sudden inadvertent stretching and this causes a more generalised muscle spasm and stiffness. There is a further complication because if muscles contract inappropriately they can damage themselves literally by pulling themselves apart (and, indeed, this is the mechanism that athletes employ to get fitter – if you damage the muscles slightly, this stimulates the production of more muscle). Further pain develops because the blood circulation through the muscles is disturbed and there is the build-up of toxic metabolites, in particular lactic acid. As I have said, lactic acid causes pain. So often we then see a particular vicious cycle with allergic muscles causing spasm, spasm causing build-up of toxic metabolites, this build-up causing more pain and the muscles reacting to pain with further spasm.

Muscle pain is one of the nastiest pains that one can experience. Indeed, labour pains are, of course, muscle pains. Biliary colic and renal colic are also muscle pains – ask any sufferer how bad that pain is. Opiate analgesics are ineffective.

Typically the problem is much worse in the morning and improves as the day progresses. Often there are good days and bad days. Gentle regular exercise, such as walking, is very helpful and indeed some patients find that they have to exercise very intensely and very regularly to keep the problem at bay (if the allergen has not been recognised). Heat, hot baths and gentle massage help to relax the muscle in the short term, as does keeping the body in one particular position, but the first movement after these interventions has to be done carefully or the pain will come straight back again. Diazepam affords some relief because, I suspect, it makes the irritable, allergic muscle less twitchy. I have two patients with 'stiff man syndrome' who have been much improved by identifying and avoiding provoking allergens. My guess is that stiff man syndrome is an extreme version of allergic muscles. Investigations, including MRI scans and X-rays, have all been normal. However, allergic muscles can obviously co-exist with other pathology, such as arthritis and osteoporosis, and may be mis-attributed to these factors.

Osteoporosis

All CFS/ME sufferers are at risk of osteoporosis because they cannot exercise. If you have had CFS/ME for more than 10 years, or you are aged over 50, then you should have a bone density scan. Conventional scans use large doses of radiation and that is undesirable. I recommend a heel bone density scan which can be done using ultrasound – this is very reliable, involves no radiation, and can be followed up within a few months to ensure progress. In the UK these are offered inexpensively by 'Bone Matters' (see bone matters.org).

I have now collected data from 17 patients who have had bone density scans done before and after a treatment programme of simple nutritional supplements. In every case the bone density has either remained the same or increased. So whilst the numbers are small the statistics are powerful. The nutritional regimes are as follows:

The Basic Package of supplements – see page 220
The healing and repair package of supplements – see page 223
High-dose vitamin D – 5,000–10,000 IU daily (Do blood tests to make sure levels are adequate – I like to see them above 100 nanograms per millilitre [ng/ml].)
Strontium – 340–680 mg daily
Pregnenolone – 50 mg daily

Note: For minerals and strontium to be absorbed, one has to be free from the fermenting gut (see Chapter 7, page 107).

Strontium is available on prescription for the treatment of osteoporosis. However, there are two problems – first, it is made up with aspartame (a toxic sweetener); second, an unnatural salt of strontium is used, namely strontium ranelate. Drug companies could not use a natural strontium salt because that cannot be patented. This unnatural preparation of strontium carries a risk of thrombosis. I can see no biologically plausible reason why natural strontium should cause thrombosis and indeed have never witnessed any such problem in the many patients I have treated. Strontium is well tolerated. You can buy strontium as drops in the form of strontium chloride, for example, or 300 mg capsules in the form of strontium citrate.

Not only do dairy products increase mortality, they make osteoporosis worse as a study published in the *British Medical Journal* in 2014 showed.[66] The reason for this is that the proportion of calcium to magnesium in dairy is 10:1, but our requirements are for 2:1. Calcium and magnesium compete for absorption and so taking dairy induces a magnesium deficiency. The key nutrient is vitamin D. This greatly improves the absorption of calcium, but more importantly it ensures deposition in bone. With good vitamin D, one does not have to worry about calcium.

The standard treatment for osteoporosis is Adcal. However, this contains high levels of calcium and no magnesium. The dose of vitamin D is so tiny as to be ineffective. It is just 400 mcg of D3 which is equivalent to about two minutes of sunshine exposure on the skin. Indeed, I suspect that products with this combination of calcium and minimal vitamin D make osteoporosis worse – that makes perfect sense for Big Pharma since patients can then be swapped to the expensive and profit-making bisphosphonates. Most of my CFS/ME patients do not tolerate these at all well, suffering nausea, muscle pain and increasing fatigue. These drugs also have the potential for serious side effects, including oesophageal cancer, atrial fibrillation and osteonecrosis of the jaw.[67]

Menstrual problems

The menstrual cycle is entirely symptomatic of hormone levels and how these change. Progesterone and oestrogen spike mid-cycle as an egg is produced by the ovary. Progesterone remains high, but if the egg is not fertilised, it then falls rapidly and this sharp fall should produce a short, light period. It is wobbly levels of hormone that cause breakthrough bleeding, heavy periods, painful periods, irregular periods and PMT. So, for example, if progesterone levels wobble, they will cause a bleed every time they fall a bit and the bleed will stop every time the levels go up or remain constant. This explains why doctors love to treat all these conditions with the Pill – this imposes absolutely regular, high, stable levels of hormone with completely predictable and light menstrual cycles. However, the Pill comes with risks. CFS/ME is twice as common in women as men – I suspect because of the Pill and HRT. In fact, the ratio could be even higher – on my Facebook Page, 'Supporters of Dr Sarah Myhill' (run independently of me by my patients Kathryn Lloyd and Craig Robinson) the statistics are 84 per cent women and 16 per cent men. Both the Pill and HRT are major risk factors for metabolic syndrome, heart disease, cancer, infection and autoimmunity. We should be asking the question why we are seeing wobbly hormone levels in the first place. In order of priority I suspect the following:

Metabolic syndrome: The rapidly fluctuating blood sugar levels have profound effects on hormones downstream. See my book *Prevent and Cure Diabetes* for much more on this.

Fermenting gut: A common gut fermenter is yeast. Yeasts have their own steroids, one of which is ergosterol. There is evidence to suggest that this hijacks and mimics the body's own hormones, resulting in fluctuating and wobbly levels. Indeed there is much evidence that links yeast problems with endometriosis (see Chapter 7, page 107).

Hypothyroidism (see Chapter 5, page 81).

Micronutrient deficiencies (see Chapter 18, page 220).

The menopause

I believe the menopause causes problems for two reasons: first, the hot flush disturbs sleep and, second, it uses energy wastefully. I do not have space to describe the mechanisms here so please visit my website: http://drmyhill.co.uk/wiki/Menopause_-_possible_causes_of_hot_flushes_and_what_we_can_do_to_mitigate_them.

Doctors love to prescribe HRT which abolishes the symptoms directly, but this is a dangerous treatment in the long term. I do not have any easy effective treatments but the causes and treatments are as above – that is, metabolic syndrome, fermenting gut, hypothyroidism and micronutrient deficiencies. The interventions listed below do help to mitigate the problems. In addition try:

Pregnenolone 50 mg
Herbal oestrogen mimics, such as dong quai (1 g twice daily), black cohosh (6.5 mg once daily), red clover (1 g three times daily)
Clonidine 50 mg at night – it works by blocking the heating effects of the spike of pituitary hormones FSH and LH.

Interventions for menopause problems

Mitigate the flushes by keeping cool

Wear clothes that keep the body warm, but with bare arms and bare legs so that heat can be quickly lost if necessary.

Try to sleep at night with minimal coverings. Choose a mattress which is not too well insulated. Position the bed directly under an open window where there is a cool down-draught of air.

Interventions to mitigate an established flush

The quicker you can lose heat, the shorter will be the flush. Suggestions include:

Drink ice-cold water from the fridge (perhaps have a small fridge next to the bed, or have a bottle of frozen ice that slowly defrosts through the night but is ice cold to drink). Just as a hot drink is one of the fastest ways of warming up, an ice-cold drink reduces body temperatures very quickly. (Be mindful that if you have heart disease, ice-cold water can slow the heart and possibly trigger a dysrhythmia.)

Use a fan.

Consider using a mild hypnotic such as valerian, melatonin or Nytol because that helps to get you back off to sleep more quickly. It is vital to combine this with a sleep dream (see page 210).

Postural orthostatic tachycardia syndrome (POTS)

POTS is a very common, if not universal, problem in people with severe CFS/ME. It means that the sufferer can only stand for a short time before having to lie down. POTS is said to result from autonomic neuropathy, but my view is that this is the response to falling blood pressure, not the cause. Let me explain.

It is much easier for the heart to pump blood on the flat (lying down) than up and down hills (standing up). Indeed, we all feel more comfortable lying down, or sitting rather than standing, because the heart has to work less hard. In severe cases of CFS/ME the heart is in a low output state, perhaps to such a degree that it cannot pump enough blood round the body when standing. So when the sufferer stands, he/she can maintain blood pressure for a certain time, but then the heart muscle becomes fatigued because energy supply to the heart is impaired as a result of mitochondrial failure, and so the blood pressure starts to fall. Initially the body tries to compensate by making the heart beat faster. However, this too is unsustainable, and a combination of weak heart with beating too fast, results in blood pressure falling precipitously. The patient has to lie down quickly to avoid blacking out.

One can test for this by a TILT test; this can be done by Dr Julia Newton at Newcastle but other hospitals within the NHS may well offer the same. Clinically, I have found that as the mitochondrial failure is treated, the symptoms of POTS resolve. (See page 78, for more on treating mitochondrial failure.)

Craig tells me of an interesting conversation that took place within the Dr Myhill Facebook Group – it transpired that a number of sufferers found it easier to think (read, concentrate, etc) whilst lying down rather than when standing or seated. Some group members reported a sudden loss of 'thread of thought' when they stood up. I think this is explained by the same process – as these sufferers stood, blood poured away from the brain, making cognitive tasks difficult, if not impossible.

CHAPTER 23 SUMMARY

Common associated problems: fibromyalgia, osteoporosis, female sex hormone imbalances

- CFS/ME can lead to many associated problems.
- Fibromyalgia can result from:
  - **Overtraining.**
  - **Mitochondrial dysfunction:** see Chapter 4 for treatment (page 78).

- **Magnesium deficiency:** use transdermal magnesium, Epsom salt baths or injections.
- **Allergic muscles:** this is where muscles become sensitised to allergens, perhaps food types such as dairy. Consuming these food types then triggers painful muscle symptoms. The best treatment is avoidance of the allergen.

- Osteoporosis is always a risk for CFS/ME sufferers because of an inability to exercise.
- Treatment for osteoporosis is:
  - The Basic Package of supplements – see page 220
  - The healing and repair package of supplements – see page 223
  - High-dose vitamin D 5,000–10,000 IU daily
  - Strontium 340–680 mg daily
  - Pregnenolone – 50 mg daily

- Menstrual problems are common in CFS/ME. The Pill and HRT are risk factors. Other causes of menstrual problems, and associated treatments, are:
  - **Metabolic syndrome:** the rapidly fluctuating blood sugar levels have profound effects on hormones downstream. See my book on *Prevent and Cure Diabetes* for much more on this.
  - **Fermenting gut:** a common gut fermenter is yeast. Yeasts have their own steroids, one of which is ergosterol. There is evidence to suggest that this hijacks and mimics the body's own hormones resulting in fluctuating and wobbly levels. Indeed, there is much evidence that links yeast problems with endometriosis – see Chapter 7, page 107.
  - **Hypothyroidism:** see Chapter 5, page 81.
  - **Micronutrient deficiencies:** see Chapter 18, page 220.

- The menopause can be particularly problematic in CFS/ME sufferers. Treatment options are:
  - Pregnenolone 50 mg
  - Herbal oestrogen mimics, such as dong quai, black cohosh, red clover

  - Clonidine 50 mg at night (It works by blocking the heating effects of the spike of pituitary hormones FSH and LH)
  - See page 267 for other methods of mitigating the symptoms of the menopause

- Postural orthostatic tachycardia syndrome (POTS). In CFS/ME, my experience is that this is caused by poor mitochondrial function, leading to poor cardiac output. POTS resolves when the underlying mitochondrial failure has been addressed – see Chapter 4, page 78.

CHAPTER 24

Catastrophe Theory and CFS/ME

Craig Robinson

Background

Before we begin, apologies are due to any students, or indeed scholars, of Catastrophe Theory, as the discussion here may well cause you to break out in a cold sweat and scream at the author for his cavalier approach to such a beautiful theory! My only defence is that age-old one of pragmatism before idealism.

The idea that Catastrophe Theory might be linked to, or perhaps a convenient and accessible way of modelling, the recovery process from CFS/ME arose during one long weekend when Dr Myhill was encouraging me to inject as much magnesium as possible in as short a time as possible. This was not pure sadism on her part but rather the result of clinical observations she had made over the years that some CFS/ME sufferers demonstrated recovery patterns and behaviour that were 'sudden' or at least certainly 'not linear'. There appeared to be a tipping point beyond which the recovery was kick-started into action.

The purpose of this final chapter is to give you, the reader, an overview of how this sudden or not linear recovery behaviour can be modelled. It is hoped that this overview will allow a greater understanding of this kind of recovery behaviour and that in so doing, it is further hoped that those who are on the recovery path will better understand what is likely to speed up this process, and likewise what actions will most likely set them back. Moreover, it is anticipated that those who are struggling to begin their recovery process may both be encouraged and also possibly gain insights into the blockages they are experiencing to beginning on such a path to recovery.

This brief summary is not an attempt to make direct linkages between the biological processes and Catastrophe Theory as explained below. However, one could easily imagine such a scenario, for example, with regard to the workings of a single mitochondrion. If, having tested a CFS sufferer – using, for example, the mitochondrial function profile test – the efficiency with which ATP is made from ADP is determined to be abnormal, then this could be indicative of a deficiency of magnesium. It may be that such a patient's system, having been stressed into a CFS state, now requires a certain minimum level of magnesium to be present in order properly to 'start' the conversion process from ADP to ATP. This minimum level would be the 'tipping point' as mentioned above.

This is, of course, a much simplified example, designed only to demonstrate the basic point rather than give the complete picture, which is, as readers will know, much more complicated and indeed unique to each CFS/ME sufferer.

Catastrophe Theory

Catastrophe Theory is a new branch of mathematics which was developed initially by the French mathematician René Thom in the 1960s and became very popular due to the efforts of Christopher Zeeman in the 1970s.

Mathematics, as applied to real world situations, had, not exclusively but largely, concerned itself up to this point with applications that were taken to be 'continuous'. An example of such continuous behaviour is the acceleration of a car. When the accelerator pedal is applied, depending on the coefficient of friction between the tire and the ground and any other forces applied to the car, such as drag, one can calculate the manner in which the velocity of the car will increase. However, we all know how cars accelerate in subjective terms. We don't need some mathematician to calculate a rather complicated equation to show the exact velocity at any given time. What we know, from our own experience, is that cars accelerate, say, from 40 mph to 60 mph in a continuous fashion. It is never the case that the car is travelling at 40 mph and then the very next instant, it is travelling at 60 mph (although it sometimes feels like this when my wife is driving!). No, the car gradually accelerates from 40 mph to 60 mph in a fairly uniform or continuous manner.

This is all well and fine, but this kind of continuous modelling fails to address very many real-life situations that mathematicians wanted to understand. For example, the apple that perhaps fell on Sir Isaac Newton's head, and enlightened him as to the nature of gravity, did so suddenly. Said apple did not gradually detach itself from the tree but rather all of a sudden it just fell.

This type of behaviour is described as 'catastrophic' in that something (here an apple) changes from one state of being (hanging attached to the tree) to another state of being (falling, not attached to the tree) in an instant. There is no gradual change of state, as there was with the car and its velocity, but rather things happen suddenly after a tipping point has been reached.

There are many examples of this type of behaviour, not only in the physical world (icebergs suddenly breaking off ice sheets is another obvious one) but also in the behavioural, psychological and relationship social sciences. Perhaps the most famous is the cornered animal. Put simply, say a dog is cornered, and a perceived threat is gradually approaching the dog. Initially the dog will display passive behaviour, or the 'fear response'. It will stay exactly where it is and hope that the perceived threat will not materialise. However, if the perceived threat continues to advance on the dog, there will come a distance (the tipping point) where the behaviour of the dog 'flips' suddenly from passive (fear response) to aggressive (fight response), and the dog will suddenly charge its perceived threat. Here the tipping point is measured simply by way of the distance between the dog and the perceived threat. In more complicated examples, it is considerably harder to determine how to measure the tipping point.

So, what has all of this got to do with CFS?

A Catastrophe Theory model: CFS and the treatment protocol

As a vast simplification, imagine that a person is in either one of two states – they either have CFS or they do not have CFS. We all know that this condition is a very wide spectrum and this fact will also be reflected in the theory below, once fully explained. Imagine also that we can describe the required ideal treatment protocol for an individual sufferer. Then we can imagine a situation as described in Figure 24.1 (page 274).

So, to describe the behaviour, we must first understand the graph. The axis going up the page (the 'y' axis if you can remember that far back!) represents increasing levels of fatigue; I have used 'fatigue' as shorthand for intensity of symptoms. The axis going along the page (the 'x' axis) represents the level of compliance with the ideal treatment protocol for this individual patient.

It will be realised that the ideal treatment protocol for an individual patient will not actually be known! It may never be known. However, the results of various medical tests, clinical signs and symptoms, a detailed history and, perhaps most importantly, a careful recording of the patient's reactions to various treatments, will all provide clues as to what constitutes such an ideal protocol.

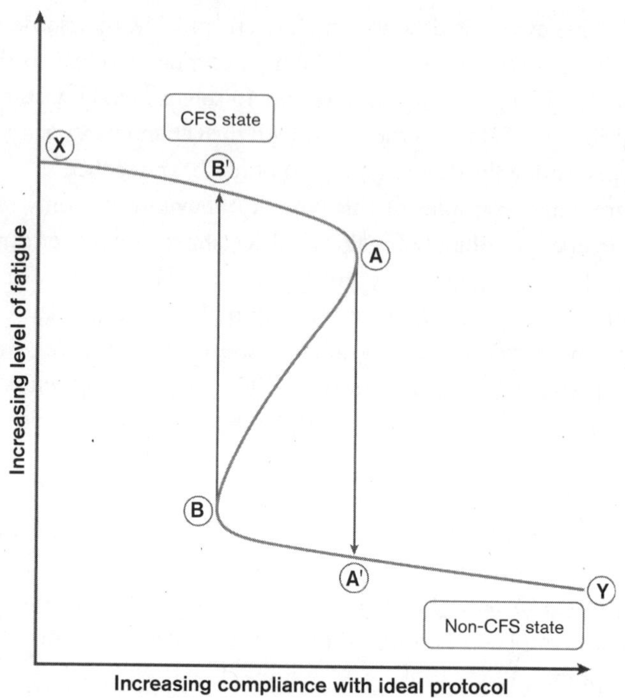

Figure 24.1. Levels of fatigue against compliance with the ideal protocol.

As such, the patient and physician will gradually move together towards the required ideal protocol by means of such methods, and also via a certain amount of trial and error, serendipity and dogged perseverance!

So we return to the graph: for example, at point X (top left of the graph) this patient has high levels of fatigue (indeed, is in a severe CFS state) and has not put in place any elements of the ideal treatment protocol. Meanwhile, at point Y (bottom right of the graph), this patient is in a non-CFS state, having relatively low levels of fatigue and has put in place much of the ideal treatment protocol. However, the interesting application of this graph is how the patient 'gets' from X to Y and also how he/she might slip back again from Y to X.

Getting from X to Y – recovery

Hint – imagine you are starting from point X on the upper part of the curve and then, in your mind's eye, move gradually to the right along this upper curve. Then follow the guide as explained in the paragraph below. Kinaesthetic learners may prefer to trace the curve with their index finger along the page, starting at point X and gradually moving to the right.

The 'good' patient, starting at point X on the upper curve, moves along the upper curve to the right, gradually increasing his (for the sake of linguistic simplicity) level of compliance with the ideal treatment protocol and in so doing does see some reduction in levels of fatigue as the upper curve comes down the page a little. This patient may feel a little despondent as he thinks to himself, 'For the effort I am putting in here (no chips, injections in the stomach every other morning), I really am not seeing that much of an improvement!' But his physician is a good one and continues to encourage and cajole him until finally the patient arrives at point A on the upper curve. At this point the patient suddenly 'falls' into a non-CFS state and arrives at point A' on the lower curve. Immediately he rings up his physician in triumph! The patient now has renewed vigour and belief in the treatment package and continues to comply more and more with the ideal protocol, moving himself further to the right of the lower curve, and eventually reaches point Y, where he wants to be.

Getting from Y to X – relapse

Hint – likewise, imagine you are starting from point Y on the lower part of curve and then move gradually to the left along this lower curve. Once again, kinaesthetic learners can trace this movement with their index finger.

The patient is now at point Y on the lower curve and after a while feels that he has recovered and so begins to lapse on the ideal treatment protocol. This slides him to the left of Y and towards, initially A' on the lower curve. This is no problem because he is still in a non-CFS state. So, the patient thinks to himself, 'I must be cured because I am now doing less of this treatment protocol and yet I still feel well – bring on the chips!' The patient is now somewhere between A' and B' on the lower portion of the curve and so is still in a non-CFS state. He continues to do less and less of the protocol until he reaches point B on the lower portion of the curve. At this point, he suddenly falls 'up' to point B' on the upper curve and reverts to a CFS state. He is despondent now and regrets his decisions to lapse on the protocol. Note also that for this patient to revert to a non-CFS state, he has to work hard to get back to point A; he can't just do a 'bit' of the protocol to revert to a non-CFS state, but rather has to move from his new state B' back to A.

Implications

The implications are clear and can be stated as below:

- It is important to recognise that we have symptoms for very good reasons – it is so that the body can protect itself from itself. Without the symptoms of pain and fatigue we would 'use' our bodies to destruction. In essence, the body can put up with only so much stress, which could be physical, mental, emotional, infectious, nutritional or whatever, but then, and suddenly, the cumulative effects of those stressors become critical and the system has to shut down into protection/hibernation mode. This results in the clinical picture of CFS (if fatigue is the main factor) or fibromyalgia (if pain is the main factor) and often both. Remember that stress is the symptom we experience when we do not have the energy reserves to cope with demands. This 'deficit' of energy reserves can be masked in the short term by the release of stress hormones, but this kind of masking is not sustainable in the long term.
- Complying with the individualised treatment protocol will yield results in the form of decreasing levels of fatigue and this will be sustained but perhaps not very marked initially.
- At a certain point of compliance with the treatment protocol, the patient arrives at a tipping point and will suddenly move from a CFS state to a non-CFS state – this is the drop from A to A' on the graph.
- After arriving at a non-CFS state, the patient can see further improvements in his/her health by continuing to comply with the protocol and will eventually arrive at a very comfortable state – point Y on the graph.
- If the patient lapses on the protocol then he/she can get away with this for quite some time. In fact, he/she can stay in a non-CFS state with less compliance to the treatment protocol than it originally took to 'flip' him/her out of the CFS state – that is, point B is to the left (and therefore less protocol compliant) than point A.
- However, eventually, continuing reductions in compliance with the protocol will bring the patient to point B and he/she will 'flip' back into a CFS state. This is the 'flip' from B to B'. Having reached point B', the patient will then require renewed vigour in protocol compliance in order to get to the point (that is, point A) where he/she will 'flip' back into a non-CFS state.
- We should all be putting in place the measures to improve health, and to stay well clear of the tipping point B so as not to risk the devastating 'flip' into CFS.

This kind of 'flipping' (both ways – from CFS to non-CFS and non-CFS to CFS) is something which Dr Myhill has observed on many occasions and the lessons are really quite simple:

Persevere. If you are complying with the protocol you are moving towards the right on the upper part of the curve, even if it doesn't feel like it at first. Any movement along the upper curve to the right gets you closer to the sought-after tipping point (point A).

Do not backtrack on the protocol if you start to feel better. This will either move you further to the left of point A on the upper part of the curve, thus getting you further away from flipping into a non-CFS state, or may even flip you back into a CFS state from a non-CFS state if you are on the lower part of the curve.

Kick-starting the system. But what of the rationale for trying megadoses of magnesium, or other micronutrients? Going for large doses, or 'flooding' the system, with particular micronutrients can sometimes give results totally out of proportion to what you might expect – if these micronutrients are key to flipping *you* from the CFS state part of the curve to the non-CFS state part of the curve, then that may be all *you* need to push *you* to point A and thus flip *you* into a non-CFS state. This was the rationale behind my taking large doses of magnesium over that long weekend. Further to this point, it seems that the large doses of whatever micronutrients are causing the blockage, which push the patient over point A on the curve to point A then also self-correct the system so that the system becomes self-perpetuating. In this way you don't need to continue with such large doses of said micronutrients for evermore. This is because the biological systems at work here have interlocking feedback systems. So that if I were 'short' on magnesium, then by flooding my system with surplus amounts of it, this blockage is overcome and the system then starts to work as it is supposed to, with micronutrients being recycled and all the other elements of the various cycles in the process kick-started. In this way, one can sometimes 'short-circuit' the long, drawn-out process of protocol implementation and compliance and get to the non-CFS state much more quickly, simply by finding the micronutrient which is causing the blockage and then flooding the patient's system with this micronutrient. Once again, this kind of short-circuiting and getting to a non-CFS state more quickly by kick-starting the system using a particular micronutrient is something that Dr Myhill has seen in her CFS patients.

Moreover, and this is difficult to represent fully here, Dr Myhill's experience is that if a patient has had CFS for a longer period of time, then his/her recovery path differs from those who have suffered for less time. The curve as described will still be valid, but it will be shifted so that it is harder to reach point A and thus flip into a non-CFS state, and likewise it will be easier to slip back to point B and flip back into a CFS state. So, CFS sufferers of longer standing have to work harder to get into a non-CFS state and also have to work harder to stay in that newly acquired non-CFS state. Their curve may look more like the one shown in Figure 24.2. Point A (tipping from CFS to non-CFS) is further to the right and so requires more work to get there, and point B (tipping from non-CFS to CFS) is also further to the right, making it easier to flip back to the CFS state with only minimal lapsing on the protocol.

The interval between B and A', in any case, can be referred to as the 'danger zone'!

'Ex-CFS sufferers' who find themselves in this danger zone, and are thus in a non-CFS state, must not be complacent and must do all they can to move to the right of the lower part of the curve so as to get away from the dreaded tipping point B which flips them back into a CFS state.

One could go further with the graphical representation of this model and have a time axis perpendicular to the page and then, by plotting the various curves for CFS sufferers at certain 'illness time lengths', one could obtain a 3-D representation of the illness curve over time as well as with respect to protocol compliance. It is not necessary to understand this finer point, but for those who may (still!) be interested, the 3-D curve might look something like Figure 24.3.

It will be recognised that this is only a model and its real intention is to give sufferers a guide as to what they might expect, a warning as to what might happen if they lapse on the protocol and an insight into why large doses of certain micronutrients may help them out of their CFS state.

Refinements

Having described the basic ideas of how Catastrophe Theory can be utilised as a tool to help patients understand their illness, there are three refinements to this basic model which can now be made.

Refinement one

It will be seen that at point A on the upper part of the curve in Figures 24.1 and 24.2, a patient will have the same degree of protocol compliance as a patient

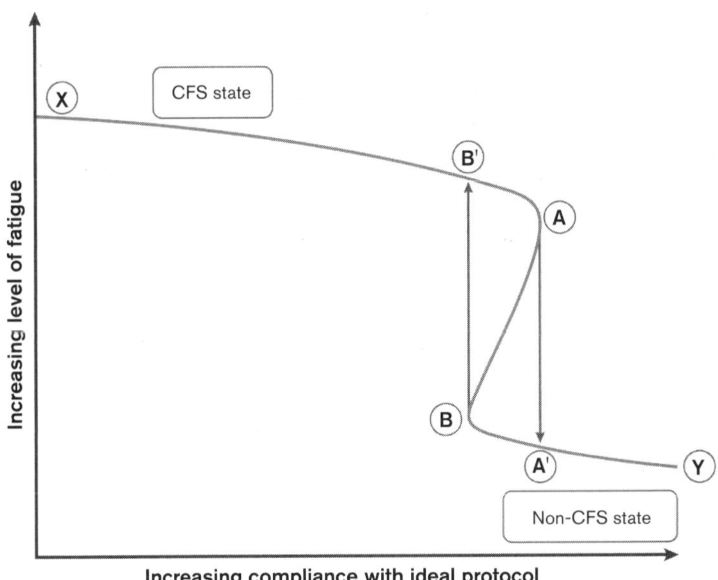

Figure 24.2. Levels of fatigue against compliance with the ideal protocol in a patient with long-term CFS.

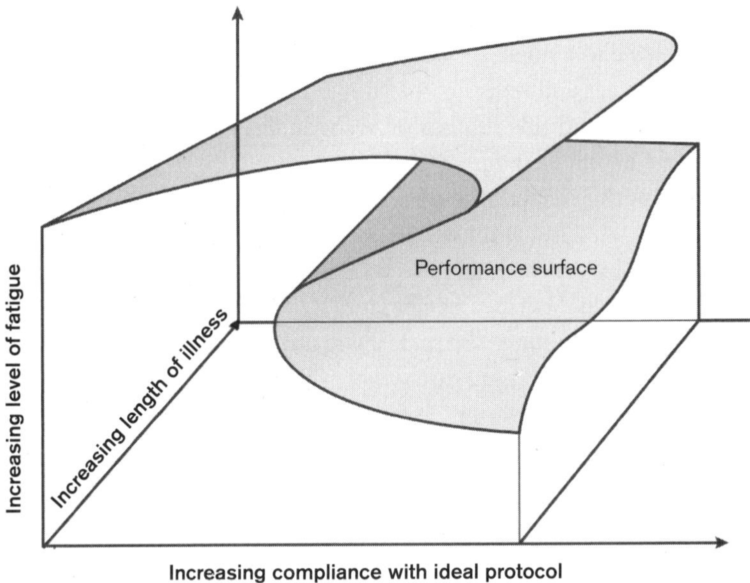

Figure 24.3. A 3-D representation of fatigue against ideal protocol against length of illness.

at point A' on the lower part of the curve. In effect the same degree of protocol compliance can result in two different patients being in two completely different states – A is a CFS state and A' is a non-CFS state. The question has to be asked as to why some patients remain 'hovering' at point A whereas other patients flip to point A' and reach a non-CFS state. To understand this, we should first consider a different example, that of the 'phantom limb'. The brain has an internal map of the body and also of what is going on in the body, and this internal map may not always reflect reality. So, a limbless person may still feel as though he/she has a (painful) limb because of this 'incorrect' internal body map that his/her brain is still relying on. In effect, the brain has not 'updated' its internal map of the body in the light of new information.

In a similar way, it is possible that the immune system has such an internal map of what is going on within itself and this map will reflect the situation as it has subsisted for some time, rather than the situation as it actually is now. So, just as the brain registers a limb, or limb pain, because that is the situation which has subsisted for some time, even though this is no longer the reality, so does the immune system register CFS because that is the situation that has subsisted for some time, even though the reality is now that the patient is in a non-CFS state.

This is not to say that the patient is unable to make the flip from a CFS state to a non-CFS state as a result of some psychological block. This is far from the truth. It is rather that patients may have to be on the cusp of flipping from a CFS state to a non-CFS state for some time before the immune system recognises this fact and registers that this is the new reality. It is possible that the physician can aid this process of recognition by using the techniques as described in Chapter 22 (page 256).

Once again, this delayed flip from a CFS state to a non-CFS state is something that Dr Myhill has witnessed in her clinical practice. Indeed, this may be the mechanism by which certain psychological techniques are effective (as well as the interventions described in Chapter 22). Moreover, if this is the case it is doubly important to address the underlying physical problems first – Dr Myhill suggests this because there are cases where such psychological techniques have made the patient much worse. This would occur if the psychological techniques were applied at a time when the body did not have the physical reserves to respond to such.

Refinement two

Just as positive interventions (such as magnesium therapy) can flip a patient from a CFS state into a non-CFS state, the opposite is also the case. So, it is possible that a bad event can suddenly flip a patient back into a CFS state without that patient doing anything or changing the protocol that he/she is currently following. For example, a (possibly ex-) CFS sufferer who has good protocol compliance and has reached a fairly comfortable non-CFS state but then is suddenly exposed to organophosphate pesticides may be pushed back to a CFS state. This gives a painful symmetry to the theory in that patients can be flipped back into CFS states not only by reducing their protocol compliance but also by such random unavoidable negative events. In addition, and crucially, this point reinforces the message that CFS patients must be careful not only to stick to their individual protocols as closely as possible but also to avoid potentially 'bad tipping factors', such as viruses, exposures to toxins and so on. For ease of reference, these bad tipping events can be referred to as 'negative events'. Sadly, Dr Myhill has treated patients such as this, where good recovery has been made and then some negative event, not related to patient protocol compliance, has pushed the patient back into a CFS state. It is important at this stage not to lose hope but rather to see this as a set back. The physician and patient will now have to work together to develop a new ideal protocol which takes into account and addresses the new stresses that have been placed on the patient's system by this negative event. Once again, the patient will progress along the curve as he/she did before, with the newly devised protocol having been fully put in place.

Refinement three

The discourse above has so far only admitted the possibility of one flip, simply from a CFS state to a non-CFS state. This is something that Dr Myhill does experience in practice. However, as was noted at the beginning of this chapter, to divide patients into two distinct sets, those who are in a CFS state and those who are in a non-CFS state, is simplistic. More often, Dr Myhill discusses with patients the probability of experiencing 'quantum leap' improvements in their condition and that these quantum leaps will most likely be many and will also be varied in their impact on symptom intensity. So, one could envisage a refinement to the generalised graph, as shown in Figure 24.4, whereby there are gradual 'stepped' reductions in fatigue levels as the patient progresses eventually to a non-CFS state. Each of these 'steps' should be regarded as very positive by both physician and patient because such a step represents an indication that the protocol has resulted in one of these mini-flips. In effect this is evidence that the patient is addressing some of the stresses on the system which are causing his/her symptom load. Nevertheless, the trick is not to sit

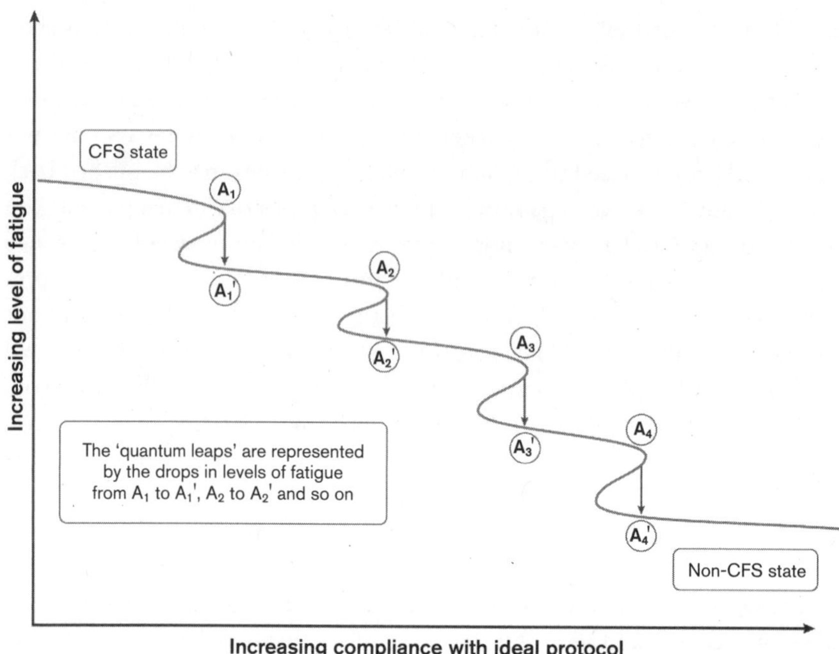

Figure 24.4. 'Stepped' graph of levels of fatigue against compliance with the ideal protocol.

back, once such a mini-flip has been secured, but rather to look for the next intervention, whilst keeping all the current protocols and interventions in place, which will result in the next mini-flip, and to continue to do so until the patient finally arrives at a non-CFS state.

CHAPTER 24 SUMMARY

Catastrophe Theory and CFS/ME

- Some CFS sufferers demonstrate recovery patterns that are 'sudden' or at least 'not linear'. There appears to be a 'tipping point' beyond which recovery is kick-started into action.
- This pattern of recovery can be modelled by looking at the basics of Catastrophe Theory.

- Catastrophe Theory is concerned with situations where small changes in circumstances can result in sudden and large changes in outcomes.
- With regard to CFS, this translates into a sudden flip from a CFS state to a non-CFS state and this happens once all elements of the individualised protocol that are needed for that particular sufferer are in place.
- The opposite is also, unfortunately, true, whereby a recovered CFS sufferer may flip themselves back into a CFS state if they lapse on the protocol, as individualised to them, or if some negative event, such as pesticide exposure or a viral attack, should befall them.
- Sometimes a single micronutrient can be the key for a particular sufferer and 'flooding' the system with this micronutrient will kick-start the system and flip that sufferer from a CFS state to a non-CFS state.
- In reality it will be a sequence of these flips (rather than one single flip) that will gradually move a sufferer from a CFS state into a non-CFS state.
- If a sufferer appears stuck on the edge of such a flip, using some of the techniques as outlined in Chapter 22 may help to induce a flip.

The key points are:

- Complying with individualised treatment protocols will yield results in the form of decreasing levels of fatigue and this will be sustained but perhaps not very markedly initially.
- At a certain point of compliance with the treatment protocol, the patient arrives at a tipping point and will suddenly move from a CFS state to a non-CFS state.
- It may be worth flooding the body with certain micronutrients, based on clinical observations of the individual sufferer, to see whether this may induce the flip from CFS state to non-CFS state.
- After arriving at a non-CFS state, the patient can see further improvements in his/her health by continuing to comply with the protocol and he/she will eventually arrive at a very comfortable state.

- If the patient lapses on the protocol then he/she can get away with this for quite some time. In fact, he/she can stay in a non-CFS state with less compliance to the treatment protocol than it originally took to flip him out of the CFS state.
- However, eventually, continuing reductions in compliance with the protocol, or an unfortunate negative event, such as pesticide exposure or a viral assault, will flip the sufferer back into a CFS state.
- If flipped back into a CFS state, the sufferer should tighten up on his/her individualised protocol and also, if necessary, deal effectively with the negative event that forced this backwards flip.
- We should all be putting in place the measures to improve health, and comply with individualised treatment protocols, so that we stay well clear of the 'backward' tipping point and do not to risk the devastating flip back into CFS.

I wish to place on record my thanks to the wonderful members of the Facebook groups 'Support Dr Sarah Myhill' and 'Support for followers of Dr Myhill's protocol' who used their very valuable, and in many cases limited, resources of energy and time to read and comment upon my initial draft of this chapter. Finally, and of course, thanks are due to Dr Sarah Myhill, who has not only been a constant source of enlightenment and encouragement for my own personal stepped recovery path but who is also someone that I am proud to call my friend.

Postscript

Western Medicine has lost its way. Doctors no longer look for the underlying causes of disease, a process which used to be called diagnosis, but rather seek a 'quick fix' response that will see the patient out of their surgery door in under 10 minutes. This quick fix response usually comprises the prescribing of symptom suppressing medications. Doctors have become the puppets of Big Pharma, dishing out drugs and working to a 'checklist' culture which is directed at the symptom, rather than the patient. Patients are seen as a collection of walking symptoms, rather than as people, each with a highly individual set of circumstances. Worse than this, not only do these prescription drugs do nothing to address the root causes of illness, but often they accelerate the underlying pathology and so drug prescribing snowballs. This leads to a vicious spiral of increasing drug costs, coupled with worsening pathologies for individual patients, whilst at the same time there is an increasing number of new, and chronic, patients, because their illnesses are never properly addressed at the root cause. It is no wonder that the National Health Service is being overwhelmed. The result is that millions suffer a painful, premature, and often lingering death from diseases which are completely avoidable and reversible.

The time has come for patients to be empowered, by taking back control of their own health. To achieve this empowerment, patients need:

1. The knowledge to work out why they have symptoms and disease.
2. Direct access to all relevant medical tests.
3. Direct access to knowledgeable health practitioners who can further advise and guide them, together with direct access to safe and effective remedies.

None of this is beyond patients who are always highly motivated to be well again, and who always know their bodies better than anyone else. It is time to break down the artificial barriers that have been placed between patients and the direct access to medical knowledge, tests and experts that they so deserve.

This three-stage process of patient emancipation is addressed in the following ways:

1. The knowledge can be found in these four books.

Sustainable Medicine. This is the starting point for treating all symptoms and diseases. It explains why we have symptoms, such as fatigue and pain, and explains how one can work out the mechanisms of such symptoms and which are the appropriate medical tests to diagnose these mechanisms. Most importantly, *Sustainable Medicine* identifies the 'Tools of the Trade' to effect a cure. These tools include diet, nutritional supplements and natural remedies.

Prevent and Cure Diabetes. All medical therapies should start with diet. Modern Western diets are driving our modern epidemics of diabetes, heart disease, cancer and dementia – this process is called metabolic syndrome. *Prevent and Cure Diabetes* explains in detail why and how we have arrived at a situation where the *real* weapons of mass destruction can be found in our own kitchens. Importantly, it describes the vital steps every one of us can make to reverse this situation so that life can be lived to its full potential.

Diagnosis and Treatment of Chronic Fatigue Syndrome and Myalgic Encephalitis. This book – which I hope you are either about to read or are reading now – further explores the commonest symptom which people complain of, namely fatigue, together with its pathological end result when this symptom is ignored. This is my life's work, having spent over 35 years in clinical practice and many months doing academic research, and co-authored three scientific papers, all directed at solving this jigsaw of an illness. This book has application not just for the severely fatigued patient but also for the athlete looking for peak performance and for anybody not feeling on top form.

The PK Cookbook. This gives us the *how* of the Paleo-ketogenic (PK) diet. This is the starting point for preventing and treating modern Western diseases, including diabetes, arterial disease, dementia and cancer. Dietary changes are always the most difficult, but also the most important, intervention. This book is based on my first-hand experience and research on developing a PK diet that is sustainable long term. Perhaps the most important feature of this diet is the PK bread – this has helped more people stick to this diet than all else! Secondly, the book introduces PK salt (named Sunshine salt because it is rich in vitamin D). This salt is comprised of all essential minerals (plus vitamins D and B12) in physiological amounts within a sea salt. This more than compensates for the mineral deficiencies that are ubiquitously present in all foods from Western agricultural systems. It is an essential and delicious addition to all modern Western diets.

2. Access to medical tests

Many medical tests can be accessed directly online:

www.bloodtestsdirect.co.uk: Here blood tests can be accessed directly without a doctor's request. Many can be done on fingerdrop samples of blood.

www.arminlabs.com/en: These blood tests (including for Lyme disease) can be accessed directly without the need for a referral from a doctor or other health practitioner.

www.biolab.co.uk: For these tests you need referral by a health practitioner – see 'NHW' below.

www.gdx.net/uk: This is the link for Genova labs – referral by a health practitioner is needed - see 'NHW' below. Tests include blood, urine, stool and saliva samples. Many blood tests can be carried out at home on a fingerdrop sample of blood, without the need for a nurse or doctor to be involved at all.

3. Direct access to knowledgeable health practitioners who can further advise and guide patients

Natural Health Worldwide (NHW) is a website where any knowledgeable practitioner (experienced patient, health professional or doctor) can offer their opinion to any patient. This opinion may be free or, for a fee, by telephone, email, or Skype. The practitioner needs no premises or support staff since bookings and payments are made online. Patients give feedback to that practitioner's reputation page and star ratings evolve. See www.naturalhealth worldwide.com.

PART IV

Appendices

APPENDIX 1

Tests and interpretations

All things are subject to interpretation; whichever interpretation prevails at a given time is a function of power and not truth.

FRIEDRICH NIETZSCHE
(15 October 1844 – 25 August 1900)

We must get to the truth if we are to progress to understanding and recovery. Tests are very helpful to eliminate some causes of fatigue and work out mechanisms of fatigue. I often see people who already have many test results. These results have either been ignored by their doctors or incorrectly interpreted. Worse than this, many patients are told by their doctor that all their tests are normal and so nothing is wrong and so they must be well. To my mind this is medical negligence. Tests ask specific questions, and in CFS/ME patients doctors are not asking the right questions. In dealing with CFS/ME doctors:

- do not ask the correct energy delivery questions
- do not ask the right nutritional questions
- do not ask the right inflammation questions
- use worthless allergy tests to tell patients they are not allergic
- use worthless stool tests to tell patients their gut is fine

Indeed, they often use tests to eliminate obvious pathology, and use these as an excuse to tell patients that nothing is wrong. They do enough to protect themselves from formal complaint in a tick box, investigation style, which fails to address any of the underlying causes. They hear the patient but do not listen. They secure their position medico-legally, then, in no uncertain terms, make it quite clear to the patient not to return. This is done either through advocating a graded exercise programme, recommending referral to a psychiatrist or intimating that the CFS/ME sufferer is an idle hypochondriac.

This progression would be hilarious if the results were not so tragic.

If the person you are talking to doesn't appear
to be listening, be patient. It may simply be that
he has a small piece of fluff in his ear.

AA MILNE in *Winnie-the-Pooh*

Incorrect test interpretation arises for several possible reasons, including:

The normal population reference ranges have changed. Now, 100 per cent of the Western population eating a Western diet are powering their bodies with sugar and starch. Eventually this results in metabolic syndrome and diabetes, with all the abnormalities that accompany such. Metabolic syndrome and diabetes are risk factors for CFS (much more of this in my book *Prevent and Cure Diabetes*). So blood sugar levels, triglycerides, HBA1Cs and inflammatory markers are all set too high because they are referenced to what is now 'normal' (for a population eating poor diets and with metabolic syndrome, etc) rather than what is 'physiologically desirable'. For example, during my medical lifetime the so-called normal range for ESR (a measure of inflammation in the blood) has moved from 1–10 mm/hr to 1–20, simply because the 'average Westerner' is now more inflamed due to lifestyle choices and diets.

Doctors ignore borderline results so long as they are in the 'normal range'. But one's *individual* normal range is not the same thing as the population reference range. This is of particular relevance in the treatment of hypothyroidism. Research done originally in the UK, and now repeated in America, clearly shows that the individual normal range of thyroid hormone levels is not the same as the population reference range.[68]

The normal range of vitamin B12 in the blood is said to be 150–700 (units). This may be sufficient to prevent pernicious anaemia, but for many CFS/ME sufferers, optimal biochemical function may not occur until levels are over 2,000. The only way to find out is a trial of B12 injections – indeed, this is such a safe and effective intervention I try this almost routinely in all my CFS/ME patients.

CFS/ME sufferers are often told that their serum magnesium is normal and so no supplements or injections are needed. Oh dear! *Serum* magnesium (that is, what is in the bloodstream) is maintained at the expense of intracellular levels because if serum magnesium falls then the heart stops in systole. (Magnesium is needed for muscles to relax.) Serum magnesium is only of practical relevance in the seriously ill ITU patient. Most doctors do not understand this difference between a serum magnesium and a red-cell magnesium. Most labs just measure serum levels and patients are told their magnesium is normal. So we have to measure intracellular magnesium via a red-cell magnesium test.

If the doctor does not know the reason for a problem, then a spurious one is given instead. So, for example, an apparently inexplicably low haemoglobin could be described as 'the anaemia of chronic disease'. No treatment is given. In fact, the patient may be anaemic because of a lack of raw materials and energy to make new blood – this is eminently treatable.

A high, or high-normal, bilirubin level is called Gilbert's syndrome – again often dismissed by doctors as an irrelevant biochemical anomaly. But in Gilbert's, the high bilirubin is a marker for the detoxification route that normally clears bilirubin from the liver. Such an overloading occurs because this route of detox – namely, glucuronidation – is genetically absent. Gilbert's is estimated to affect perhaps 10 per cent of the population. It is a risk factor for CFS because these people cannot detoxify efficiently and are easily poisoned. I treat this with additional glutathione (250 mg daily) to support the alternative glutathione detox pathway – it should be taken for life.

Tests may be interpreted as answering a question when they do not. The best example has to do with adrenal gland fatigue, which is almost universal in CFS because CFS sufferers have been chronically stressed, perhaps for years, and the adrenal gland is exhausted. Doctors use a 'short synacthen test' to test adrenal function. Whilst this may diagnose complete adrenal failure, as occurs in Addison's disease, it does not diagnose partial adrenal fatigue. However, this test result is often used to tell CFS patients that the adrenal gland is normal.

Absence of evidence is not evidence of absence.

CARL SAGAN, American astronomer (1934–1996)

Carl Sagan is one of the heroes of Craig, my Editor and sometime co-Author – Sagan's *Cosmos* series was aired during Craig's formative years. As a result Craig specialised in planetary and rocket motion in his final year at university – essentially 'rocket science'. Craig applied for only two jobs – NASA and Price Waterhouse. The Fates determined an accountant's life for Craig, as he lost out at the last hurdle to the non-US citizen test for NASA employees.

So let's go through common tests and how I would interpret and act on them. Please note this list is not a comprehensive interpretation of all possible abnormalities and reasons for such.

Table A1.1. Standard tests, interpretations and actions required

Key: Dx = diagnosis; Px = prescription; Ix = investigation

Test	Normal range	Interpretation if high or border-line high	Interpretation if low or borderline low	Action
Haemo-globin	11–16	Smoking		Px: Stop smoking!
		Carbon-monoxide poisoning		Ix: CO blood test Look for possible source of poisoning
		Polycythaemia – a premalignant condition		Refer to haematologist
		Haema-chromatosis? (metabolic problem with iron excretion)		
			Blood loss, e.g. heavy periods	Refer to gynaecologist
			Blood loss, e.g. from the gut ▪ inflammation? ▪ malignancy?	Ix: Faecal occult blood test Ix: Faecal calprotectin
			Lack of raw materials, e.g. iron or zinc Dietary deficiency? ▪ Malabsorption due to hypo-chlorhydria and fermenting gut	Ix: Measure ferritin See Chapter 7 fermenting gut, page 107
			Poor energy delivery to the bone marrow	Read the rest of this book!
Size of red cells		Deficiency of vitamin B12 (poor methylation)		Px: Methylation package of supplements (see Chapter 20, page 233)
		Deficiency of folic acid (poor methylation)		Px: Methylation package of supplements (see Chapter 20, page 233)

Test	Normal range	Interpretation if high or borderline high	Interpretation if low or borderline low	Action
		Hypothyroidism		See Dx, Ix and Px of hypothyroidism – Chapter 5, page 81
			Deficiency of iron	Ix: Measure ferritin
			Thalassaemia or other such	Refer to a haematologist
White cell count	4–11 The ref range is negatively skewed.* I suspect this is to allow doctors to ignore intercurrent infection (assumed but unknown). I reckon a normal WCC is 4–7	General reaction to stress Immune system is active: (Persistently high WCC is much more significant. If in doubt, repeat the test.)		Look for infection. See Chapters 11 (page 151) and 12 (page 161)
Lympho-cytes		Viruses		Ix for viruses
Neutrophils		Bacteria		Ix for bacteria
		Fungi		Ix for fungi
			Immune system exhausted by lack of energy or lack of raw materials from increased demand	Fermenting gut (Chapter 7, page 107) Chronic infection (Chapters 11, page 151, and 12, page 161)
Platelets	150–400	Thrombocythaemia – premalignant condition		Refer to a haematologist
			Autoimmunity	Refer to a haematologist
			Immune system exhausted by lack of energy or lack of raw materials	Read the rest of this book!

Test	Normal range	Interpretation if high or borderline high	Interpretation if low or borderline low	Action
Inflammatory markers, e.g. CRP ESR Plasma viscosity	<10 mm/hr	Immune system busy due to infection, allergy, autoimmunity. If in doubt keep repeating the test		A normal result does not exclude allergy, autoimmunity or infection Read the rest of this book!
Urea		Dehydration Poor kidney function		Drink more water Ix: Kidney function
			Poor protein intake	Eat more protein Check for malabsorption
Creatinine		High protein diet High muscle mass Poor kidney function		Eat less protein Ix: Kidney function
			Low muscle mass (common in CFS) Low protein intake	Wait until recovered Eat more protein
Sodium	135–144 mmol/L	Dehydration Salt poisoning		Drink more water Eat less salt
			Lack of salt intake Excessive water drinking Very low sodium (<130) is a medical emergency – Get help urgently!	Eat more salt Diuretics? Ketogenic diet requires 5 g (1 teaspoon) of salt a day
			Excessive sweating	Correct the cause
			Kidney failure Adrenal failure Excess diuretics	Urgently refer to specialist Ix: Addison's Ix: Kidney failure
Potassium	3.5–4.8	Kidney failure Many drugs Adrenal failure		Refer to specialist
			Inadequate intake of vegetables	Correct the cause

Test	Normal range	Interpretation if high or borderline high	Interpretation if low or borderline low	Action
			Severe diarrhoea	Ditto
			Many drugs	Ditto
Total cholesterol (TC) and HDL cholesterol	The percentage of HDL to TC is the critical measurement	>40%		Good low GI diet Excellent! Carry on
		20–40% suggests early metabolic syndrome		Room for improvement. Read our book *Prevent and Cure Diabetes*
			<20% is typical of metabolic syndrome	Arterial damage. Read our book *Prevent and Cure Diabetes*
High cholesterol	>7.0	Vitamin D deficiency		Ix: Measure vitamin D
		Hypothyroidism		Ix: Free T4, free T3 and TSH levels (see Chapter 5, page 81, on hypothyroidism)
Calcium (must be a corrected calcium to be valid)	2.15–2.6 pmol/l	Hyper-parathyroidism Nasty diseases!		Medical emergency – urgent referral or hospital admission if >3.3. Ix: Measure parathormone
			Vitamin D deficiency	Ix: Measure vitamin D
			Kidney failure	Refer to specialist
			Hypo-parathyroidism	Ix: Measure parathormone
				Normal calcium does not exclude osteoporosis
Serum magnesium	1.7–2.3 mg/dl	Nearly always normal		Ix: Red cell magnesium is a better reflection of body stores

Test	Normal range	Interpretation if high or borderline high	Interpretation if low or borderline low	Action
Vitamin D	70–200 nmol/l (NHS reference range is set too low at 30–60)	Over-dosing with D3		No problem with up to 10,000 IU per day
			Lack of sunshine	Take vitamin D Sunbathe
Bilirubin	<19	Gilbert's syndrome		Glutathione 250 mg daily for life See page 237
Alkaline phosphase	20–150 IU/l	Tissue damage – usually liver or bone		Ix the cause
			Low phosphate The Pill and HRT	Correct the cause
Alanine transferase	Female: <34 IU/l Male: <53 IU/l	Liver damaged by infection, toxin(s) (e.g. drugs, alcohol, possibly products of fermenting gut) Muscle damage		Correct the cause (see Chapter 20, page 233)
Gamma GT		Liver damage by infection Enzyme induction by toxin (e.g. alcohol, drugs or from fermenting gut)		Correct the cause (see Chapter 20, page 233)
Lactate dehydrogenase	140–280 UI/l	Any tissue damage (e.g. muscle, heart, liver, kidneys, blood, brain)		See Chapter15, page 183
Thyroid tests		A normal result does not exclude a thyroid problem		See Chapter 5, page 81, on thyroid function

Test	Normal range	Interpretation if high or border-line high	Interpretation if low or borderline low	Action
Adrenal	Short synacthen test	A normal result does not exclude an adrenal problem		See page 92, on adrenal function
Allergy tests		A positive result may be helpful	False negatives common	I never do allergy tests and do not trust the results anyway. Good detective work needed
Female sex hormones		Menopausal		
FSH (follicle stimulating hormone) and LH (Luteinis-ing hormone)	FSH 1–18 mIU/ml LH 2–18 mIU/ml Low day 3–5 of menstrual cycle; spikes mid cycle.	Menopausal		If not due to menopause then consultant opinion needed
			Females: polycystic ovarian syndrome Males: low sperm count	Further investigation
Oestrogen and progesterone	I rarely measure these	Problems arise with wobbly hormone levels		See page 266 – problems with female sex hormones
Stool tests	Standard NHS tests often inadequate			See Chapter 7, page 107, the fermenting gut
Urine tests for infection		>10,000 microbes per ml is a positive test	One can get symptoms with much lower counts if allergic to microbes	May need antibiotics D-mannose (2 g, 2–4 times daily) Ketogenic diet

Test	Normal range	Interpretation if high or border-line high	Interpretation if low or borderline low	Action
Urine dip sticks (these can be purchased online)	Protein, blood, white cells, nitrites	Inflammation (infection, allergy, autoimmunity) Kidney damage, kidney stones		Ref for further Ix
DNA tests, SNIPs	I never request these tests	The results give potential genetic weaknesses which have minor clinical relevance and rarely affect management		

* In negative skew, the left tail of the graph is longer and the mass of the distribution is concentrated to the right. For WCC, readings to the right are often ignored as 'normal' on the basis that there is an 'intercurrent infection' – that is, an assumed but unknown infection involved. Taking this approach is potentially dangerous as important immune system reactions may be missed. Figure A1.1 is the negative skew graph.

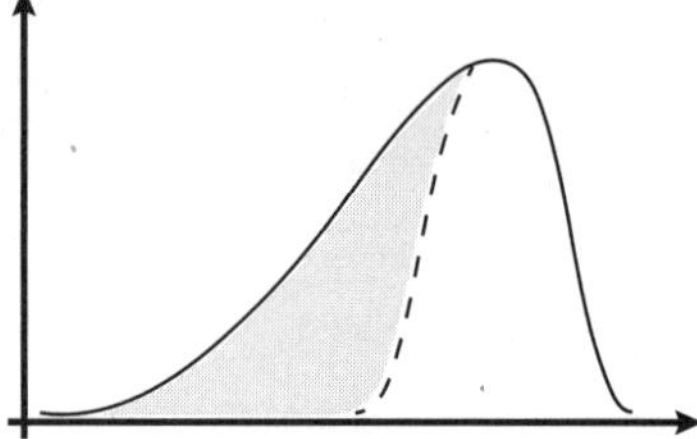

Figure A1.1.

APPENDIX 2

Exercise – the right sort

Humans, along with all other mammals, evolved living physically active lives. One needs exercise as one needs food and water: in just the right amount. Too much risks injury and muscle damage; too little and we degenerate.

CFS sufferers do not have the energy for physical exercise. Many of those who are severely affected dare not 'exercise' (by which I mean virtually any physical activity for some sufferers) because the slightest exertion triggers major relapse. Whatever exercise one chooses to do, the amount is determined by how one feels the next day. Delayed fatigue is a characteristic of severe CFS.

If any exercise is possible, then we need to choose that type which gets us fit and strong for the least possible time and effort. Again, Nature holds all the answers. I do not see badgers and foxes trotting round my hill every morning to get fit. Most of the time wild animals are in hiding or feeding quietly. However, once a week there will be a predator-prey interaction – the predator must run for his life to get his breakfast, the prey must run for his life to escape being breakfast. In doing so, both parties will achieve maximum lactic acid burn. This is all that is required to get fit and stay fit.

The underlying principles

We are taught that there are two types of fitness – viz, muscle power and cardiovascular fitness. Not so. What drives cardiovascular fitness is muscle strength. When muscle strength is used to its full capacity, it creates a powerful stimulus to the energy supply mechanism. This includes mitochondrial function and heart function. The heart pumps blood to send fuel and oxygen round the body where it is picked up by mitochondria which convert that to ATP, the currency of energy in the body. This means that if muscle strength is correctly developed, then this automatically translates into cardiovascular fitness and increased numbers of mitochondria. More mitochondria derive from better cardiovascular fitness. Most importantly, there is an excellent research base to show that only 12 minutes a week exercise is needed to achieve this.

What this means is that cardiovascular fitness *is the same thing* as mitochondrial fitness. Getting fit is actually about supplying the right stimulus to mitochondria to get them geared up to speed and to increase their numbers. If the mitochondria can supply the energy, then the muscle can work at a high level and maintain that. There is a virtuous circle:

> *better cardiovascular fitness → increased numbers of mitochondria → better mitochondrial fitness and better mitochondrial fitness → better muscle power → better cardiovascular fitness, and then we return to the start of our circle . . .*

But the important point about lactic acid is that it provides a powerful stimulus to our energy supply system. Lactic acid stimulates mitochondria to grow and divide and mitochondria make up 20 per cent of muscle weight and 25 per cent of the weight of the heart. More mitochondria mean bigger muscles (each heart cell has 2,000–3,000 mitochondria occupying most of the cell). Big muscles mean lots of mitochondria, which means good cardiovascular fitness. I think this explains why CFS sufferers do not have obvious muscle wasting though they should because they are obliged to rest. However, they constantly switch into anaerobic metabolism with the production of lactic acid and this helps maintain numbers of mitochondria.

Pattern of recovery – cautionary note

Before any type of exercise is tried, one must be sure that one is at the right stage of recovery for this to be commenced. Please read these various stages *carefully*:

Stage 1 – Windows of improvement

You start to see windows of time when you feel better (but cannot do more). These may just be a few hours initially, or a day or two. At this stage, do not be tempted to do more activity – that will just postpone your recovery and complicate things. The trouble is the very personality that often gets people into CFS does not help them to get out of it. Many CFS sufferers have a little devil on their shoulder that beats them up every time they try to rest.

Stage 2 – Feel fine, doing nothing

The sufferer must feel completely well whilst doing absolutely nothing. The reason why it is so important to get to this stage is because that is the best test of how the body is functioning. The blood test for a cell-free DNA is a measure of tissue damage and this (cell-free DNA) is potentially a disease-amplifying process. The reason for this is that when there is lots of cellular debris swilling around the body, the immune system makes antibodies against it and this has the potential to set up either allergies or possibly autoimmunity. When there is lots of immune activity there is excessive production of free radicals and this puts an extra stress on the antioxidant system. The bottom line is that feeling ill puts a great stress on the body, energy is expended uselessly in coping with this stress and the whole business of recovery is further delayed.

Stage 3 – Feel fine doing nothing every day

This stage is arrived at when you feel absolutely fine doing absolutely nothing (and of course this never really happens in true life because life has a habit of getting in the way) *and* this level of wellness is maintained for some days or, even better, weeks. That is to say, your level of wellbeing becomes established, more robust and less susceptible to the fluctuations of everyday life. Suddenly you start to have a future and your horizons expand. Then you can move into stage 4 . . .

Stage 4 – Activity programme

IT IS ABSOLUTELY ESSENTIAL THAT STAGE 3 HAS BEEN REACHED BEFORE ATTEMPTING THIS. Carefully start a very gradual graded activity programme. The deal is that you are allowed to increase your activity, which may be mental or physical, on the grounds that you feel fine the next day. I do not mind people feeling tired at the end of the day – that is physiological and helps you to have a good night's sleep. However, if the fatigue is delayed and so you wake up the next morning feeling exhausted as a result of the previous day's exertions, then you have overdone things and must pull back. **IT IS ESSENTIAL THAT YOU LISTEN and DO PULL BACK – OTHERWISE YOU RISK A RELAPSE AND RETURNING TO AN EARLIER STAGE OF THE PROCESS.**

This explains why there is no standard activity programme to follow because however much you can or cannot do depends entirely on how you feel. I suppose one way around this would be to do daily blood tests for cell-free DNA, but this would be rather impractical.

So long as you continue to feel well and do not get delayed fatigue then the graded activity programme can be continued. But always go very gradually so as not to risk the gains that have been made.

However, during all this time it is *very* important to hold the whole regime of diet, sleep, supplements, pacing, detoxing or whatever in place.

Stage 5 – A programme of exercise that increases the number of mitochondria

Once you get to a stage where you feel well all the time, and activity levels are acceptable, then you can start to do exercises. **AGAIN, DO NOT ATTEMPT THIS UNTIL STAGE 4 HAS BEEN WELL ESTABLISHED, OTHERWISE, A RELAPSE MAY BE A RISK. And again, IT IS ESSENTIAL THAT YOU LISTEN and DO PULL BACK** if necessary. These exercises are now detailed below.

So what sort of exercise?

To increase muscle bulk and improve cardiovascular fitness one needs to do the right sort of exercise.

- The exercise has to be very slow but powerful – this prevents damage to muscles and joints.
- The window of time to exercise a group of muscles needs to be 45–90 seconds.
- At the end of this window, the muscles being worked must be burning with lactic acid and weak – that is to say, the exercise cannot be sustained any longer. This provides the maximum stimulus for improved energy supply (and therefore cardiovascular fitness) and enlarging muscles. Since over half of muscle weight is mitochondria, big muscles mean more mitochondria. What makes muscles fatigue is not lack of muscle filaments, but inability to supply energy to them. When body builders show off their muscles, actually they are showing off their mitochondria!
- Only do this once – repeating the exercise just causes muscle damage.
- After exercising a group of muscles, they must be rested for a week. This allows time for healing and repair to upgrade mitochondria and make more of them.
- There is no gain to be had by repeating these exercises more often than once a week – the heart and mitochondria only need one good kick

to upgrade their performance. Indeed, repeat exercises are likely to be counter-productive by causing too much tissue damage.
- It really is a case of 'no pain, no gain', but the good news is that with correct exercise the pain is only short lived.

Indeed, I use the above techniques of exercise to keep my horses fit. Once a week they go for a jolly ride, warm up, and towards the end of the ride they gallop a mile up a gradually increasing slope. They love this gallop, I never have to ask them to go faster, they always give 100 per cent and race each other up the hill. At the top they can barely walk and are puffing and blowing. My mare Louisa is the fastest horse on the team-chasing circuit, winning the 2016 National Intermediate speed championship competition as lead horse.

What are the actual exercises?

(Thank you to my friend Daniel Gray for putting together these exercises which require no special equipment.)

Arms and upper body – do press-ups

Depending on how strong you are, choose an appropriate starting position and then go from there, down the following list, as you get stronger:

- Start with standing upright facing a wall, feet apart, one stride away from the wall. Put your arms out with hands against the wall; then, keeping your body straight, bend your arms so your nose nearly touches the wall and push yourself back upright again.
- Do the same against a solid table – that is, with your body at 45 degrees to the ground, so that your arms are pushing against the top of the table.
- Lying on your front, do 'lazy' press-ups, keeping your knees on the floor but body straight as you push your hands against the floor.
- Do full press-ups from the toes.
- Do full press-ups with a weight (e.g. small rucksack) on your back.

Allow a 45–90 second window of time; this should be filled by 15–25 press-ups. Then rest until the lactic burn has gone.

Legs and lower back – use squats

Depending on how strong you are, choose an appropriate starting position and then go from there, down the following list as you get stronger:

- Use your legs to squat from haunches on ankles to standing upright. Keep your back straight at all times. Always hold onto something solid to keep your balance while doing this. Again choose an appropriate starting position:
  - Hold onto a firm object with your arms – for example, a chair each side to help a little and to balance. Do not go down fully onto your haunches but just bend knees to 90 degrees.
  - As above, but go lower using your arms to help a little.
  - As above, but with no help from your arms. Just hold a chair or table for balance.
  - Drop down to haunches with each squat.
  - Carry a weight on your back in a rucksack (this is the only piece of equipment you need).

Again, allow a 45–90 second window of time; this should be filled by 15–25 squats. Then rest until the lactic burn has gone.

Tummy muscles – sit-ups

Depending on how strong you are, choose an appropriate starting position and then go from there, down the following list as you get stronger. The key point to remember here is that the back must be flexed throughout this exercise – do not go flat to the floor or this will straighten the back and stress the intervertebral discs so you risk popping one out!

- Sit on the floor, knees bent to 90 degrees, shoulders and back rounded forwards almost in a foetal position and toes tucked under a solid piece of furniture – a sofa or large armchair is ideal. Put a large cushion behind you so you cannot lie flat on the floor.
- Keep your back rounded, tip backwards rotating on your hips until your tummy muscles pull, then sit up.
- Do the same, each time going further back until your shoulder blades touch the cushion, then sit up again. I repeat, do NOT go completely flat.
- Do the same but with your arms clasped behind your head.
- Do the same with a weight clasped onto your chest.
- Increase the weight.

If at any time you get back pain, then stop – it may be because you are not rounding your back sufficiently and putting strain on your intervertebral discs and psoas muscles. Again allow 45–90 seconds. This window of time should be filled by 15–25 sit ups. Then rest until the lactic burn has gone.

Back and extensor neck muscles – forward bends from the hips

Depending on how strong you are, choose an appropriate starting position and then go from there, down the following list as you get stronger. For this exercise, your back must be in the opposite shape compared to sit-ups. It must be arched or extended – again this is to prevent pressure on the intervetebral discs and stop them popping out with the pressure.

- Keep your back arched at all times – again all the movement should come from your hips.
- Keep your legs straight – you may feel slight pulling down your hamstrings as you bend.
- Don't pause between bends to relieve the lactic acid burn – keep the pain slowly increasing.
- Just bend to 90 degrees.
- Bend further.
- Do the same with your hands clasped above your head.
- Do the same with a weighted rucksack on your back.
- Move the rucksack higher so it lies between your shoulders and neck.

Again, allow 45–90 seconds. This window of time should be filled by 15–25 forward bends. Then rest until the lactic burn has gone.

Conclusion

The CFS/ME sufferer must observe the following:

- Do the 'to your limit' exercises once a week to increase your numbers of mitochondria and improve cardiovascular fitness.
- Do very gentle daily mobilisation exercises to put every joint and muscle through its full range of movement to stay supple.
- Anything else should be done, whenever you like, for pure fun in such a way that you do not risk injury or exhaust the system or develop delayed fatigue. For me this is my daily walk with my adored Patterdale terrier, Nancy. [Editor's note: Local rabbits should watch out on these daily walks!]

APPENDIX 3

Record keeping

Craig Robinson

Weekly activity sheet for pacing and keeping records

There are many ways of keeping records to help with pacing. Here is one such low-tech way:

Produce a handwritten spreadsheet with 7 rows and 12 columns as shown in the example on page 310. Each column represents one hour and each row is a day.

This spreadsheet enables you to record seven days' worth of activity versus rest.

It is obviously a bit rough and ready but this is how it can work.

The 12 boxes across the page are for a waking day – say 12 hours. You could split this into smaller time intervals (for example, quarters of an hour). You can vary this to suit your situation.

When you rest – and this means doing absolutely nothing for most of that hour – colour that hour's box with a yellow highlighter.

When you do a cognitive activity (such as reading, watching TV or listening to the radio) for the majority of an hour, colour that hour's box with a blue highlighter.

When you do a physical activity (such as sitting in the garden) for the majority of an hour, colour that hour's box with a green highlighter.

Then, as the month comes to a close, you can get a very quick idea of how much time was spent doing each type of activity and how much time was spent resting.

One important point is that if you increase activity hours by *one* hour then, by definition for that day, you reduce resting hours by *one* hour too and so then the difference between them increases by *two* hours. So doing an extra hour has more of an effect than you might imagine as you are both doing more and also have less time to recover from that level of increased activity.

Figure A3.1, page 310, is an example of a weekly activity sheet, with divisions for quarter of an hour slots of activity / rest.

> *'When you wake up in the morning, Pooh,' said Piglet at last, 'what's the first thing you say to yourself?'*
> *'What's for breakfast?' said Pooh. 'What do you say, Piglet?'*
> *'I say, I wonder what's going to happen exciting today?' said Piglet.*
> *Pooh nodded thoughtfully. 'It's the same thing,' he said.*
>
> AA Milne in *Winnie-the-Pooh*

Page-to-a-day diary record of activities, protocol compliance, diet and symptoms

There are many ways of keeping a daily record of diet, activity, symptoms and protocol compliance. Here is one possible method:

- Buy a 'page-to-a-day' diary and divide each page into rough quarters.
- Then each day record as follows:

Top left – food eaten and drinks drunk. So a typical entry might be 'Full English breakfast'

Top right – supplements taken. You will know what regime you are on and so usually this takes the form of anything 'new' you are trying or anything you forgot to take that day. So, a typical entry might be 'Started pregnelone at 25 mg' or 'Forgot to inject magnesium'

Bottom right – activities. This will vary from sufferer to sufferer. For some, a typical entry might be 'Managed to get to the toilet unaided' or 'Washed my hair' whereas for others a typical entry might be 'Went to theatre to see *The Small Hand*'. Include here a record of last night's sleep.

Day/Hour	7–8				8–9				9–10				10–11				11–12			
Sunday																				
Monday																				
Tuesday																				
Wednesday																				
Thursday																				
Friday																				
Saturday																				

Figure A3.1. Weekly activity record sheet. This example is for a CFS sufferer waking at 7.00 am and retiring at 7.00 pm.

Bottom left – symptoms. So a typical entry might be, 'Lower calf muscles burny' or 'Weepy'.

- Then, write a very brief review at the end of every week, summing up how you feel that week has been, compared with a kind of subjective 'rolling average' at the current time.
- In addition, at the front of the diary keep a list of 'positives', that is, times when you felt happy. So, a typical entry here might be 'Really enjoyed going to see Wycombe Wanderers play' or 'Had a good chat with my daughter'.
- When you feel below par physically, look over these records for:

Am I doing too much? (activity corner)

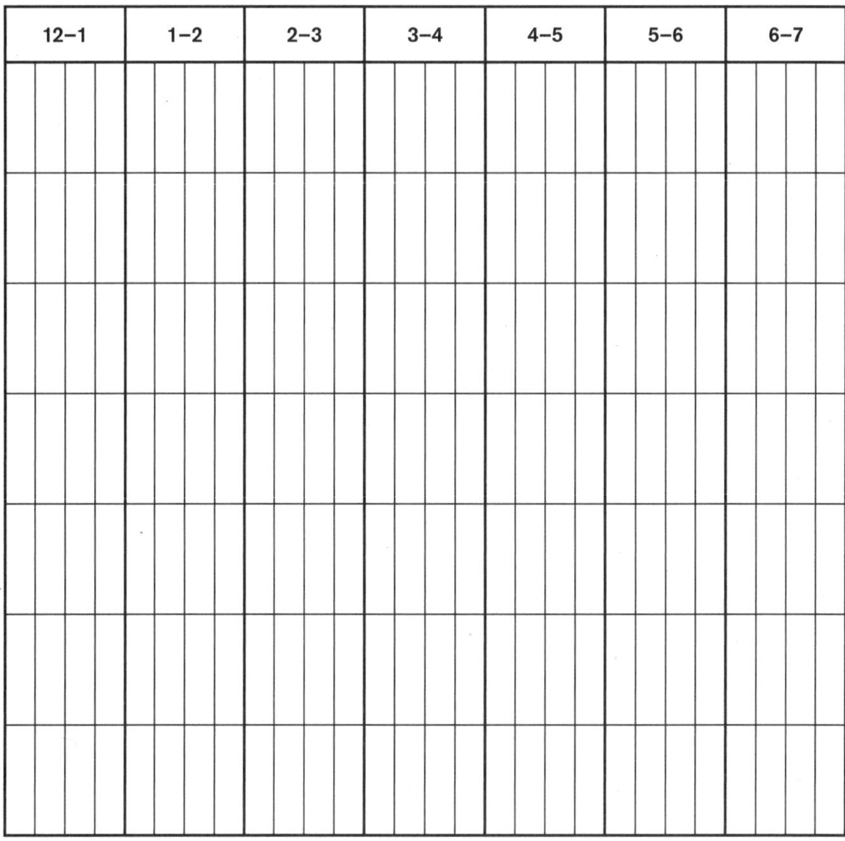

12–1	1–2	2–3	3–4	4–5	5–6	6–7

Am I not sleeping enough? (activity corner)
Am I eating the wrong stuff/ or have I started eating something new? (food/drink corner)
Have I lapsed on the protocol? (supplements corner)

- When you feel below par physically *and* emotionally, do as above *plus* read through all the positives or times when you felt happy at the front of the diary – sometimes look at last year's positives and happy times too – and try to pick one such positive or happy time and relive it in your mind. These tactics will help to ascertain why you are feeling below par and also give an idea as to how to deal with it both via changes to supplement intake, diet and activity levels and also emotionally by remembering that your life has good things in it too.

APPENDIX 4

Chemicals that can switch on CFS/ME and multiple chemical sensitivity

The chemicals which in my clinical practice I have seen switch on CFS/ME and multiple chemical sensitivity are pesticides, VOCs and heavy metals.

Pesticides

Pesticides include organophosphates (OPs), organochlorines, glyphosate, synthetic pyrethroids and formaldehyde. These can derive from sources and activities such as those listed below:

- sheep dipping
- spraying agricultural chemicals (farming, market gardening)
- being sprayed by tractor or helicopter and spray drift (adjacent homes)
- insect control 'squeeta betas' (a system for spraying pesticides from a motorised vehicle)
- contamination of water supplies
- working in a chicken farm (fumigation, control of parasites)
- working in the sea with factory-farmed salmon in Scotland (where chemicals are used to control fish lice)
- repeated head lice treatments
- house fumigations for flea control or bed bugs

- insect control in hot countries with DDT, OPs, etc
- control of sand flies (Gulf War syndrome)
- greenhouse fumigations
- working in a research plant centre where chemicals were weekly used to prevent cross contamination
- high school student doing a biology project with pesticides
- carpet factory where fleeces are washed after sheep have been dipped
- lorry driver delivering OPs to farmers
- government inspectors in sheep markets
- dairy farmers daily exposed to OPs for fly control in the milking parlour
- poisoning through exposure to dumped cans of sheep dip
- welders working in a factory which was manufacturing OPs
- timber treatments in houses
- handling treated timbers
- treatment of external parasites in dogs, cats, cows (OP pour-ons) and so on
- firefighters poisoned by burning chemicals
- formaldehyde leaking from cavity wall insulation
- flower industry (lots of chemicals on flowers)
- airline pilots exposed to OPs used in engine oils (which allow oils to work at high temperatures) – see www.aerotoxic.org
- cabin staff on airplanes using pesticides to prevent inadvertent import of foreign insects
- DDT used to treat infestations (possibly misdiagnosed as polio)

Volatile organic compounds (VOCs)

This is poisoning from un-burnt hydrocarbons such as oil, gas, coal and wood. Free-standing gas heaters are a particular hazard. These poisonings go under the misnomer 'carbon monoxide poisoning'.* Actually the carbon monoxide is just

---

* **Historical Note:** This is not an exclusively modern problem. See 'The carbon monoxide poisoning of two Byzantine emperors'.[69] I suspect that the misnomer of 'CO poisoning' is being used again here. This paper concludes:

> *In this paper, two possible cases of acute carbon monoxide poisoning previously not identified in the medical and historical literature are discussed. The first concerns the famous Byzantine Emperor Julian the Apostate, who may have suffered mild carbon monoxide poisoning from which he quickly and completely recovered. The*

a small part of the problem. Yes – this certainly causes acute symptoms, but the long-term poisoning arises from the toxic VOCs from unburnt hydrocarbons.

- Aerotoxic syndrome – this arises because cabin air is pulled in over the engines and possibly contaminated with unburnt fuel and OPs used as oil improvers. (See www.aerotoxic.com)
- Vehicle exhaust fumes
- Solvents used in carpets – new carpets are particularly pernicious. This together with poor ventilation is probably the main cause of sick building syndrome.
- Paints
- Glues
- Printing inks
- Cleaning agents – bleach
- Disinfectants – these often include formaldehyde or other such related compounds.
- Sterilising agents – e.g. 'Milton'
- Perfumes
- Cosmetics – many are toxic, especially hair dyes.

Heavy metals

- Mercury from dental amalgam is the biggest single heavy metal problem.
- Nickel we often see blocking biological enzymes (commonly from stainless steel saucepans, and from jewellery). Nickel is a problem because it 'looks' like zinc. Zinc deficiency is very common in people eating Western diets, and so if the body needs zinc and it is not there, it will use look-alike nickel instead, but nickel does not do the job and, indeed, gets in the way of normal biochemistry.
- Vaccinations are a mixture of heavy metals with viral/bacterial particles and I see many cases of ME following vaccination.
- Lead, cadmium, antimony, arsenic.
- Depleted uranium in Gulf War veterans.

---

second case involves his successor, Jovian, who may have succumbed to severe carbon monoxide poisoning. Both cases were in all likelihood due to the burning of coal in braziers, a usual method of indoor heating during that epoch.

APPENDIX 5

How to reduce your chemical exposures

Do a good chemical clean-up: chemicals make you fat and fatigued

We live in an increasingly polluted world containing an increasing number of chemicals which are toxic to our genes, to our brains, to our internal metabolism and to our immune system. These nasty chemicals almost certainly account for our ever increasing incidence of cancer and birth defects and our declining fertility due to lifetime exposure. I believe they also make us more susceptible to CFS because they are toxic to the immune system, to the brain, to our hormonal control and to our internal metabolism. All these systems are implicated in CFS, as discussed throughout this book.

It is impossible to completely avoid every chemical; if I did blood tests I would find a wide range of organochlorine pesticides in everybody. However, anything which can be done to reduce the chemical load will be helpful in allowing our bodies to recover.

I was very interested by a book published in 2002 called *The Detox Diet* by Dr Paula Baillie-Hamilton which explains how chemicals in foods and the air interfere with internal metabolism to make us fat and lethargic – indeed, she points out that farm animals are deliberately fed hormones, antibiotics and pesticides to make them fat and lethargic, and therefore they do not have to eat so much in order to put on weight (cheap meat!).[70] Many chemicals are persistent and become concentrated as they move up through the food chain

– it is very likely that if we were the farm animal then we would be declared too toxic to eat; we are right at the top of the food chain and so we have accumulated more toxins than most species. I suspect the mechanism of this has to do with metabolic syndrome and insulin resistance.

The issues listed below need to be addressed to reduce your chemical exposure.

Foods

- Find the best quality food you can afford.
- If organic food is available, go for it. Organise a regular, delivered, organic food box.
- Eat foods as unprocessed as possible – most foods in tins or packages contain preservatives or have been irradiated.
- Eat foods which have not been plastic-wrapped – the plasticiser gets into the food.
- Avoid foods wrapped in aluminium foil, or in aluminium cans.
- Eat fresh foods – if they have to be stored, deep freezing is probably the least harmful.
- Contact the Soil Association (www.soilassociation.org) or Henry Doubleday Research Association, now known as Garden Organic (www.gardenorganic.org.uk).

Water

- A clean water supply is essential. The water companies are largely interested in bacterial counts, but there are many possible chemicals in water. The two I have most concerns over are fluoride and chloramine (see the Chloramine Information Center here chloramineinfocenter.com for details of problems with chloramine.) I consider bottled (ideally in glass) or filtered water an essential for regular use.
- The terms 'Natural Mineral Water', 'Spring Water' and the labelling of 'Bottled Water' are all legally defined in England in 'The Natural Mineral Water, Spring Water and Bottled Drinking Water (England) Regulations 2007 (as amended)'.[71] As a rough guide, check the labels and be especially careful with products marked 'Bottled Water' – these can come from a variety of sources, including municipal supplies.
- Perhaps remember the words of Pliny the Elder:

. . . waters vary with the land over which they flow
and the juices of the plants they wash . . .

PLINY THE ELDER (23 AD – 25 August 79 AD)

Clean air

- If you can smell it, it can make you ill. The olfactory nerve in the nose responsible for smell is a direct extension of the brain. If you can smell something then the chemical is in your brain. The obvious offenders are air fresheners, sprays, perfumes and cleaning agents but there are a host of other chemicals also in everyday use.
- New paints and carpets (especially rubber-backed, stuck down) give out toxic fumes for months after being installed; use water-based paints wherever possible.
- Pesticides – dog and cat flea treatments, fly repellents, house fumigations and timber treatments all contain toxic pesticides which persist for months and even years.
- Gas central heating and gas cookers can trigger multiple chemical sensitivity in the susceptible.
- Carbon monoxide poisoning can present with CFS.

Occupational exposures

Occupational exposures are described in Appendix 4 (page 312).

Cosmetics

Nearly all deodorants contain aluminium, which, when applied to skin, especially warm sweaty areas, is readily absorbed. Aluminium is extremely toxic and has a known association with Alzheimer's disease. Perfumes and 'smellies' can be a real problem, especially with multiple chemical sensitivity. Read the report prepared by The Campaign for Safe Cosmetics entitled 'Not So Sexy: The Health Risks of Secret Chemicals in Fragrance'.[72]

Garden chemicals

Many of these are extremely toxic. Children should not be allowed to play on treated lawns for at least six weeks after spraying.

Drugs

Most CFS/ME sufferers know that alcohol makes them feel awful. This is also true of many prescription drugs, such as beta blockers, antidepressants, cholesterol drugs, diuretics and hypnotics. If prescribed, first ask the question 'Why? Does this address the underlying mechanism that is causing my health problems?' (For more on this see my book *Sustainable Medicine.*) Any drug should be tried with great caution. Many prescription drugs are detoxified in the liver so these add to the total chemical load the liver has to deal with.

Many head lice treatments contain pesticides. Lice can be easily controlled with wet combing or electric 'zappers' though it does take a fair amount of time and persistence, especially if hair is long.

Outdoor air pollution

Many industries discharge pollutants directly into the local air, water and soil. The worst offenders are power stations which burn toxic waste, manufacturing industry, nuclear power stations leaking radiation and the chemical industry. Busy roads create traffic fumes. Nasty chemicals are dumped at toxic waste sites where they pollute ground water and soil. You need local knowledge to identify these issues. For further information go to Friends of the Earth (www.foe.co.uk). Ask specifically about:

- Heavy metals – arsenic, cadmium, nickel, copper, lead, aluminium, etc
- Radioactive waste
- Pesticide residues – organochlorines and dioxins, organophosphates, pyrethroids, etc
- Small particulate matter – many polluting industries hide their waste by discharging it in such small particles that they cannot be seen. These PM1 particles, or smaller, cannot be filtered out by the nose and bronchi but pass directly into the lungs and are well absorbed into the bloodstream. PM1 particles are much more dangerous than PM10. We now have problems with nanoparticles that are even worse.
- Volatile organic compounds (VOCs) – solvents, benzene compounds
- Polluting gasses – SOx, NOx, COx, that is, sulphur, nitrogen and carbon compounds

APPENDIX 6

Studies showing that viral infection is a major cause of post-viral CFS

Dr Lerner worked for over 25 years researching and treating, primarily, post-viral CFS. In 2007 the CFS Foundation was set up as a repository for all his published work and also as a mechanism to conduct a major new study, bringing together all of his papers into one definitive report. This definitive report took 18 months to complete and looked at Dr Lerner's studies and papers since 1993. A bullet point précis of that report is reproduced below.

The CFS Foundation officially closed in 2011 but maintains a website complete with all of Dr Lerner's work and studies – please see: www.treatmentcenterforcfs.com/CFS_Foundation.

Please see in particular the section on CFS publications: www.treatmentcenterforcfs.com/cfs_publications/index.html, which lists Dr Lerner's 15 published studies on CFS, along with 3 other publications. Some of these papers are discussed in more detail following.

Dr Lerner's definitive study, 2010[73]

Bullet-point précis of definitive study

- EBV was causally involved in 81 per cent of the CFS cases studied, sometimes with human cytomegalovirus (HCMV) or human herpes virus 6 (HHV-6) as co-infections.
- EBV-CFS was effectively treated with long-term valacyclovir.
- Dr Lerner used the validated Energy Index Point Score® (EIPS) to monitor the severity of CFS cases in this study.

There are many ability scales for CFS – some are linear while others are exponential or sigmoidal ('S-shaped') in nature. The choice of scale used has a lot to do with what outcomes and physiological markers you are measuring. I use the one developed by Dr Bell – see Appendix 10, page 344.

Four studies showing that long-term antivirals work

Dr Lerner showed that the Epstein-Barr virus could be treated effectively with the anti-viral valacyclovir and that if there is co-infection with HCMV or HHV-6 then some trials used valgancyclovir in addition to the valacyclovir. He reported good responses to treatment.

Below are details of four studies using this combination of drugs; all reported long-term patient improvements. In these groups, between 10 and 25 per cent of patients required full-dosage, long-term therapy to maintain an EIPS value of more than 7. Valacyclovir has been continued for seven years in patients without ill effects. Dr Lerner commented that patients appreciated the good prognostic omen of an early Herxsheimer response to drug treatment.

Study 1, 2002[74]

Basic summary

Valacyclovir works well for CFS patients who have high titres (test results) to EBV but not as well for CFS patients who have high titres to both EBV and HCMV.

Bullet-point précis

- The design of the study was to determine the safety and efficacy of a six-month trial of valacyclovir.

Table A6.1. Dr Lerner's Energy Index Point Score. (Note: this is very different from the one I use – the Bell disability score)

CHRONIC FATIGUE SYNDROME	
0	Bedridden, up to bathroom only
1	Out of bed 30–60 minutes a day (sitting in chair is out of bed)
2	Out of bed sitting, standing, walking 1–2 hours per day
3	Out of bed sitting, standing, walking 2–4 hours per day
4	Out of bed sitting, standing, walking 4–6 hours per day
5	Perform with difficulty sedentary job 40 hours a week, daily naps
RECOVERY	
6	Daily naps in bed, may maintain a 40-hour sedentary work week plus light, limited housekeeping or social activities
7	No naps in bed. Up 7.00 am to 9.00 pm. Able to work a sedentary job plus light housekeeping
8	Full sedentary work week, no naps, some social activities plus light exercise
9	Same as (8) above plus exercise approximately 1/2 to 2/3 normal without excessive fatigue, awakens next morning refreshed
10	Normal

- The Phase I treatment group was 10 CFS patients who met the detailed diagnostic criteria for the study, which included high titres to EBV. The control group in Phase 1 was nine CFS patients who met the detailed diagnostic criteria and who additionally had high titres to HCMV. Phase 1 patients had been ill for less than one year.
- Both the parallel treatment and control CFS groups in Phase I received valacyclovir for six months.
- In Phase II, six additional CFS patients who met the detailed diagnostic criteria (but did not have high titres to HCMV) were added. This group had been ill for a mean of 55.8 months (about five years).
- The CFS Energy Index Point Score (Table A6.1) was used to record each CFS patient's functional capacity at baseline and after one, three and six months of valacyclovir. Various other physiological measurements were taken.
- The 16 CFS patients (included in both phases of this study) who had EBV-persistent infection (but no high titres to HCMV) were improved after six months of valacyclovir treatment.
- The nine patients (Phase 1) who had high titres to CMV were not as improved after treatment with valacyclovir.

- The conclusion was that valacyclovir was a safe and efficacious treatment for CFS sufferers who had high titres to EBV but that such treatment with valacyclovir alone did not significantly improve CFS patients who additionally had high titres to HCMV.

Study 2, 2004[75]

This study aimed at addressing the patient cohort who have high titres to HCMV, as well as meeting the detailed diagnostic criteria (which includes high titres to EBV), and who do not recover well with valacyclovir treatment alone.

Basic summary

Valacyclovir and valgancyclovir used together work well for CFS patients who have high titres to both EBV and HCMV.

Bullet-point précis

- Patients initially were treated with just valacyclovir, but after six months those patients with co-infection were also given valgancyclovir.
- Many physiological and other measurements were taken, including the CFS Energy Index Point Score (EIPS) and also a 'symptom score'. The CFS Energy Index Point and symptoms scores were taken at 30-day intervals for 18 months.
- There were 11 CFS patients who received treatment and the control group consisted of 21 (mainly CFS) patients.
- Higher symptom scores indicate the presence of more symptoms, with a score of 1.0 being the highest.
- At baseline, the mean symptom score was 0.81 for the 11-patient cohort receiving treatment. When assessed six months after initiation of treatment with intravenous valgancyclovir, this cohort of 11 patients had a mean symptom score of 0.38. At month 12 of the study, the mean cumulative symptom score was 0.28, and at month 18, the mean symptom score was 0.19.
- The conclusion of the study was that the use of valacyclovir and valgancyclovir together, reduces symptom severity in CFS patients who have chronic viral presences of both EBV and CMV.

Study 3, 2007[76]

Basic summary

Valacyclovir works well in an EBV subset of CFS patients.

Bullet-point précis

- The hypothesis of this study was that there is a subset of CFS patients whose illness has a chronic infection of EBV as its cause.
- Group 1 patients consisted of the EBV subset of CFS patients.
- Group 2 patients were CFS patients who did not belong to the EBV subset.
- After six months, Group 1 CFS patients receiving valacyclovir experienced an increased mean EIPS point score of 1.12, while the Group 1 placebo cohort experienced an increased EIPS point score of 0.42.
- Some patients resumed normal activities from Group 1.
- Group 2 patients had increased EIPS but at lower levels.
- The conclusion was that valacyclovir administration in the EBV subset improved recovery rates.

Study 4, 2010[77]

Basic summary

Valacyclovir works very well on an EBV subset of CFS patients. Valacyclovir and valgancyclovir used together work well on an EBV/HCMV/HHV6 subset of CFS patients.

Bullet-point précis

- The hypothesis of this study was that CFS is caused by single or multiple Epstein-Barr virus (EBV), and co-infection with cytomegalovirus (HCMV) or human herpes virus 6 (HHV6) infection.
- To determine this cause, long-term subset-directed valacyclovir or valganciclovir was administered to two groups of patients.
- Group A patients (106 patients) had no co-infections (EBV only).
- Group B patients (36 patients) did have co-infections. (EBV and HCMV and HHV6).
- Data were collected at physician visits every 4 to 6 weeks from these 142 CFS patients at one clinic from 2001 to 2007.
- To be included in this study, patients had to be followed for at least six months.
- The data captured included over 7,000 patient visits and over 35,000 fields of information.
- The Group A CFS patients (no co-infections) returned to a near-normal to normal life.
- The long-term EIPS value increased with subset-directed long-term valacyclovir or valgancyclovir therapy.

- Secondary endpoints (cardiac, immunologic and neurocognitive abnormalities) improved or disappeared.
- Group B CFS patients (herpes virus plus coinfections), although improved, continued to have CFS.

Conclusion

The treatment regimes trialled in these studies work well. Treatment with long-term valacyclovir used to be an expensive therapy. Dr Lerner's costing for valacyclovir tablets for 1 gram every six hours was of the order 25–30,000 USD per year. The cost has recently come down significantly because the patent has run out. I can now obtain 42 valacyclovir at 500 mg for £22.20 (April 2016). This gives a monthly cost of around £133.20. Valgancyclovir remains costly at present. There is no doubt that valacyclovir is a very useful treatment for a subset of patients. My recommendation at present is to reserve this for those who do not respond to the standard nutritional work-ups.

APPENDIX 7

Overview of the entire protocol

The energy equation

Fatigue is the symptom we perceive when energy demand exceeds energy delivery. This is the all-important energy equation that dominates the management of CFS/ME. It is attention to both sides of this equation that will deliver a result clinically. This equation is easily summarised as:

Available energy = Energy delivery *minus* Energy demand

CFS occurs when energy demand chronically outstrips energy delivery.
ME occurs when we have CFS *plus* inflammation.

Table A7.1. The energy **delivery** side of the equation

Fuel in the tank	Diet, hypoglycaemia, micronutrients and gut function	Chapter 6 – Diet the whys? Chapter 17 – Diet the bare essentials Chapter 18 – Basic Package of nutritional supplement Chapter 7 – The fermenting gut
Regular servicing	Sleep	Chapter 16 – Sleep
The engine	Mitochondria	Chapter 4 – It's mitochondria, not hypochondria
Oxygen and fuel delivery	Heart, lung, blood supply	Appendix 1– Tests
Accelerator pedal	Thyroid gland	Chapter 5 – The thyroid
Gear box	Adrenal gland	Chapter 5 – The adrenal glands
Exhaust system	Liver, kidney, detoxing	Appendix 1 – Tests Chapter 20 – Detoxing
The driver of the car	The brain – to keep the energy equation in credit	Chapter 15 – Pacing

Table A7.2. The energy **demand** side of the equation

Normal energy expenditure: Housekeeping duties Physical activity Mental activity	Basic metabolism: heart, gut, liver, kidney, lung, hormonal function	Chapter 8 – Basal metabolism
Wasteful energy expenditure: Immunological holes	Inflammation for healing and repair	Chapter 15 – Pacing Chapter 9 – General anti-inflammatory treatments
	Inflammation from acute infection	Chapter 19 – Avoid infection
	Inflammation from chronic bacterial infection	Chapter 12 – Lyme disease and co-infections
	Inflammation from chronic viral infection	Chapter 11 – Treating chronic viral infection Appendix 6 – Ditto
	Useless inflammation in allergy and autoimmunity	Chapter 10 – Allergy and autoimmunity Chapter 13 – Reprogramming the immune system
Emotional holes		Chapter 21 – The emotional holes in the energy bucket

Table A7.3. If you have no time or energy just go to these sections of the book

Which tests to start off with	Appendix 1 – Tests
What to eat	Chapter 17 – Paleo-ketogenic diet
Which supplements to take	Chapter 18 – The Basic Package and The Bolt-on-Extras The mitochondria package The healing and repair package The detox package
Get off to sleep	Chapter 16 – Sleep
You must pace	Chapter 15 – Pacing
Get help and money	Appendix 9 – Help, welfare benefits . . . Appendix 10 – . . . and support
Then you will have some energy . . .	. . . to read the rest of the book!

APPENDIX 8

Growing your own probiotics

Let medicine be thy food and food be thy medicine.

HIPPOCRATES (c. 460 BC – c. 375 BC)

Probiotics have many health benefits and indeed people who eat them live longer. Those health benefits include:

- protection from infection
- protection from the fermenting gut
- normal immune programming
- protection from constipation
- improved absorption of micronutrients

The best results of probiotics come from live cultures. The joy of this is that they can be easily and inexpensively grown at home on a range of substrates. Different people are suited to different cultures and substrates and so there is much scope for trial and error. The two that I most commonly use are kefir grown on soya or coconut milk, or *Lactobacillus rhamnosus* grown on the same – this microbe has been used to switch off allergy. For those who are interested in this immune switching off ability, please see www.doctormyhill.co.uk/wiki/Oral_immunotherapy:_switching_off_food_allergies_using_food.

The joy of using live microbes is that one culture can last a lifetime. Because dairy products are not evolutionarily correct foods, kefir should be grown on non-dairy foods such as soya milk or coconut milk.

How to grow live cultures

Start off with one litre of, say, long-life soya milk in a jug, add the kefir sachet, keep warm (22–23 degrees Centigrade). Within 12–24 hours it should have a semi-solid, junket-like consistency. Do not expect it to look like commercial yoghurt, which has often been thickened artificially.

Store the culture in the fridge, where it ferments further. This slower fermentation seems to improve the texture and flavour. However, it can be used at once as a substitute in any situation where you would otherwise use cream or custard. I often add a lump of creamed coconut (for the recipe, see my cookbook) which further feeds the kefir, imparts a delicious coconut flavour and thickens the culture.

Once the jug is nearly empty, add another litre of soya milk, stir it in and away you go again. I don't even bother to wash up the jug – the slightly hard yellow bits on the edge I just stir in to restart the brew. This way the kefir culture lasts for life.

Stir in ground almonds or other ground-up nuts or seeds which absorb fluid and thicken the culture. Delicious! I use kefir to swallow my daily vitamins and minerals – this keeps it turning over so I do not forget to use it; otherwise it might go off by mistake.

APPENDIX 9

Sources of support

These are sources of support that members of the two Facebook support groups (listed below) have found useful.

1. CFS/ME specific support organisations

The list that follows is far from exhaustive and is intended to give readers a 'starting guide' as to where to look for information and support on CFS/ME-related issues. These issues could, for example, include advocacy, help with welfare benefits or general information on possible causes of and treatments for CFS/ME. In addition, there is a significant bias towards UK organisations as this is the geographical location of the vast majority of my CFS patients.

Two Dr Myhill 'support' Facebook groups

Support Dr Sarah Myhill

Website: www.facebook.com/groups/108048875899603
Number of members – approximately 3,180 (May 2016)

ADMINS OF GROUP
Kathryn Lloyd – ACTIVE ADMIN
Craig Robinson – ACTIVE ADMIN
(Ruth Myhill – SLEEPING ADMIN)
(Jo Chamberlain – SLEEPING ADMIN)
(Nadine Hooper – SLEEPING ADMIN)
(Isaac Segal – SLEEPING ADMIN)

History: This group was set up by Jo Chamberlain in April 2010. It is a support group for patients but it is an *open* group and so posts can be seen by all users of Facebook. It is now a forum where patients can discuss issues arising from following Dr Myhill's protocol and also where the admins post new items of interest as Dr Myhill develops her protocol further.

Support for followers of Dr Myhill's protocol

Website: www.facebook.com/groups/435645003161721
Number of members – approximately 2,130 (May 2016)

ADMINS OF GROUP

Kathryn Lloyd – ACTIVE ADMIN
Craig Robinson – ACTIVE ADMIN
(Isaac Segal – SLEEPING ADMIN)
(Ruth Myhill – SLEEPING ADMIN)

History: This was set up jointly by Craig Robinson and Kathryn Lloyd in November 2012 as there was perceived to be a need for a forum where people could discuss the protocol and any questions they might have in a closed and more private environment – posts in this group can only be seen by other group members. It serves exactly the same purpose as the above mentioned group but does so in a 'closed' environment. Membership of either of these groups is via approval from either Craig Robinson or Kathryn Lloyd.

Dr Myhill 'support' Facebook page

Supporters of Dr Sarah Myhill

Website: www.facebook.com/pages/Supporters-of-Dr-Sarah-Myhill/230752230289407
Number of members – approximately 1,630 (May 2016)

ADMINS OF PAGE

Kathryn Lloyd – ACTIVE ADMIN
Craig Robinson – ACTIVE ADMIN

Brief description: This is a page where notices concerning Dr Myhill's website and work are posted. Also, any changes to protocol guidance are posted here. Membership of this page is via approval from either Craig Robinson or Kathryn Lloyd.

Dr Myhill Twitter feed

@Myhill News

Website: twitter.com/MyhillNews
Number of followers – approximately 1,440 (May 2016)

Brief description: This is a very useful feed to keep abreast of new developments concerning Dr Myhill's website and work, and also to be notified of any changes in protocol guidance. Craig Robinson administers this feed.

Dr Myhill official YouTube channel

Website: www.youtube.com/watch?v=NhlGM4kNIsI&list=PLJGxkcH41f8m9HwHlDor56bpd4E44fynS

Brief description: There is a collection of useful YouTubes about Dr Myhill's protocol from various media outlets. Kathryn Lloyd and Craig Robinson administer this channel.

Other recommended sources of help

25% ME Group

Address: 21 Church Street, Troon, Ayrshire KA10 6HT, UK
Tel: +44 (0)1292 318611
Advocacy helpline: +44 (0)141 570 2938
Website: www.25megroup.org

Brief description: This group is a unique and independent support group set up to help people who suffer from severe ME and to break the isolation that it brings to their lives. Their twice-yearly magazine contains a wealth of information, support and practical tips. Upon subscribing you receive a full contact list of all other members.

Action for ME

Address: PO Box 2778, Bristol BS1 9DJ, UK
Tel: +44 (0)845 123 280
Website: www.actionforme.org.uk

Brief description: Action for ME funds research. This organisation has a helpful section to assist CFS sufferers to gain benefits.

Blue Ribbon for the Awareness of ME (BRAME)

Address: 30, Winner Avenue, Winterton-on Sea, Gt Yarmouth, Norfolk NR29 4BA, UK
Tel: +44 (0)1493 393717
Website: www.brame.org

Brief description: BRAME was launched to create awareness and understanding that ME is a very real and debilitating illness and to highlight the consequences of living with ME.

Co-Cure

Website: Please go to listserv.nodak.edu/archives/co-cure.html to search the archives and sign up to receive new updates.

Brief description: This is an online resource where one could sign up to to receive email updates concerning new research and advocacy issues as they happen. Co-Cure describes itself as an information exchange forum. Subscription is free.

Get Well from ME

Website: getwellfrom.me.uk/about-me

Brief description: Giles Meehan has produced a series of YouTube clips which can be seen at this website. Many sufferers have found this to be a useful resource.

The Grace Charity for ME

Address: The Grace Charity for ME, 20 Dickens Close, Langley, Maidstone, Kent ME17 1TB, UK
Website: www.thegracecharityforme.org

Brief description: The Grace Charity has produced a variety of helpful information and in particular a (perhaps unique) *Hospital Booklet* for ME sufferers. The website is extensive and the Grace Charity makes a very positive statement of its aims on the Homepage: 'Please note: we DO NOT promote or encourage GET (Graded Exercise Therapy) or CBT (Cognitive Behavioural Therapy) for ME sufferers. Neither do we promote the Lightning Process, Mickel Therapy, or the Reverse Therapy. However, we DO PROMOTE a biomedical perspective of ME.'

The Hummingbirds' Foundation for ME (HFME)

Website: www.hfme.org

Brief description: The mission statement for this organisation is 'The HFME is dedicated to fighting for the recognition of Myalgic Encephalomyelitis based on the available scientific evidence, and for patients worldwide to be treated appropriately and accorded the same basic human rights as those with similar disabling and potentially fatal neurological diseases such as Multiple Sclerosis.' There is a wide variety of useful resources concerning illness definition and research studies, etc.

Invest in ME Research

Address: PO Box 561, Eastleigh, Hampshire SO50 0GQ, UK
Tel: +44 (0)2380 251719 or (0)7759 349743
Website: www.investinme.org

Brief description: This is an independent UK charity campaigning for biomedical research into myalgic encephalomyelitis, as described by WHO ICD 10 G93.3.

Let's Do It For ME

Website: ldifme.org

Brief description: Let's Do It for ME is a patient-led organisation that has the remit of raising funds for Invest in ME research's studies. They can be found on Facebook by searching for 'Let's Do It for ME'.

ME Alliance Northern Ireland (MEANI)

Email: Mrs McParland at joanmcparland@live.co.uk

Brief description: This is a new alliance of patient organisations in Northern Ireland.

ME Association

Address: 7 Apollo Office Court, Radclive Road, Gawcott, Bucks MK18 4DF, UK
Tel: +44 (0)1280 818964 (9.30 am to 3.00 pm)
Website: www.meassociation.org.uk

Brief description: The ME Association provides information to its members via a newsletter and funds research projects. Perhaps most useful is the very full referencing in Charles Shepherd's book, *Living with ME,* sold through the ME Association. Although some readers may find this book a little negative, it is nonetheless a good one-stop-shop for referencing material. The ME Association also provides useful leaflets on UK welfare benefits.

ME Research UK

Address: ME Research UK, The Gateway, North Methven Street, Perth PH1 5PP, UK
Tel: +44 (0)1738 451234
Website: www.meresearch.org.uk

Brief description: ME Research UK is a medical research charity based in the United Kingdom with the principal aim of commissioning and funding scientific (biomedical) investigation into the causes, consequences and treatment of CFS/ME.

ME Society of America

Website: web.archive.org/web/20140401062754/http://www.cfids-cab.org/MESA

Brief description: The ME Society of America is a research-information website that was run by Maryann Spurgin PhD until her retirement in 2007. In 2013 the website was archived and can no longer be found in a usual internet search. This statement appears on the home page of the Society's website: 'The M.E. Society of America is an organization that seeks to promote understanding of the disease known as myalgic encephalomyelitis (ME/CFS), a multi-system disease adversely affecting the cellular mitochondria and the heart, brain, neuroendocrine, immune, and circulatory systems. M.E. was first described in the 1950's following the recognition of many cases around the world, including a number of cases at the Royal Free Hospital in England. Many different viruses, bacteria, or toxins in combination with genetic factors may be involved in the etiology of the disease, which usually begins in childhood or early adulthood with an acute infection. Studying research-based subsets is the key to scientific progress in this area of investigation. In a number of publications, Dr A. Melvin Ramsay outlined a definitional framework for M.E. that described abnormal muscle metabolism, circulatory impairment, and cerebral involvement.'

ME-CFS Community.com

Website: cfsknowledgecenter.ning.com

Brief description: This is a global organisation designed to break the isolation of the illness and facilitate information exchange. New research and advocacy matters are reported.

MEActionUK

Website: www.meactionuk.org.uk

Brief description: This is an online organisation which provides advocacy information as well as some detailed papers regarding the 'politics' of ME and research into ME.

Pesticide Action Network (PAN) UK

Address: The Brighthelm Centre, North Road, Brighton BN1 1YD, UK
Tel: +44 (0)1273 964230
Website: www.pan-uk.org

Brief description: This is a useful network for those sufferers who feel that their condition was either caused by or has been worsened by pesticide exposure.

PAN UK works to replace hazardous chemical pesticides with sustainable and equitable alternatives in agriculture, urban areas, homes and gardens. It seeks change in policy and practices at home and overseas, and supports projects bringing real economic, health and environmental benefits to the developing world.

Salus Fatigue Foundation

Email: info@salus.org.uk
Tel: +44(0)121 3556853
Website: www.salus.org.uk

Brief description: This organisation says: 'At Salus we take a self-management approach, providing support, advice and education for people affected by CFS. All our services are free within our specialised centre based in the West Midlands, providing educational workshops, counselling, pacing groups, relaxation, yoga, Qi gong. We offer a closed Facebook page allowing remote support and for people who live outside the Birmingham area to have access to positive support. The Salus team, through their own personal experiences with recovery from CFS, are here to inspire and share their knowledge to help you improve your health and wellbeing.'

Stonebird

Website: www.stonebird.co.uk

Brief description: Stonebird is a web resource that seeks to share some of the experience of living with ME. The 'Stonebird' represents the idea that you don't have to do anything to be of beauty and value in the world. The site has information and comments about matters relating to severe ME.

The Young ME Sufferers Trust (TYMES)

Address: PO Box 4347, Stock, Ingatestone CM4 9TE, UK
Tel: +44 (0)845 003 9002
Website: www.tymestrust.org

Brief description: This is a national charity dedicated to supporting young people with ME, their families and professionals.

2. General support organisations

Carers UK

Tel: +44(0)808 808 7777 (Weds and Thurs 10 am–12 pm and 2 pm–4 pm)
Website: www.carersuk.org

Citizens Advice

Website: www.adviceguide.org.uk

Disability Rights UK

Tel: +44(0)300 555 1525 (Mon and Thurs 9 am to 1 pm)
Website: www.citizensadvice.org.uk

Brief description: This organisation produces a wide variety of factsheets. The Independent Living Advice Line provides advice on arranging care in the UK through Direct Payments including appeals against funding decisions by social services.

UK ME & Chronic Illness Benefits Advice Group (Facebook)

Website: www.facebook.com/groups/278260135547189

Brief description: This is an excellent group for ME sufferers who are claiming welfare benefits. There are superb resources in the 'Files' section of the group and it is very well run by a great team of admins.

3. Local self-help groups

This list is far from exhaustive but does represent local UK groups that members of Dr Myhill's Facebook support groups have found useful. They are listed in no particular order. Where more information is provided, this does not necessarily mean that this group is more active than other groups listed with fewer details; it merely means that more information was provided to Kathryn and Craig at the time when they compiled the list. It is recommended that, if you are interested, contact be made with the group so that further details can be elucidated. In addition, please note that some of these groups are free, whereas others make a charge.

Dorset ME Support Group

Website: www.dorsetmesupport.org.uk

CFS/ME Support Group Surrey (Facebook)

Website: www.facebook.com/groups/393742460836314

Brief description: A new, free support group for people with CFS/ME who live in Surrey. This is a place to share ideas and tips on coping with living with the condition whilst getting better. Admin of this Facebook group is Emma Joy.

Fibromyalgia Action UK

Head office tel: +44(0)844 826 9033 (open from 10 am–2 pm)
Helpline: +44(0)844 887 2444
Website: fmauk.org

Brief description: A national fibromyalgia charity.

Fibromyalgia conference

Email: Jeanne Hambleton at jeanne@follypogsfibro.org
Tel: +44(0)8433 828 829

Brief description: A fibromyalgia conference is run each year by FollyPogs Research charity, which is linked to Fibromyalgia South East Support.

Fibromyalgia South East Support (FMSSES)

For information on local groups in the South East area contact the group's coordinator Teresa White.

Email: tjswhite1954@live.co.uk
Tel: +44(0)1243 670783

FM/ME/CFS & Carer's Support Group West Wales

Website: fmmecfswestwales.jimdo.com

Hampshire Friends with ME

Address: The Community Centre, Brinton Lane, Hythe, Southampton SO45 4DU, UK
Tel: +44(0)845 834 0325
Website: www.friendswithme.org.uk

Brief description: Regular newsletters by post or email, containing medical and research information, practical tips, group activities and news, members' poetry pages, fun pages and more. Members contact list. Telephone support line. Local branches across the county, organising regular meet-ups, events, outings (usually with subsidised electric scooters), meditation sessions and pub meals. Lively, fun and supportive members' Facebook group. Home visit service for the severely affected (currently in transition). Well-stocked library with wide variety of books, CDs and DVDs. 'Group ethos: emphasis on social and emotional support, friendship and fun – as far as the illness allows. Aspiration to expand support for the housebound and severely affected.'

Isle of Wight Fibromyalgia Support Group

Group leader Karen Smith can be contacted by:
Email: iwfmsg.fibromates@gmail.com
Tel: +44(0)844 887 2346

Brief description: Meet on the second Tuesday of the month at All Saints Church, Ryde, corner of Queens Road and West Street, in the hall at the back. From 1.30 pm to 4 pm. Free designated parking is available. Between meetings the group organises social get-togethers, and a newsletter is sent by email at the end of each month. Members receive an FMS/CFS information pack (for as long as funds allow!). Newcomers are greeted by a 'Fibro Buddy'. A sub of £3 is charged per meeting which includes refreshments. Membership is £6 per annum, payable on second meeting. The group has a range of speakers, and has a close relationship with the pain clinic, and Dr Gary Lee who is currently heading a research programme with Southampton University, and many of the group members are participants; the current phase involves 'active' MRI scans of the brain. The group has developed close links with other community groups and healthcare professionals, such as The Health Trainer Service, Community Action IW, The Isle of Wight Anxiety and Panic Attack Support Group IW, and The Independent Living Centre, etc. The group is a registered FMAUK local group.

Leeds ME Network

Website: leedsmenetwork.yolasite.com

Brief description: This is a self-help group for patients sharing information of interest to people with CFS/ME in the Leeds area. There are monthly meetings.

Lincoln ME Friendship Group (Facebook)

Website: www.facebook.com/groups/1596074597279301

Brief description: As well as being a means for local people to support each other online, we have regular meetings for coffee and chat (at the moment roughly once a month). This is all arranged via the Facebook Group.

ME Association Sussex

Website: www.meassociation.org.uk/2009/09/sussex

ME Leicester

Address: 36 Scraptoft Lane, Leicester LE5 1HU, UK

ME North East

Website: www.menortheast.org (large website – worth a look.)

ME North Notts

Address: 3 Roderick Avenue, Kirkby in Ashfield, Notts, UK

MEDALS

Address: ME Doncaster, 10 Thellusson Ave, Scawsby, Doncaster DN5 8QN, UK
Tel: +44(0)1302 787353

MEND

Address: ME North Derbyshire, 46 Edinburgh Road, Chesterfield, Derbyshire S41 7HE, UK

OMEGA – Oxfordshire Support Group for ME/Chronic Fatigue Syndrome and Related Conditions

General email: enquire.omega@gmail.com
Email for South Oxon Support Group:
Tessa Keys – tessamary_keys@yahoo.co.uk
Email for Wantage and Grove Support Group:
Annie Kingsbury – anniekingsbury@talktalk.net
Email for website queries/problems: omega.webmaster0@gmail.com
Tel. for Wantage and Grove support group: +44(0)1235 763813
Website: omegaoxon.org

Brief description: OMEGA is the Oxfordshire Myalgic Encephalomyelitis Group for Action. It is a self-help group for people with ME or chronic fatigue syndrome, and their carers. Members can benefit from contact with other people who recognise and understand the illness. Members give each other friendship and support, exchange information about treatments, and learn from each other about management.

reMEmber

Address: PO Box 1647, Hassocks, West Sussex BN6 9GQ, UK
Email: me_cfs@hotmail.com
Website: www.remembercfs.org.uk

Sheffield ME Group

Address: The Circle, Rockingham Lane, Sheffield S1 4FW, UK
(Tuesday to Thursday 10 am–4 pm)
Tel: +44(0)114 2536700
Website: www.sheffieldmegroup.co.uk

Brief description: This group seeks to raise the general awareness of CFS/ME and to educate the general public through the promotion and dissemination of knowledge about the illness. It runs a variety of services, such as an information service, regular and special meetings, a library and newsletter, a listening ear, and social meetings. They have lots of information and help for anyone who needs it.

Sheffield Yoga for ME/CFS

Website: www.sheffieldyogaforme.org.uk

Shropshire ME Group

Website: www.shropshiremegroup.org.uk

Solihull and South Birmingham ME Support Group

There is no official address, but anyone interested in joining should contact Jenny.
Email: jennylg@live.co.uk
Tel: +44(0)121 689 0777
Text: 07817 561 216
Website: ssb4mesupport.weebly.com

BRIEF DESCRIPTION:

Meetings: The group has 10 meetings a year. The timetable of these is on the website. They take place either in the evening in Shirley or in the afternoon in Stirchley. Sometimes the meetings are just general social meet-ups, sometimes they have relevant speakers at the meetings. People with ME, CFS and FMS, their carers and their families are welcome. You do not have to be a member to attend the meetings.

Newsletters: The group has its own newsletter which is full of the latest research and info into the illness, alongside lighter stuff like jokes. Jenny mainly does the newsletter but any member of the group can submit something to Jenny to be included. You have to be a member to get the newsletter, but membership is cheap.

Group library: A variety of audio books, paper books, CDs and DVDs are available for the group to borrow for free. Most are related to the illness, some are more general.

Information service: There are a certain amount of information leaflets and packs available for anyone who wants to look at them.

Contact list service: Optional Contact List service which enables members to get in touch with each other for friendship and support. You do not have to be on this list if you do not wish to be.

Facebook page: A closed group where members post socially and to provide support and information. You can only join the group if you are a member, or if you contact Jenny and request to join.

South East London ME Support Group

Website: www.selmesg.org

Sussex & Kent ME/CFS Society

Website: www.measussex.org.uk

tamesidefibromyalgia

Website: fibro-warriors.co.uk

Tyne and Wear ME/CFS Support Group

(Previously Sunderland and South Tyneside ME/CFS support group)
Email: me-cfs@blueyonder.co.uk
Tel: +44(0)191 4556959
Website: www.mecfs.co.uk

Brief description: This organisation provides free membership, monthly meetings, quarterly newsletter and monthly updates; it has a dedicated telephone information line.

Worcestershire ME Social Group

Address: 1 The Old School House, Church Lane, Martley, Worcester WR6 6QA, UK
Tel: Chairman, Ian Logan – +44(0)1886 888419
Website: worcsmegroup.weebly.com
Area contacts:

- Bromsgrove: Edwina Evans – +44(0)1527 832245
- Droitwich: Stephen Woodfield – +44(0)1905 798671
- Hagley: Warwick Davis – +44(0)1384 892442
- Pershore/Evesham: Phil Moss – +44(0)1386 423463
- Malvern & Worcester: Ian Logan – +44(0)1886 888419
- Redditch: Jackie Elston – +44(0)1527 458840
- Wyre Forest: Audrey Hammond – +44(0)1562 822834

Brief description: There is a newsletter; there are monthly meetings, sometimes with guest speakers.

Yoga for ME (and Fibromyalgia) in Brighton and Hove, Sussex

Tel: +44(0)7939 830096 (Mondays at 2.30pm–3.45 pm)
Website: www.cornerstone-hove.org.uk

Brief description: Very gentle and supported yoga classes for those with ME or fibromyalgia. It is led by a qualified yoga teacher who understands ME and fibromyalgia and its limitations. There is an opportunity for a cup of tea and a chat afterwards.

The York ME Community

Email: Bill Clayton – bill@York-ME-Community.org
Website: www.york-me-community.org

Brief description: Bill's introduction to the website – 'My name is Bill Clayton and I live in Fulford, York. I am aware of many national websites and forums dealing with ME, but I feel there is a need for something more local, allowing us to get a true feel for what support there is in the area, and fostering a greater togetherness in our efforts to improve that support for the people of York. This site will only be as good as the support given by those that visit it, adding their ideas and experiences, so please spread the word that we are here to help each other and raise awareness of ME in York. I would like to give a huge thanks to my brother Ian who has put this site together for me, with me adding the content, but now it's pretty much over to you to bring it to life.'

APPENDIX 10

The Bell CFS Ability Scale – a measure of where you are

The fatigue in CFS is both mental and physical. For some sufferers, the physical is the greatest burden, and for others the mental fatigue is most troublesome. This scale was developed by Dr David Bell as a clinically useful way to assess response to treatment – it combines physical and mental activity with levels of wellness. This is not entirely satisfactory because different people suffer in different ways but it does give an idea of the level of disability.

100: No symptoms with exercise. Normal overall activity. Able to work or do house/home work full time with no difficulty.

90: No symptoms at rest. Mild symptoms with physical activity. Normal overall activity level. Able to work full time without difficulty.

80: Mild symptoms at rest. Symptoms worsened by exertion. Minimal activity restriction needed for activities requiring exertion only. Able to work full time with difficulty in jobs requiring exertion.

70: Mild symptoms at rest. Some daily activity limitation clearly noted. Overall functioning close to 90 per cent of expected except for activities requiring exertion. Able to work and do housework full time with difficulty. Needs to rest in day.

60: Mild to moderate symptoms at rest. Daily activity limitation clearly noted. Overall functioning 70 to 90 per cent. Unable to work full time in jobs requiring physical labour (including just standing), but able to work full time in light activity (sitting) if hours are flexible.

50: Moderate symptoms at rest. Moderate to severe symptoms with exercise or activity; overall activity level reduced to 70 per cent of expected. Unable to perform strenuous duties, but able to perform light duty or desk work* for four to five hours a day, requiring rest periods. Has to rest or sleep one to two hours daily.

40: Moderate symptoms at rest. Moderate to severe symptoms with exercise or activity. Overall activity level reduced to 50 to 70 per cent of expected. Able to go out once or twice a week. Unable to perform strenuous duties. Able to work sitting down at home for three to four hours a day, but requires rest periods.

30: Moderate to severe symptoms at rest. Severe symptoms with any exercise. Overall activity level reduced to 50 per cent of expected. Usually confined to house. Unable to perform any strenuous tasks. Able to perform desk work* for two to three hours a day, but requires rest periods.

20: Moderate to severe symptoms at rest. Unable to perform strenuous activity. Overall activity 30 to 50 per cent of expected. Unable to leave house except rarely. Confined to bed most of day. Unable to concentrate for more than one hour a day.

10: Severe symptoms at rest. Bedridden the majority of the time. No travel outside of the house. Marked cognitive symptoms preventing concentration.

0: Severe symptoms on a continuous basis. Bedridden constantly, unable to care for self.

* 'Desk work' includes everyday tasks such as sitting at a table to eat or read.

GLOSSARY AND WEBSITE LINKS

Acquired metabolic dyslexias

As we age, we get less good at aspects of the metabolic process. This can affect the production of hormones, for example.

Aerotoxic syndrome

The poisoning of airline pilots, cabin crew and passengers is possible in any air flight! Over the past few decades there has been a fundamental design fault in the majority of airplanes used to move people around the world. The engines compress and heat outside air which is then mixed with fuel and burned in order to propel the aircraft. As the air is already compressed and warmed, it makes a cheap way of supplying breathing air to the cabin. However, it is subject to contamination from the engines particularly if engine design is faulty or if engine seals become worn. Indeed, all jet engines leak oils and fumes to a certain extent and these chemicals get in to cabin air. Because jet engines run at such high temperatures, additives are put into oil so they can work better. Therefore depending on the design, the age and the recent service history of the engine, occupants of any aircraft will be more or less poisoned by these fumes.

http://www.drmyhill.co.uk/wiki/Aerotoxic_syndrome
http://www.aerotoxic.org/

Allergic muscles

Allergy never ceases to surprise and amaze me for the multiplicity of symptoms that it can cause. It is now clear to me that any part of the body can react allergically. Irritable bowel syndrome is partly due to allergy in the gut, migraine is allergy in the brain, asthma is allergy in the lungs, so why not allergic muscles? The more I look for this condition the more I find it, and it is obvious when you look for it.

The natural progression of allergy is for allergens to start producing symptoms in one target organ and move on to another. So the typical history through life of the dairy allergic person would be to start with colic as a baby, then move on to other manifestations such as toddler diarrhoea, catarrh, ear infections and sore throats, irritable bowel syndrome, migraine, arthritis, fatigue and allergic muscles.

How do allergic muscles start? What seems to happen is that muscles get sensitised as a result of mechanical damage. Tearing or bruising the muscle means that it comes in direct contact with blood, which may be carrying food antigens. I suspect the allergy is switched on at that time and the pain which follows the muscle damage and which persists long term is mis-attributed to damage, when actually it is sensitisation. So a torn muscle in the back from, say, lifting a heavy load could sensitise to, say, dairy products and it is the consumption of dairy subsequently which keeps the problem on the boil.

http://drmyhill.co.uk/wiki/Allergic_muscles

Anaesthetic action – theories of

Ferments such as alcohol, esters, aldehydes and other lipid-soluble substances have a general anaesthetic-like effect on membranes of the brain. This probably manifests by inhibiting energy delivery mechanisms to the brain. The consensus is that general anaesthetics also exert their effects (analgesia, amnesia, immobility) by modulating the activity of membrane proteins in the neuronal membrane. However, the exact location and mechanism of these actions are still largely unknown. Much research has been done and there are a number of theories that attempt to explain anaesthetic action but none so far has been categorical in fully explaining the action.

Anaesthetics and CFS

Anaesthetics are a problem for people with CFS for many possible reasons.

CFS sufferers are much more likely to get idiosyncratic (that is, unusual) reactions to drugs compared with the normal population. This may be because they are often slow detoxifiers. This may be a congenital problem or secondary to micronutrient deficiency or because their detox system is already overwhelmed by internal toxic stress (such as from the fermenting upper gut) or overwhelmed by external toxic stress. One example of this is that nearly all my CFS patients react badly to any amount of alcohol and to normal doses of antidepressants. So anaesthetics may result in slow recovery time with a flare of fatigue and other symptoms associated with that fatigue.

Many CFS sufferers have a problem because of multiple chemical sensitivity. These patients react in an allergic way to chemicals. Thankfully it is very rare for this to manifest with life-threatening reactions such as anaphylaxis.

The problem in CFS is poor energy delivery at the cellular level. This means energy delivery to organs is slow and so organ function is impaired. So, for example, in severe CFS the heart is in a state of low cardiac output often bordering on heart failure. This means there is less scope to react to stressful situations.

A related problem is that CFS and hospitals do not combine easily. The nutritional quality of food in hospitals is often poor, with little provision for allergy problems or fermenting gut problems. The beds can be uncomfortable, there is no peace from light, noise, heat and disturbance (least of all at night), there are all sorts of chemical smells, but worst of all there is an almost complete lack of understanding for the problems of CFS patients, with 'helpful' nurses encouraging you to 'do it all yourself' and 'start exercising as soon as possible'.

http://www.drmyhill.co.uk/wiki/CFS_and_Anaesthetics

Antioxidants

What allows us to live and our bodies to function are billions of chemical reactions in the body which occur every second. These are essential for the production of energy, which drives all the processes of life such as nervous function, movement, heart function, digestion and so on. If all these enzyme reactions invariably occurred perfectly, there would be no need for an antioxidant system. However, even our own enzyme systems make mistakes and the process of producing energy in mitochondria is highly active. When mistakes occur, free radicals are produced. Essentially, a free radical is a molecule with an unpaired electron; it is highly reactive and to stabilise its own structure, it will literally stick on to anything. That 'anything' could be a cell membrane, a protein, a fat, a piece of DNA, or whatever. In sticking on to something, it denatures that something so that it has to be replaced. This means having free radicals is extremely damaging to the body and therefore the body has evolved a system to mop up these free radicals before they have a chance to do such damage and this is called our antioxidant system. There are many substances in the body which act as antioxidants, but the three most important frontline antioxidants are:

Coenzyme Q10 (co-Q10) is the most important antioxidant inside mitochondria and also a vital molecule in oxidative phosphorylation (see page 55). Co-Q10 deficiency may also cause oxidative phosphorylation to go slow because it is the most important receiver and donor of electrons in oxidative phosphorylation. People with low levels of co-Q10 have low levels of energy.

Superoxide dismutase (SODase) is the most important superoxide scavenger in muscles (zinc and copper SODase inside cells, manganese SODase inside mitochondria and zinc and copper SODase outside cells).

Glutathione peroxidase is an enzyme dependent on selenium and glutathione, a three-amino acid polypeptide, and a vital free radical scavenger in the blood stream.

These molecules are present in parts of a million and are in the frontline process of absorbing free radicals. When they absorb an electron from a free radical, both the free radical and the antioxidant are effectively neutralised, but the anti-oxidants reactivate themselves by passing that electron back to **second line antioxidants** such as vitamins A and beta-carotene, some of the B vitamins, vitamin D, vitamin E, vitamin K and probably many others. These are present in parts per thousand. Again, these are neutralised by accepting an electron, but that is then passed back to the ultimate repository of electrons, namely vitamin C. This is present in higher concentrations.

http://drmyhill.co.uk/wiki/Antioxidants

Arrhythmias

See Dysrhythmias page 355.

Arthritis

'Arthritis' simply means pain in the joints. It names a symptom and is not a diagnosis; it therefore begs the question: what is causing it? Although arthritis has been classified into two types, inflammatory and degenerative, most sufferers usually have a bit of both. Regardless of the type of arthritis one has, my treatment is the same. In addition to my standard package for good health (see Paleo-ketogenic diet [Chapter 17], nutritional supplements [Chapter 18], sleep and exercise [Appendix 2]), I recommend:

- physiotherapy/osteopathy to sort out problems with posture, etc
- additional nutritional supplements, including my own 'Joint Mix'

- keeping joints warm

http://drmyhill.co.uk/wiki/Arthritis_-_Nutritional_treatments

Autoimmunity

Autoimmunity occurs when the immune system has made a mistake. The immune system has a difficult job to do, because it has to distinguish between molecules which are dangerous to the body and molecules which are safe. Sometimes it gets its wires crossed and starts making antibodies against molecules which are safe. For some people this results in allergies, which is a useless inflammation against safe foreign molecules. For others this results in autoimmunity, which is a useless inflammation against the body's own molecules. These are acquired problems – we know that because they become much more common with age. It is likely we are seeing more autoimmunity because of Western lifestyles, diets and pollution. Chemicals, especially heavy metals, get stuck onto cells and change their 'appearance' to the immune system and thereby switch on inappropriate reactions.

http://drmyhill.co.uk/wiki/Autoimmune_diseases

Brain fog

What I mean by brain fog is:

- poor short-term memory
- difficulty learning new things
- poor mental stamina and concentration – there may be difficulty reading a book or following a film story or following a line of argument
- difficulty finding the right word
- thinking one word, but saying another

What allows the brain to work quickly and efficiently is its energy supply. If this is impaired in any way, then the brain will go slow. Initially, the symptoms would be of foggy brain, but if symptoms progress, we end up with dementia. We all see this in our everyday life, with the effect of alcohol being the best example. Short-term exposure gives us a deliciously foggy brain – we stop caring, we stop worrying, it alleviates anxiety. However, it also removes our drive to do things, our ability to remember; it impairs judgement and our ability to think clearly. Medium-term exposure results in mood swings and anxiety (only alleviated by more alcohol). Longer-term use could result in severe depression and then dementia – examples include Korsakoff's psychosis and Wernike's encephalopathy. (Incidentally, these two examples also illustrate how most drug side-effects result from nutritional deficiencies – look them up on Wikipedia!)

The cellular form of energy, ATP, along with DNA, is an ancient molecule. It multitasks. It also functions as a neurotransmitter – to be precise a co-transmitter. Other neurotransmitters will not work unless they are accompanied by a molecule of ATP. Improve ATP and you improve all aspects of brain function. Improving ATP delivery is the best treatment for low mood and depression.

http://www.drmyhill.co.uk/wiki/Brain_fog

Candida

See Yeast problems, page 381.

Carbon monoxide and multi-sensitivity syndrome (MUSES)

I see a great many people who are hypersensitive. Sometimes the hypersensitivity is exquisite and is to light, noise, touch, smells (multiple chemical sensitivity) and often to electromagnetic radiation (electrical sensitivity). I had always wondered if there is an underlying mechanism and it appears there is! Alberty Donnay, President of the MCS Referral and Resources (www.mcsrr.org), has produced a convincing case that this is evidence of past or current carbon monoxide (CO) poisoning, which may come from outside the body or be made by the body itself as a stress response. This switches on a hypersensitivity and hypervigilance, which amounts to chronic anxiety and possibly psychiatric symptoms. The good news is that this is curable with oxygen treatment administered according to the protocol developed by Donnay. In the short term, CO displaces oxygen from haemoglobin and sticks more avidly so all organs are oxygen deprived. This can result in a multiplicity of symptoms but notably 'flu-like symptoms, headache, fatigue, weakness, muscle pains, cramps, nausea, vomiting, upset stomach, diarrhoea, confusion, memory loss, dizziness, incoordination, chest pain, rapid heartbeat, difficult or shallow breathing and changes in sensitivity of hearing vision, smell, taste, touch. There is an obvious vicious cycle here – the stress causes the CO and the CO causes the hypersensitivity. As well as impairing oxygen delivery, CO can destabilise blood sugar levels and dysregulate the autonomic nervous system to disturb heart rate, respiration and blood vessel tone, upset mental function (learning and memory), disturb sexual function and sensitisation to smells, light, sound, touch, etc.

http://drmyhill.co.uk/wiki/Carbon_monoxide_poisoning_and_multi-sensitivity
For safety advice: http://www.co-gassafety.co.uk

Cell-free DNA

Cell-free DNA is a substance we can measure as an indication of cell damage. If cells are healthy and intact there should be negligible cell-free DNA in the blood stream.

Chelation therapy

This can be used either orally or intravenously to reduce heavy metal load and is of proven efficacy. A 'chelating agent' (see DMSA and DMPS) is used, which mops up heavy metals and is eliminated from the body taking them with it. There are some concerns about some of the chelating agents mobilising mercury into the brain rather than out of it, which I suspect explains why chelation has slightly fallen out of favour in some circles.

Chemical poisoning

The diagnosis of chemical poisoning is suspected from a history of exposures resulting in typical clinical syndromes and confirmed by the appropriate medical tests. There is a series of criteria to be fulfilled to make a confident clinical diagnosis of poisoning by chemicals. The criteria are:

1. The subject was fit and well prior to chemical exposures.
2. There is evidence of exposure to the putative chemicals and toxins.
3. The subject initially developed local symptoms which became worse with repeated exposures.
4. With repeated exposures a typical clinical picture emerges characterised by chronic fatigue syndrome, immune disruption (allergies, autoimmunity, susceptibility to infections), accelerated ageing (so the sufferer gets diseases before their time), neuro-degeneration, diabetes and cancer.
5. Similar patterns of disease are seen in other people working under similar conditions.
6. There is similar factual evidence from other subjects who have been poisoned, such as the Gulf War veterans, sheep-dip poisoned farmers, aerotoxic pilots.

7. There is laboratory evidence of poisoning and effects of that poisoning.
8. There are no other possible explanations for this pattern of symptoms.
9. There is a response to treatment with clinical improvements as a result of detoxification, nutritional and immune support.

http://drmyhill.co.uk/wiki/Chemical_poisoning_-_general_principles_of_diagnosis_and_treatment

Coenzyme Q10

See Antioxidants, page 349.

Delayed fatigue

Delayed fatigue is a key diagnostic symptom of CFS. Acute fatigue symptoms persist for 24–96 hours if the sufferer overdoes things, with the result that an active day is 'paid for' by one or more days when the sufferer has no energy to do anything. This is because when mitochondria are stressed, all the energy molecules (ATP, ADP and AMP) are drained out and cells have to wait for between one and four days for new energy molecules to be made.

Detoxification

As part of normal metabolism, the body produces toxins which have to be eliminated, otherwise they poison the system. Therefore, the body has evolved a mechanism for getting rid of these toxins and the methods that it uses are as follows:

- Antioxidant system – for mopping up free radicals. See Antioxidants (page 349).
- The liver – detoxification by oxidation and conjugation (amino acids, sulphur-compounds, glucuronide, glutathione, etc) for excretion in urine.
- Fat-soluble toxins can be excreted in the bile. The problem here is that many of these are recycled because they are reabsorbed in the gut.
- Sweating – many toxins and heavy metals can be lost through the skin.
- Dumping chemicals in hair, nails and skin, which is then shed.

This system has worked perfectly well for thousands of years. Problems now arise because of toxins which we are absorbing from the outside world. This is inevitable since we live in equilibrium with the outside world. The problem is that these toxins (such as alcohol) may overwhelm the system for detoxification, or they may be impossible to break down (such as silicone and organochlorines), or they may get stuck in fatty organs and cell membranes and so not be accessible to the liver for detoxification (such as many volatile organic compounds). We all carry these toxins as a result of living in our polluted world.

http://drmyhill.co.uk/wiki/Detoxification
http://drmyhill.co.uk/wiki/Detoxing

DMSA

This is the chelating agent 2-3-dimercapto-succinic acid magnesium salt, used for heavy metal detox. It binds with metals in the body and takes them with it when excreted.

http://drmyhill.co.uk/wiki/Heavy_metal_poisoning

DMPS

This is the chelating agent 2-3-dimercapto-1-propane-sulphonic acid sodium salt, used for heavy metal detox. It binds with metals in the body and takes them with it when excreted.

http://drmyhill.co.uk/wiki/Heavy_metal_poisoning

DNA adducts

This test measures chemicals that have stuck on to DNA. I now use this test regularly for patients who have either been exposed to chemicals or developed cancer. Almost invariably I find toxic chemicals with the most common being lindane, nickel, PBBs (used as fire retardants) and other heavy metals. It is possible to get rid of these toxins, either by using high doses of the beneficial minerals, or by using chelation therapy, or by doing sweating detox regimes, or a combination of these factors.

http://drmyhill.co.uk/wiki/DNA_adducts

Dysrhythmias

A normal person's heart should beat somewhere between 65 and 80 beats per minute, with the rate slightly speeding up as one breathes in and slightly slowing down as one breathes out. Fit athletes have a slower pulse because as a result of training the heart beats more powerfully at rest. A regular beat is achieved by the pacemaker, which is comprised of cells at the top of the heart – that is, within the atria.

Our natural, in-built pacemaker generates an electrical pulse, which firstly flows down the top of the heart thereby making the atria contract; there is a small delay whilst the electrical wave flows into the bottom half of the heart, which makes the two ventricles contract. It is this alternate contraction of the atria which fires blood into the ventricles to fill them up, followed by a contraction of the ventricle, which fires blood out of the heart and sends it on its way round the body.

One can, therefore, get irregular heart rate or lack of coordination between the atria and the ventricles, or lack of coordination of the ventricles, as a result of disturbances of the pacemaker or the tissues that conduct the wave of electricity away from the pacemaker to the rest of the heart. Disturbances of the pacemaker and conducting tissue cause a whole variety of heart dysrhythmias, from the heart going too slow or going too fast, to missed beats, irregular beats, or a complete disassociation of heart activity such as atrial fibrillation or even ventricular tachycardias or fibrillations.

However, whatever the nature of the disturbance, the fundamental causes are pretty much the same. Many of these disturbances, such as ventricular ectopics, are fairly harmless and do not cause too much trouble. However, you should see them as a warning sign to change your lifestyle and address the underlying factors that are causing them in order that they do not progress to anything more serious. Electrical disturbances of the heart are caused by: poor blood supply, micronutrient deficiencies, poor energy supply at the cellular level, thyroid disease and toxic stress. All these need to be investigated and addressed. My general guidance for good health, as outlined throughout this book, may be sufficient. Should you have established dysrhythmias requiring prescription medication, then no changes should be made to medication without informed discussion with your GP and ideally your cardiologist. All dysrhythmias need medical input from your GP or cardiologist but the following interventions may be additionally helpful.

http://drmyhill.co.uk/wiki/Heart_Dysrhythmias,_Irregular_Pulse,_Missed_beats_and_Palpitations

Enzyme-potentiated desensitisation (EPD)

EPD is a vaccine which can be used to desensitise patients to foods, inhalants and chemicals. It has some bacterial antigens. The vaccine has been developed and refined by Dr Len McEwen over the past 30 years. It is supplied to the doctor who mixes the appropriate dose in a sterile environment, immediately prior to dosing. EPD works by manipulating the normal immune processes for creating and turning off allergies.

http://drmyhill.co.uk/wiki/Enzyme_Potentiated_Desensitisation_(EPD)

Fibromyalgia

Like fatigue, fibromyalgia is a symptom – it just means pain in the muscles. It occurs very commonly with chronic fatigue syndrome, because I suspect the underlying causes are similar.

http://drmyhill.co.uk/wiki/Fibromyalgia

Gilbert's syndrome (GS)

GS is a common genetic liver disorder found in 3 to 12 per cent of the population. It produces elevated levels of unconjugated bilirubin in the bloodstream. In otherwise healthy people, this normally has no serious consequences. Mild jaundice may appear under conditions of exertion or stress. The cause of GS is the reduced activity of the enzyme glucuronyltransferase. There are a number of variants of the gene for the enzyme, so the genetic basis of the condition is complex.

Gout

Gout is one of those conditions that never really made sense to me until I learned that uric acid is an important antioxidant in the bloodstream. What this means is that if levels of other antioxidants fall low, then the body compensates for this by pushing out more uric acid. That is absolutely fine, but the trouble is that if the level of uric acid gets too high, then, being rather insoluble, it precipitates out as crystals in the joint to cause an acute attack of gout. This is very tiresome because acute gout is extremely painful! The immune system does not like these gritty crystals in the joints and produces lots of inflammation to get rid of it and it is this that causes the heat, pain, swelling, redness and loss of function. The diagnosis is made by the characteristic clinical picture of acute severe joint pain, but one can also get a low grade generalised arthritis from gout. Blood tests will show high serum uric acid and it is this that gives the game away. Improving antioxidant status in the blood is therefore the best approach to treatment (see Antioxidants, page 349). Acute attacks are often precipitated by dehyration, so drinking plenty of fluids should help.

http://drmyhill.co.uk/wiki/Gout

Gulf War syndrome (GWS)

GWS is the archetypal environmental illness caused by a combination of factors, including:

- Immune insult caused by many different vaccinations (up to 14 in some soldiers) given on the same day
- Chemical warfare – organophosphate chemical weapons were used in the Gulf, notably sarin
- Biological warfare – infectious agents were sprayed onto the troops; the organism was Mycoplasma incognito
- Pyridostigmine – this is the 'antidote' to organophosphate poisoning but is toxic in its own right
- Organophosphate pesticides, used for control of sand flies and other insects, were weekly sprayed onto tents
- Fumes from oil-well fires
- Uniforms were dipped in organophosphates
- Depleted uranium resulting in radioactive exposures
- Water from drinking and showering was often stored in tanks usually used for oil and diesel

This was the most environmentally polluting war in history.

Veterans tell me that the chemical alarms were constantly going off but the usual response was to switch the alarm off!

Many of the soldiers who came back from the Gulf War with GWS are suffering, amongst other things, from a chronic infection caused by Mycoplasma incognito. This was developed as part of germ warfare and it may be that many thousands of the veterans are infected. Treatment is with high-dose doxycycline 200 mg daily for six weeks, with further cycles given subsequently. To find out more about mycoplasmal infections and how to test for them, visit the website of the Institute of Molecular Medicine (immed.org).

The symptoms of GWS are identical to those of CFS. Recently the Ministry of Defence has admitted that GWS can be caused by organophosphate poisoning. This is not at all surprising to me because the clinical features of GWS are identical to those in my 'sheep dip 'flu' farmers. By taking a careful history I often find evidence of pesticide exposure in CFS patients – often they had not connected the chemical exposure to their symptoms. Examples include woodworm timber treatments, house fumigation, excessive use of fly sprays/ Vaponas and pet flea-treatments.

http://drmyhill.co.uk/wiki/Gulf_War_Syndrome

Hyperventilation

Before I read Buteyko's book *Freedom from Asthma* I had never understood why humans evolved such an inefficient system of breathing. We inhale most of our recently exhaled air, which to me seemed a nonsense: it is much more efficient to have a one-way flow of air over a surface, like fish do with water over gills. However, there is a good reason.

Life evolved over millions of years in an atmosphere rich in carbon dioxide, the waste gas of respiration. Carbon dioxide became essential for normal cell metabolism because cells used carbon dioxide to maintain their optimal pH (acidity). When levels of carbon dioxide in the atmosphere fell, cells had to develop a mechanism for artificially bathing themselves in the right level of carbon dioxide for their efficient metabolism. And so lungs evolved.

Lungs are necessary to keep carbon dioxide levels high in inhaled air and therefore in the blood. The blood is very efficient at gathering oxygen and all arterial blood is 100 per cent saturated with oxygen. But here comes the crunch – oxygen is only readily released from red blood cells to supply oxygen to the tissues in the presence of high levels of carbon dioxide. So what does this mean in practice?

Many patients, particularly asthma patients, but also CFS patients, have a sensation that they are not getting enough oxygen to their tissues. Their response to this is to breathe more deeply. However, blood cannot become more than 100 per cent saturated with oxygen. All that happens is that more carbon dioxide is washed out of the blood. This makes oxygen cling more fiercely to haemoglobin in red blood cells and therefore oxygen delivery to the tissues is made worse. Paradoxically, to improve oxygen supply to the tissues you have to breathe less!

Breathing less increases carbon dioxide levels and improves oxygen delivery. Lowering carbon dioxide levels in the blood has other dire effects. It upsets the acidity of the blood and causes what is known in medical jargon as a respiratory alkalosis. This causes all sorts of awful symptoms such as panic attacks, pain, fatigue, feeling spaced out and dizzy, brain fog and so on.

Again, taking the evolutionary approach, humans used to live a far more active existence. Because we are now so sedentary, we do not need the oxygen supply our lungs have evolved to deliver. We do not produce enough of the waste gas carbon dioxide either. The system is underused and so there is an in-built tendency to breathe too much. This is worsened by stimulants such as excitement (sitting in front of an exciting film, but not using any oxygen up), caffeine, computer games and so on. Hyperventilation is probably extremely common and we could all benefit from breathing less. We have simply got into bad habits and have to re-learn how to breathe.

http://drmyhill.co.uk/wiki/Hyperventilation

Hypochlorhydria

Hypochlorhydria arises when the stomach is unable to produce sufficient hydrochloric acid. It is a greatly overlooked cause of problems. The stomach requires an acid environment for several reasons:

- digestion of protein
- emptying the stomach correctly, and failure to do so results in gastro-oesophageal reflux disease
- sterilisation of the stomach and kill bacteria and yeast that may be ingested
- absorption of certain micronutrients, in particular divalent and trivalent cat-ions such as calcium, magnesium, zinc, copper, iron, selenium, boron and so on

As we age, our ability to produce stomach acid declines, but some people are simply not very good at producing stomach acid, sometimes because of pathology in the stomach (such as an allergic gastritis secondary to food intolerance), but sometimes for reasons unknown. The stomach is lined with cells that are proton pumps – that is to say they pump hydrogen ions from the blood stream into the lumen of the stomach. Stomach acid is simply concentrated hydrogen ions. There is a natural tendency for these hydrogen ions to diffuse back from where they came but this is prevented by very tight junctions between stomach wall cells. However, if the gut becomes inflamed for whatever reason, a 'leaky gut' (see page 364) develops and hydrogen ions leak back out. A common cause of inflammation and leaky gut is allergy.

Short-term treatment includes taking acid supplements, such as cider vinegar; high-dose ascorbic acid with meals; or betaine hydrochloride capsules. Often in the longer term, with the correct diet (low glycaemic index, low allergy potential, smaller meals), getting rid of *Helicobacter pylori*, and correcting gut flora, this cures the chronic gastritis and the stomach is again able to produce acid normally.

http://drmyhill.co.uk/wiki/Hypochlorhydria

Hypoglycaemia

'Hypoglycaemia' is the term used for blood sugar being at too low a level. To explain how this happens it is necessary to describe how sugar levels are controlled. It is critically important for the body to maintain blood sugar levels within a narrow range. If the blood sugar level falls too low, energy supply to all tissues, particularly the brain, is impaired. However, if blood sugar levels rise too high, then this is very damaging to arteries and the long-term effect of arterial disease is heart disease and strokes. This is caused by sugar sticking to proteins and fats to make AGEs (advanced glycation end-products) which accelerate the ageing process. Normally, the liver controls blood sugar levels. It can create the sugar from glycogen stores inside the liver and releases sugar into the blood stream minute by minute in a carefully regulated way to cope with body demands, which may fluctuate from minute to minute. Excess sugar flooding into the system after a meal can be mopped up by muscles but only so long as there is space there to act as a sponge. This occurs when we exercise. This system of control works perfectly well until we upset it by eating the wrong thing or not exercising. Eating excessive sugar at one meal, or excessive refined carbohydrate (which is rapidly digested into sugar) can suddenly overwhelm the muscle and the liver's normal control of blood sugar levels.

We evolved over millions of years eating a diet that was very low in sugar and had no refined carbohydrate. Control of blood sugar therefore largely occurred as a result of eating this Paleo-ketogenic diet and the fact that we were exercising vigorously, so any excessive sugar in the blood was quickly burned off. Nowadays the situation is different: we eat large amounts of sugar and refined carbohydrate and do not exercise sufficiently to burn off this excess sugar. The body therefore has to cope with this excessive sugar load by other mechanisms. When food is digested, the sugars and other digestive products go straight from the gut in the portal veins to the liver, where they should all be mopped up by the liver and processed accordingly. If excessive sugar or refined carbohydrate overwhelms the liver, the sugar spills over into the systemic circulation. If not absorbed by muscle glycogen stores, high blood sugar results, which is extremely damaging to arteries. If we were exercising hard, this would be quickly burned off. However, if we are not, then other mechanisms of control are brought into play. The key player here is insulin, a hormone secreted by the pancreas. This is very good at bringing blood sugar levels down and it does so by shunting the sugar into fat. Indeed, this includes the 'bad' cholesterol LDL. There is then a rebound effect and blood sugars may well go too low – in other words, hypoglycaemia occurs. Low blood sugar is also dangerous to the body because the energy supplied to all tissues is impaired.

Subconsciously, people quickly work out that eating more sugar alleviates these symptoms, but of course they invariably overdo things; the blood sugar level then goes high and they end up on a roller-coaster ride of blood sugar level going up and down throughout the day. Ultimately, this leads to 'metabolic syndrome' or 'syndrome X' – a major cause of disability and death in Western societies, since it is the forerunner of diabetes, obesity, cardiovascular disease, degenerative conditions and cancer.

http://drmyhill.co.uk/wiki/Hypoglycaemia

Hypothyroidism

Underactive thyroid is a very common problem in CFS, often as a knock-on effect of a general suppression of the hypothalamic-pituitary-adrenal axis – that is, the coordinated functioning of those three glands.

The thyroid gland can be underactive for three reasons – the gland itself fails (primary thyroid failure), the pituitary gland which drives the thyroid gland into action under-functions, or there is failure to convert inactive thyroxine (T4) to its active form (T3). The symptoms of these three problems are the same, but blood tests show different patterns:

- In **primary thyroid failure**, blood tests show high levels of thyroid-stimulating hormone (TSH) and low levels of T4 and T3.
- In **pituitary failure**, blood tests show low levels of TSH, T4 and T3.
- If there is a **conversion problem**, TSH and T4 may be normal, but T3 is low.

There is another problem too, which is that the so-called 'normal range' of T4 is probably set too low. I know this because many patients with low normal T4 often improve substantially when they are started on thyroid supplements to bring levels up to the top end of the normal range.

http://drmyhill.co.uk/wiki/Hypothyroidism

Inflammation

Inflammation is an essential part of our survival package. From an evolutionary perspective, the biggest killer of *Homo sapiens* has been infection, with cholera claiming a third of all deaths ever. The body has to be alert to the possibility of any infection, to all of which it responds with inflammation. However, inflammation is metabolically expensive and inherently destructive. It has to be, in order to kill infections by bacteria, viruses, parasites or whatever. For example, part of the immune defence involves a 'scorched earth' policy – tissue immediately around an area of infection is destroyed so there is nothing for the invader to parasitise. The mechanism by which the immune system kills these infections is by firing free radicals at them. However, if it fires too many free radicals, then this 'friendly fire' will damage the body itself. Therefore, for inflammation to be effective it must be switched on, targeted, localised and then switched off. This entails extremely complex immune responses; clearly, there is great potential for things to go wrong. Inflammation is also involved in the healing process. Where there is damage by trauma, there will be dead cells. Inflammation is necessary to clear away these dead cells and lay down new tissues. Inflammation is characterised by heat and redness (heat alone is antiseptic), combined with swelling, pain and loss of function, which immobilises the area being attacked by the immune system. This is necessary because physical movement will tend to massage the infection to other sites.

If one looks at life from the point of view of the immune system, it has a very difficult balancing act to manage. Too little reaction and we die from infection; too much reaction is metabolically expensive and damaging. If switched on inappropriately, the immune system has the power to kill us within seconds, an example of this being anaphylaxis.

http://drmyhill.co.uk/wiki/Inflammation

Kefir

Kefir is a fermented milk drink made with kefir 'grains' (a yeast/bacterial fermentation starter) and has its origins in the north Caucasus mountains around 3000 BC. It is a useful probiotic because it is rich in lactobacillus, which keeps the lower gut slightly acidic, displaces unfriendly bacteria, is directly toxic to yeast and is anti-inflammatory to the gut. Production of traditional kefir requires a starter community of kefir grains, which are added to the liquid one wishes to ferment.

Kefir grains cannot be produced from scratch, but the grains grow during fermentation, and additional grains are produced. Kefir grains can be bought from or donated by other growers. The joy of using kefir is that one sachet can last a lifetime. Furthermore, the best results for probiotics come from using live cultures.

I have been growing kefir and it grows well at room temperature. Because dairy products are not evolutionarily correct foods, kefir should be grown on non-dairy foods such as soya milk, rice milk or coconut milk, and who knows what else! Start off with one litre of soya milk in a jug, add the kefir sachet and within about 12–24 hours it should have semi-solid, junket-like consistency. Do not expect it to look like commercial yoghurt, which has often been thickened artificially. Then keep the culture in the fridge, where it ferments further. This slower fermentation seems to improve the texture and flavour. However, it can be used at once as a substitute in any situation where you would otherwise use cream or custard. I often add a lump of creamed coconut which further feeds the kefir, imparts a delicious coconut flavour and thickens the culture. Once the jug is nearly empty, add another litre of soya milk, stir it in, keep it at room temperature and away you go again. I don't even bother to wash the jug – the slightly hard yellow bits on the edge I just stir in to restart the brew. This way a sachet of kefir lasts for life! One idea I am playing with is the possibility of adding vitamins and minerals to the culture. The idea here is that they may be incorporated into the bacteria and thereby enhance the absorption of micronutrients. You could try this if you do not tolerate supplements well.

http://drmyhill.co.uk/wiki/Kefir

Leaky gut

Normally one expects foods to be completely broken down into amino acids (from protein), essential fatty acids and glycerol (from fats) and single sugars, or 'monosaccharides' (from carbohydrates). The undigested foods stay in the gut and the small digested molecules pass through the gut wall into the portal blood stream and on to the liver where they are dealt with. However, leaky gut means food particles get absorbed before they have been properly digested. This means large food molecules get into the blood stream. These large molecules are 'interesting' to the immune system, which may mistake them for viruses or bacteria. In this event, it may attack these harmless molecules, either with antibodies or directly with immune cells. This causes inflammation. Inflammation in the gut causes diseases of the gut. Inflammation elsewhere can cause almost any symptom you care to mention. It may switch on allergy or autoimmunity – that is, it is potentially a disease-amplifying process.

Another problem with small digested molecules or polypeptides getting in to the bloodstream is that these molecules may be biologically active. Some of them act as hormone mimics, which can affect levels of glucose in the blood or blood pressure. This is akin to throwing a handful of sand into a finely tuned machine – it makes a real mess of homeostatic (balancing) mechanisms of controlling body activities.

http://drmyhill.co.uk/wiki/Leaky_gut_syndrome

Lipids, fats and essential fatty acids

The vast majority of cell metabolism takes place on, in or around cell membranes. The structure of cell membranes is identical throughout the animal kingdom. They are made up of fatty molecules which have a water-loving end and a fat-loving end; these combine in a sandwich so the fat-loving end forms the core of the membrane and the water-loving end the outside of the membrane. The structure of the membrane and how liquid it is depends on the fats that are in it. If the composition of membranes changes, then they will either become more stiff or more liquid.

There are a great many effects which result from this, for example increased irritability and sensitivity, which of course could explain many CFS symptoms, such as intolerance of chemicals and foods, intolerance of heat, light and touch, low pain threshold, cardiac arrhythmias and so on. Indeed, a great many drugs work because of their effects on changing membrane structure, such as general anaesthetics, tranquillisers, pain killers and anti-inflammatory drugs.

Mitochondrial membranes are different from cell membranes because they have to be a little stiffer in order to hold still the bundles of enzymes called cristae on which oxidative phosphorylation (see page 55) takes place. They have an additional fat – namely, 'cardiolipin' – to create this extra stiffness. Having the correct oils in the diet is essential for energy supply to the brain. Poor energy supply means foggy brain.

http://drmyhill.co.uk/wiki/Lipids,_fats_and_essential_fatty_acids

Magnesium

Red blood cell levels of magnesium are almost invariably low in patients with CFS. Furthermore, very many patients with CFS benefit from magnesium by injection. I believe that a low red cell magnesium is a symptom of mitochondrial failure. It is the job of mitochondria to produce ATP for cell metabolism and about 40 per cent of all mitochondrial output goes into maintaining calcium/magnesium and sodium/potassium ion pumps. I suspect that when mitochondria fail, these pumps malfunction and therefore calcium leaks into cells and magnesium leaks out. This, of course, compounds the underlying mitochondrial failure because calcium is toxic to mitochondria and magnesium is necessary for normal mitochondrial function. This is just one of the many vicious cycles we see in patients with fatigue syndromes. The reason for giving magnesium by injection is in order to reduce the work of the calcium/magnesium ion pump by reducing the concentration gradient across cell membranes.

http://www.drmyhill.co.uk/wiki/Magnesium

Maintaining and restoring good health

I describe my general approach throughout the book, but in summary it consists of:

- Eating a Paleo-ketogenic diet
- Taking nutritional supplements, including a daily dose of sunshine
- Getting a good night's sleep on a regular basis
- Getting the right balance between work, rest and play
- Doing a good chemical clean-up of your environment
- Detox regimes – either regular exercise or far-infrared sauna-ing
- Looking after your friendly bacteria on the skin, gut and perineum.

http://drmyhill.co.uk/wiki/The_general_approach_to_maintaining_and_restoring_good_health

Malabsorption

The job of the gut is to absorb the goodness from food. To do this, it first has to reduce food particles to a size which allows the digestive enzymes to get at them; then it has to provide the correct acidity for enzymes to work, produce the necessary enzymes and emulsifying agent (bile salts), and move the food along the gut. Finally, the large bowel allows growth of bacteria for a final digestive/fermentative process and water extraction. The gut has a particularly difficult job because it has to identify foods that are safe from potentially dangerous microbes (most are not dangerous but positively beneficial). This explains why 90 per cent of the immune system is gut associated. The inoculation of the gut with the good microbes takes place in the gut in the first few minutes following birth. Anything which goes wrong with any of these processes can cause malabsorption. Malabsorption means that the body does not get the raw materials for normal everyday work and repair. Consequently, there is the potential for lots of things to go wrong.

http://drmyhill.co.uk/wiki/Malabsorption

Mercury poisoning

The early symptoms of mercury poisoning can be very variable but may include loss of short-term memory, a metallic taste in the mouth (this is difficult since taste is relative and dental amalgam is constantly present) and fine tremor. Mercury may also cause personality changes (like the Mad Hatter from *Alice in Wonderland*, which was written at a time when hatters used mercury in hat-making). It is also toxic to the nerves of the heart and may be a cause of electrical dysrhythmias (palpitations).

Dental amalgam is the commonest source of mercury poisoning. Professor Fritz Lorscheider's work over many years has looked at whether mercury leaches out from dental amalgam. At room temperature, mercury is a liquid and in dental amalgam it is not chemically bound into the amalgam, but there as a liquid, albeit a very tough and stiff liquid. He took some sheep, filled their molars with dental amalgam which was radioactively labelled and four months later scanned the sheep to see if the mercury had moved to other parts of the body; he discovered that it had deposited in their bones, kidneys and brain. He then looked at what mercury does in the brain. He found that, at concentrations lower than would be found in the saliva of a person with amalgam fillings, nerve fibres collapsed because they could not build their essential structure. (For more detail see the link below.)

The pathology he found is similar to Alzheimer's disease, in which neurofibrillary tangles are formed. Essentially, Lorscheider's findings tell us that mercury causes Alzheimer's disease. Alzheimer's is also associated with aluminium poisoning. The main source of aluminium is from antacids, antiperspirants and cooking foil, pots and pans. In California, Sweden, Germany and Norway mercury amalgam has been banned.

http://drmyhill.co.uk/wiki/Mercury_-_Toxicity_of_Dental_Amalgam_-_Why_you_should_have_your_dental_amalgams_removed

Minerals

You could argue that we all die ultimately from mineral and vitamin deficiencies. People who traditionally live to great ages are often found living in areas watered by streams from glaciers. Glaciers are lakes of ice which have spent the previous few thousand years crunching up rocks. Therefore the waters coming from the glaciers are very rich in minerals. This is used not just to drink but to irrigate crops and to bathe in. These people therefore have had excellent levels of micronutrients. Given the right raw materials, things do not go wrong in the body and ageing is slow. For example:

- Low magnesium and selenium is a risk factor for heart disease.
- Low selenium increases risk of cancer.
- Copper is necessary to make elastic tissue – deficiency causes weaknesses in arteries leading to aneurysms.
- Low chromium increases the risk of diabetes.
- Good antioxidant status (vitamins A, C, E and selenium) slows the ageing process.
- Superoxide dismutase enzymes require zinc, copper and manganese to function.
- Iodine is necessary to make thyroid hormones and is highly protective against breast disease.
- The immune system needs a huge range of minerals to work well, especially zinc, selenium and magnesium.
- Boron is highly protective against arthritis.
- Magnesium is required in at least 300 enzyme systems.
- Zinc is needed for normal brain development; a deficiency at a critical stage of development causes dyslexia.
- Any deficiency of selenium, zinc, copper or magnesium can cause infertility.
- Iron prevents anaemia.
- Molybdenum is necessary to detox sulphites.

The secret of success is to copy nature. Civilisation has brought great advantages, but at the same time is responsible for escalating death rates from cancer and heart disease. I want the best of both worlds. I like my warm kitchen, fridge, wood-burning cooker, computer and telly, but I want to eat and live in the environment in which primitive man thrived.

http://drmyhill.co.uk/wiki/Minerals

Multiple chemical sensitivity (MCS)

MCS is an inevitable part of modern Western lifestyles. Chemicals have huge potential to do harm, and if the body senses this it will set up an early warning system. It achieves this by giving you symptoms when you are exposed to such a chemical. In low doses, chemicals can be detoxified in the body and do not cause problems. If our defences are overwhelmed, the chemical will cause a poisoning. The body recognises this and remembers the chemical, so in the future, when there are tiny, non-poisonous exposures, the alarm bells ring with symptoms. This is fine if it is just one or two chemicals causing minor symptoms – for example, if I smell perfume I will sneeze, but with larger doses I suffer a foggy brain. The mechanism of this is the same as the mechanism for viral infection and subsequent immunity. Problems arise when there is sensitivity to many chemicals and the warning symptoms are severe. Some people can have anaphylactic reactions to chemicals, with collapse. For some it involves a sudden and major flare of their fatigue, muscle symptoms, migraine or whatever. What this means in practice is that chemical sensitivity and toxicity go together. People with chemical sensitivity have been 'poisoned' somewhere in the past and are likely to have an ongoing toxic load. This is why detox regimes are part of the treatment I advocate for CFS.

http://drmyhill.co.uk/wiki/Multiple_Chemical_Sensitivity_(MCS)_-_Principles_of_Treatment

Muscle stiffness

Muscle stiffness is a symptom seen when muscles cannot move quickly without accompanying pain or spasm. Sufferers have to move slowly. They quickly work out that after the muscle has not been used for some time – for example, on rising from sleep, or from having sat in one position for some time – their first movement has to be particularly slow, gentle and tentative. Moving too quickly brings about acute pain and possibly spasm. Thanks to the work of Dr McLaren-Howard, we know the possible mechanisms for this stiffness include:

1. For muscles to relax they require magnesium and for muscles to contract they require calcium. Any imbalance of this – that is, too much calcium or too little magnesium – very much increases the tendency to spasm and contraction. Modern diets are low in magnesium and high in calcium and this will increase the tendency to spasm.
2. Other dietary indiscretions will also raise intercellular calcium levels. Calcium is held inside cells via a binding protein and this is stimulated by cyclic AMP and insulin. The two dietary problems which induce these enzymes are caffeine and carbohydrates respectively. Therefore, a Western diet will tend to predispose towards muscle stiffness.
3. Rheumatic patches may well present with the symptom of stiff muscles.
4. We have the issue of allergic muscles (see page 347).
5. Once a person has developed a tendency to muscle spasm and pain, we then get a learned response. The brain anticipates that the muscle will go

into spasm if moved too quickly and therefore all movements are generally slowed down to prevent this from happening. It may well be that therapies known to be effective for stiff muscles, such as Pilates, Bowen technique, massage and other such manipulations, are re-educating the brain into realising that it is now 'safe' to move freely. However, they will be much more effective if the underlying physical causes are also addressed.

6. There is clearly a neuro-psychological element. The brain is also responsible for muscle tone and neurological problems such as Parkinson's disease will result in muscle stiffness or even spasticity. Psychological stress will also tend to increase muscle tension and worsen an underlying tendency. Diazepam is one of the most useful muscle relaxants.
7. Exercise – the right type may well be a factor.

http://drmyhill.co.uk/wiki/Muscle_Stiffness

Naltrexone

The idea behind using low-dose naltrexone is to stimulate the production of endogenous (the body's own) opiates. These have disease-modifying effects in a wide range of conditions and there is now good evidence for this. Naltrexone on its own has very little effect on the body. Typically, it is used to reverse the effects of poisoning by opiates such as morphine, and is the perfect antidote to, for example, morphine or a morphine-like substance which may be used for darting and tranquillising wild animals. They will wake up within a few minutes if injected with naltrexone. The usual dose of naltrexone to treat opiate poisoning is 50 mg. The daily dose of naltrexone for our purposes is 4 mg. Naltrexone is available in the UK on prescription, either from your GP or from a private practitioner. It comes in several forms – as capsule, liquid or transdermal cream.

http://drmyhill.co.uk/wiki/Low_dose_naltrexone

Nickel

Nickel (Ni) is a nasty toxic metal and a known carcinogen. It is one of the metals we see most commonly in toxicity tests – it appears stuck onto DNA, stuck onto translocator protein and is often present in blood at high levels. Nickel is a problem because it 'looks' like zinc. Zinc deficiency is very common in people eating Western diets, so if the body needs zinc and it is not there, it will use look-alike nickel instead. But nickel does not do the job and, indeed, gets in the way of normal biochemistry. Zinc is an essential co-factor in 300 enzyme systems that we know of and maybe others we do not know of, so there is enormous potential for harm from nickel. Nickel sensitivity is very common and often diagnosed from rashes from jewellery, zips, watches, etc. What we know from people with chemical sensitivity is that they often have toxic loads of those things they are sensitive to. So nickel sensitivity often equates with nickel toxicity. Nickel is unavoidable if you live a Western lifestyle! Many industrial processes release nickel into the atmosphere.

- Stainless steel – contains 14 per cent nickel; this includes cookware and eating utensils! Use cast iron pans, glass or ceramic.
- Jewellery – used because it is such a versatile, malleable metal. Well absorbed with piercing.
- Catalytic converters in cars release fine particulate nickel into the atmosphere – so fine that it cannot be filtered out by the lining of the bronchus, so it is well absorbed by inhalation and easily gets into blood vessels. Here it triggers inflammation and arterial disease.
- Cigarette smoke.
- Medical prostheses.

http://drmyhill.co.uk/wiki/Nickel_-_a_nasty_toxic_metal

Organophosphate (OP) poisoning

Different people have different symptoms of OP poisoning. Symptoms depend partly on how much OP they have been exposed to, whether they have had single massive exposure, or chronic sub-lethal exposure, whether it has been combined with other chemicals and how good their body is at coping with toxic chemicals. Symptoms divide into the following categories:

No obvious symptoms at all – A government-sponsored study at the Institute of Occupational Medicine that looked at farmers who regularly handled OPs but who were complaining of no symptoms, showed that they suffered from mild brain damage. Their ability to think clearly and problem solve was impaired.

Sheep dip 'flu (mild acute poisoning) – This is a 'flu-like illness which follows exposure to OPs. Sometimes the farmer just has a bit of a headache, feels unusually tired or finds he/she can't think clearly. This may just last a few hours to a few days and the sufferer recovers completely. Most sufferers do not realise that they have been poisoned and put any symptoms down to a hard day's work. It can occur after dipping, but some farmers will get symptoms after the slightest exposure, such as visiting markets and inhaling OP fumes from fleeces.

Acute organophosphate poisoning – This is the syndrome recognised by doctors and Poisons Units. Symptoms occur within 24 hours of exposure and include collapse, breathing problems, sweating, diarrhoea, vomiting, excessive salivation, heart dysrhythmias, extreme anxiety, etc. Treatment is with atropine. You have to have a large dose of OP to have this effect (such as, drink some of the dip!) and so this syndrome is rarely seen.

Intermediate syndrome – This occurs 1–3 weeks after exposure and is characterised by weakness of shoulder, neck and upper leg muscles. It is rarely diagnosed because it goes unrecognised.

Long-term chronic effects – These symptoms develop in some susceptible individuals. They can either occur following a single massive exposure, or after several years of regular sub-lethal exposure to OPs. The treatment follows the same principles as for any chemical poisoning (see Chemical poisoning, page 353).

Fortunately, most farmers are intelligent and realise the above state of affairs, but the lack of street credibility and help from government agencies makes this illness a social and financial disaster area.

http://drmyhill.co.uk/wiki/Organophosphate_Poisoning

Osteoporosis

Osteoporosis is a modern disease of Western society. Primitive societies eating Paleo-ketogenic diets do not suffer from osteoporosis. So the underlying principle for avoiding osteoporosis is that we should mimic primitive cultures eating a Paleo-ketogenic diet and living a toxin-free life. This does not mean you need to run around half naked in a rabbit-skin loin cloth depriving yourself of the pleasures of twenty-first-century Western life. We need to cherry pick from the good things of both civilisations.

Medical professionals would have us believe that the only important constituent of bone is calcium. Actually bone is made up of many different minerals including, in order of proven importance, magnesium, calcium, strontium, boron, silicon, selenium, zinc, chromium and maybe others. For its formation it also requires a whole range of vitamins, essential fatty acids and amino acids. All these nutrients are supplied liberally by a Paleo-ketogenic diet based on meat, fish, eggs, nuts, seeds and vegetables. Western civilisation now gets 70 per cent of its calories from four foods, namely grains, dairy, potato and sugar – sugar is already a refined food, and most grains are eaten refined, as are potatoes. The refining process strips out many essential micronutrients and these are further depleted by storage, cooking, packing and light. In addition to this, many other substances we consume have a diuretic effect, in particular tea, coffee and alcohol, and this further strips essential micronutrients from the body. There are a great many studies which show that modern Western diets are markedly deficient in these essential micronutrients. By following my standard recommendations for supplements combined with a Paleo-ketogenic diet and exercise, you will prevent osteoporosis.

http://drmyhill.co.uk/wiki/Osteoporosis_-_a_long_term_complication_of_CFS

http://www.drmyhill.co.uk/wiki/Osteoporosis

Pacing

Pacing involves the '80 per cent rule' – work out what you can do in a day without becoming exhausted and then do just 80 per cent of it. Rest is the single most important factor in allowing CFS sufferers to get better. An invariable feature of the history is that exercise (either mental, physical or emotional) makes the symptoms worse. Indeed, this distinguishes CFS from depression – exercise tends to improve the symptoms of people who are simply depressed. In CFS, the desire is there but the performance is lacking. However, all CFS sufferers tend to push themselves to their particular limit every day and therefore do not give themselves a chance to get better. Most also compare themselves with what they were like before their illness began. This is hopeless as it makes sufferers unrealistic about their current situation and prevents rest and pacing.

http://drmyhill.co.uk/wiki/Getting_enough_rest

Pain

Although pain seems like 'a pain', actually it is essential for our survival. Pain protects us from ourselves. It prevents us from damaging our bodies. Indeed, people who are born with no pain perception look as if they have been traumatised – they are covered in cuts, bruises and sores, because they do not realise that they are damaging themselves. Pain is the local method of avoiding damage – it makes us protect the affected part of the body and makes us keep it still so that healing and repair can take place. If pain becomes more generalised then pain is accompanied by fatigue.

What this means is that chronic pain and chronic fatigue go hand in hand and therefore so should treatment. We learn through experience what is painful; this makes us avoid those painful experiences and therefore protects our bodies. Although it is desirable to learn about pain, this can also cause problems because if the underlying causes of the pain are not identified we 'learn' more pain.

In the ideal situation, we damage our bodies with, say, a cut or bruise and the local pain makes us care for that damaged area by protecting it and keeping it still so that healing and repair can take place. With healing, the pain goes. If the root source of the pain is not identified, it creates a problem because then the pain increases. The body naturally thinks that increasing pain means we will take more care, identify the source of the pain, keep the limb more still and therefore the body winds up the pain signal to try to elicit the appropriate response. Effectively we learn to feel more pain because there is an upgrading of this pain response. This is not a psychological effect – this actually occurs within the cells themselves. This makes it very important to identify causes of pain and allow time for healing and repair, otherwise the pain will get worse.

http://drmyhill.co.uk/wiki/Pain

Pancreatic function

The pancreas is a large gland which lies behind the stomach and upper gut. It has two major functions of clinical importance. Firstly, it acts as an endocrine organ to produce insulin and other hormones essential for the control of blood sugar. Secondly, it has an exocrine function to produce enzymes essential for the digestion of food. These enzymes include those to digest proteins, fats and starches and to work best they need an alkali environment. This alkali environment is provided by the liver, which produces bile containing bile salts and bicarbonate. When food is present in the duodenum and jejunum, the gall bladder contracts, sending a bolus of bile salts and bicarbonate which meet up downstream with pancreatic enzymes to allow digestion to take place in the duodenum and jejunum. If the pancreas does not produce sufficient digestive enzymes, then foods will not be digested. This can lead to problems downstream. Firstly, foods may be fermented instead of being digested and this can produce the symptom of bloating due to wind, together with metabolites such as various alcohols, hydrogen sulphide and other toxic compounds. Secondly, foods are not fully broken down so that they cannot be absorbed and this can result in malabsorption. Where there is severe pancreatic dysfunction it is obvious because the stools themselves become greasy and fatty, foul smelling, bulky and difficult to flush away. Where there is malabsorption of fat, there will be malabsorption of essential fatty acids such as the omega-3 and omega-6 fatty acids, and there will be malabsorption of fat-soluble vitamins such as vitamins A, D, E and K.

If foods are poorly digested, this results in large antigenically interesting molecules appearing downstream, which alerts the immune system and could switch on allergies – that is, poor digestion of food is a risk factor for allergy.

http://drmyhill.co.uk/wiki/Pancreatic_exocrine_function

Patent foramen ovale

The idea here is that if mitochondria go really slow, the heart does not beat strongly. This can result in an opening of the foramen ovale, a hole between the left and right atria (which normally closes as a flap at birth), so blood bypasses the lungs and does not pick up oxygen as it should. This means arterial oxygen levels will drop precipitously and CFS/ME patients suddenly dive into a much worse state.

http://www.drmyhill.co.uk/wiki/Patent_foramen_ovale

Plastic rose syndrome

A man walks into an allergy clinic complaining of an allergy to roses. The doctor puts a plastic rose under his nose. The man sneezes. Is this a psychological or physical reaction? It is both. The new buzz word to explain this is 'psycho-neuro-immunology' (of the mind, the physical brain and the immune system). If you take a rat and scratch his skin, then rub in bacteria, he will develop inflammation. If you repeat this daily, he will develop inflammation every day. After several weeks of this, you just scratch the skin, but don't rub in bacteria. The rat will develop inflammation just as if bacteria had been rubbed in. The immune system has learned to expect bacteria and reacts appropriately.

http://drmyhill.co.uk/wiki/Plastic_Rose_Syndrome

Postural orthostatic tachycardia syndrome (POTs)

This is a very common problem in people with severe CFS. It means the sufferer can only stand for a short time before having to lie down. POTs is said to result from autonomic neuropathy, but my view is that this is a response to falling blood pressure, not the cause. Let me explain.

It is much easier for the heart to pump blood on the flat (lying down) than up and down hills (standing up). Indeed, we all feel more comfortable lying down or sitting rather than standing because the heart has to work less hard. In severe cases of chronic fatigue syndrome, the heart is in a low output state, perhaps so much so that it cannot pump enough blood round the body when standing. This means that when the sufferer stands, he/she can maintain blood pressure for a certain time, but then the heart muscle becomes fatigued because energy supply to the heart is impaired as a result of mitochondrial failure, so the blood pressure starts to fall. Initially the body tries to compensate by making the heart beat faster. However, this too is unsustainable and weak heart beats that are too fast result in blood pressure falling precipitously. The sufferer has to lie down quickly to avoid blacking out.

http://drmyhill.co.uk/wiki/Postural_orthostatic_tachycardia_syndrome_or_POTs

Pregnancy and CFS

As I see it, there are three issues to consider when thinking about CFS and pregnancy:

1. **Pre-conception care:** By paying attention to diet, supplements, toxic stress and hormonal imbalances, you can ensure the best possible outcome to pregnancy. Healthy babies can only be achieved through attention to the above factors and there is never a more important time in your life to be disciplined about these things than prior to pregnancy. If the problem is just CFS and nothing more (as if that were not enough!), then you should have already in place the nutritional supplements that I recommend as standard, you should be working hard at getting a good night's sleep on a regular basis, eating essentially a Paleo-ketogenic diet which is of low glycaemic index and be aware of the toxic problems which can contribute to CFS and can certainly be a problem pre-pregnancy. If the mitochondrial support regime has been started, then this should be continued unchanged throughout pregnancy. None of these supplements have any deleterious effects in pregnancy – indeed, one would expect them to improve matters!
2. **The effect of pregnancy on energy levels generally:** This I find is completely unpredictable. Some women feel at their best when they are pregnant and some at their worst. I simply have no way of predicting how any individual will react. The most important thing to bear in mind is that for those people who need thyroid supplements, their thyroid requirements

will increase during pregnancy. Since the level of thyroxine in the blood has profound effects on the developing baby, then it is essential that this is monitored closely and I recommend blood tests at least every month initially until levels are stable. Indeed, for anybody considering pregnancy, it would be a good idea to get thyroid function checked before conception.

3. **Energy requirements:** Obviously, the business of being pregnant, giving birth and caring for a new baby is going to greatly increase energy demands. It is so important to be realistic about what can and cannot be done and put plans in place for help. I have had one patient who was very severely afflicted who was able to get help from Social Services so that she could cope with her baby.

Also, be prepared to be very disciplined with the baby. Modern parents are far too indulgent. Lay down strict rules about sleep, rest and feeding regime so that you can get your break from the baby. Be very prepared to use a playpen so that you do not spend your life chasing round after the toddler and making sure that he/she does not get into trouble.

http://drmyhill.co.uk/wiki/CFS_and_Pregnancy
http://drmyhill.co.uk/wiki/What_to_do_to_ensure_a_healthy_child

Prion disorders

I think of prion disorders as protein cancers. Prions are proteins which are normally present in the body and perform essential functions. However, if they come into contact with a particular toxin or heavy metal or another twisted prion (rotten-apple effect), then they too twist and distort. When they twist in such a way that they cannot be broken down by the body enzyme systems, they cause problems because the body cannot break them down so it dumps them. Pathologically this is known as amyloid. This results in deposition of these indigestible proteins and this can be anywhere in the body.

Cancers, of course, are simply cells which replicate themselves and build up to cause problems. Viruses are strips of DNA which replicate themselves and build up in the body to cause problems. Difficulties arise when they literally get in the way of the body and stop it functioning normally. Although amyloid can occur anywhere in the body, the biggest problem is in the brain, perhaps because it is a closed box and therefore there is not any room for all this excess protein to be dumped and partly because each part of the brain is unique and any loss of function is quickly noticed. So these protein cancers tend to cause problems which may take many years to develop and so far the medical profession has no method of slowing down this process. The conditions they cause include Alzheimer's disease, Parkinson's disease, Creutzfeldt-Jacob's disease and motor neurone disease. We are currently seeing an epidemic of these conditions – the number of people suffering from them is increasing fast. Not my words but the words of Professor Colin Pritchard, Professor of Epidemiological Medicine at Southampton University. They are an inevitable part of Western lifestyles and diets high in sugar and refined carbohydrate. Indeed, Alzheimer's has been dubbed 'diabetes of the brain'.

http://www.drmyhill.co.uk/wiki/Prion_disorders

Probiotics

In a normal situation free from antiseptics, antibiotics, high-carbohydrate diets, bottle feeding, hormones and other such accoutrements of modern Western life, the gut flora is safe. Babies start life in mother's womb with a sterile gut (although interestingly there is some evidence that their gut becomes inoculated before birth through transfer of microbes across the placenta!). During the process of birth, they become inoculated with bacteria from the birth canal and perineum. These bacteria are largely bacteroides which cannot survive for more than a few minutes outside the human gut. This inoculation is enhanced through breast-feeding because the first milk, namely colostrum, is a highly desirable substrate for these bacteria to flourish. We now know that this is an essential part of immune programming. Indeed, 90 per cent of the immune system is gut associated. These essential probiotics programme the immune system so that they accept them and learn what is beneficial. A healthy gut flora therefore is highly protective against invasion of the gut by other strains of bacteria or viruses. The problem is there is no probiotic on the market that supplies bacteroides for the above reasons. If we eat probiotics which have been artificially cultured, for a short while the levels of these probiotics in the gut do increase. However, as soon as we stop eating them, levels taper off and disappear. For bacteria to be accepted into the normal gut and remain, they have to be programmed first through somebody else's gut (in this case, mother's).

So, when it comes to repleting gut flora, there are two ways that we can go about this – either we can take probiotics very regularly (and the cheapest way to do this is to grow your own probiotics) or to take bacteroides directly. Indeed, this latter technique is well established in the treatment of *Clostridium difficile* (a normally fatal gastroenteritis in humans) and interestingly in idiopathic diarrhoea in horses. In the latter case horses are inoculated with the bacteria from the gut of another horse. These ideas have been developed further by Dr Thomas Borody with his ideas on faecal bacteriotherapy, which can provide a permanent cure in cases of ulcerative colitis, severe constipation, *Clostridium difficile* infections and pseudomembranous colitis. The reason this technique works so well is because the most abundant bacteria in the large bowel, bacteroides, cannot survive outside the human gut and cannot be given by any other route. The gut flora is extremely stable and difficult to change. Therefore if you are going to take probiotics, you have to be prepared to take them long term. Many preparations on the market are ineffective. Those found to be most effective are those milk ferments and live yoghurts where the product is freshly made. It is not really surprising. Keeping bacteria alive is difficult and it is not surprising that they do not survive dehydration and storage at room temperature. So your best chance of eating live viable bacteria is to buy live yoghurts or drinks. These can be easily grown at home, just as one would make home-made yoghurt. If you cannot grow easily from a culture, then it suggests that the culture is not active, so this is a good test of what is and is not viable. I have tried to culture on milk and soya from dried extracts with very poor success rates – suggesting that the dried extracts are not terribly viable.

The use of probiotics is already established practice in animal welfare and probiotics are actively marketed to the horse industry for this very reason. Furthermore, probiotics are routinely used in the pig industry to prevent post-weaning diarrhoea. Anyone who has to take antibiotics for any reason should take these cultures as a routine to prevent 'super-infection' with undesirable bugs. These cultures are also an essential part of re-colonising the gut following gut eradication therapy.

http://drmyhill.co.uk/wiki/Probiotics

Retroviruses

Retroviruses are composed of RNA rather than DNA. They have an enzyme, called reverse transcriptase, that gives them the unique property of transcribing their RNA into DNA after entering a cell. The retroviral DNA can then integrate into the chromosomal DNA of the host cell, to be expressed there. So, a retrovirus enters a host cell as RNA and then transcribes into DNA once inside the cell and then integrates into the host's DNA. In order to make this transcribing possible, the exact sequence of a retrovirus's RNA changes often. This makes it harder for retroviruses to be attacked by drugs.

Superoxide dismutase (SODase)

SODase is one of the most important antioxidant enzymes which mop up free radicals. It is the most important superoxide scavenger in muscles. Deficiency can explain muscle pain and easy fatiguability in some patients. Normal levels of SODase are dependent on good levels of copper, manganese and zinc.

http://www.drmyhill.co.uk/wiki/SODase_(superoxide_dismutase)_studies

Syndrome X

A pre-diabetic state, also known as 'metabolic syndrome', when blood sugar levels see-saw between too high and too low in the presence of excessively high levels of insulin. See Hypoglycaemia, page 361.

Toxins

Modern Western lifestyles mean we are inevitably exposed to chemicals. See my website for a checklist of toxins and their sources:

http://drmyhill.co.uk/wiki/Chemical_poisons_and_toxins

Transdermal micronutrients

I see many patients for whom we know what the micronutrient deficiency is that causes their problem, but giving those micronutrients by mouth does not help, or indeed makes them worse. What I suspect is getting in the way is the gut. For micronutrients to get into the body to do good they must first get there! To achieve this we need the ability to digest and absorb them and the energy to do this. I suspect the latter is a problem for many of my severe CFS patients. Food allergy, the fermenting gut and poor stomach, liver and pancreatic function may all be problems. This may explain why so many of my sick patients do well on injections of micronutrients. To get round this problem I have put together some transdermal preparations to be sprayed onto the skin. A key ingredient is DMSO – this passes through skin like a knife through butter and carries through everything dissolved within it. DMSO is a naturally occurring organic sulphur-containing molecule, derived from tree bark and closely related to MSM (a useful treatment for arthritis).

The early clinical feedback has been most encouraging. However, once on the Paleo-ketogenic diet the need for transdermal minerals goes away as the fermenting microbes are starved out.

http://drmyhill.co.uk/wiki/Transdermal_micronutrients

Vitamin D and sunshine

Western cultures have become almost phobic about any exposure of unprotected skin to sunshine with the well-recognised association between skin cancer and exposure to sunshine. Indeed, the US Environmental Protection Agency is currently advising that ultraviolet light, and therefore sunlight, is so dangerous that we should 'protect ourselves against ultraviolet light whenever we can see our shadow'. However, a certain amount of sun exposure is essential for normal good health in order to produce vitamin D – and partly as a result of current recommendations, we are seeing declining levels of vitamin D and a rise in the problems that go with its deficiency.

Human beings evolved over hundreds of thousands of years in equatorial areas and were daily exposed to sunshine. Dark skins evolved to protect against sun damage. However, as hominids migrated north, those races which retained their dark skins were unable to make sufficient vitamin D in the skin and did not survive. Only those hominids with paler skins survived. Thus the further away from the Equator, the paler the skin became. Races in Polar areas survived because they were able to get an alternative source of vitamin D from fish and seafood.

There is an interesting inverse correlation between sunshine exposure, vitamin D levels, and incidence of disease as one moves away from the Equator. Even correcting for other factors such as diet, there is strong evidence to show that vitamin D protects against osteoarthritis, osteoporosis, bone fractures (vitamin D strengthens the muscles thereby improving balance and movement and preventing falls), cancer, hypertension, hypercholesterolaemia, diabetes, heart disease, multiple sclerosis and vulnerability to infections. Multiple sclerosis is a particularly interesting example of a possible vitamin D deficiency disease. Indeed, mice bred for susceptibility to multiple sclerosis can be completely protected against development of this disease by feeding them high doses of vitamin D.

http://drmyhill.co.uk/wiki/Vitamin_D_and_Sunshine

Yeast problems and candida

Yeast problems are a problem of Western lifestyles. They are triggered by high carbohydrate diets, antibiotics (which kill the good gut bugs and allow yeast to flourish) and the Pill or HRT (immunosuppressive). It is often a combination of these factors. The underlying problems include:

1. Yeast overgrowth in the gut – gut flora contains 1 per cent yeast so some yeasts are normally present in the gut. Problems seem to arise either when

they flourish in the wrong place (i.e. the upper gut – which should be sterilised by stomach acid) or there is a general overgrowth of them. Wherever numbers build up, one starts to ferment foods instead of digesting them. Fermentation causes symptoms of bloating and bubbling in the gut; sometimes this is very obvious. If fermentation occurs within minutes of eating, it is occurring in the stomach.

2. Alcohol production – yeasts ferment sugars to alcohol and this causes problems in its own right. The main one is that it tends to lower the blood sugar level, thereby destabilising levels and making the sufferer crave sugars. This is a very clever evolutionary ploy that yeasts have stumbled upon to make their host eat the very foods that the yeast wants! So sufferers often crave carbohydrates and sugars, but the more they eat, the worse they become.
3. Allergy to yeast – if the levels of yeast build up in the gut then they can switch the immune system on so that one gets allergy reactions against the yeast. This can cause low grade inflammation of the gut. Low grade inflammation will result in leaky gut. Leaky upper gut causes hypochlorhydria (see page 360) and all the problems that go with that.
4. Leaky gut – an overgrowth of the yeast in the gut can cause leaky gut (page 364). What this means in practice is that large antigenically interesting molecules get from the gut into the bloodstream where they should not be. This may elicit an immune response, which could switch on an allergy to that substance (food allergy), or, worse, an antibody could be formed which cross-reacts with the body and switches on autoimmunity.
5. Yeast cells are tiny compared to human cells and where there is leaky gut they can leak out into the bloodstream to cause allergy reactions. Eventually these yeast cells spill over into the kidneys and the urine and can be a major cause of irritable bladder syndrome or allergic bladder or allergic perineum (vulval irritation).
6. Yeast problems which become more systemic may result in yeast infections such as thrush, nail infections, tinea corporis, athlete's foot and so on.
7. If we switch on yeast sensitivity in the gut, this can cause cross-sensitivity to moulds and yeasts in the environment. This may explain why some people do not feel so well on damp days and feel very much better in hot, dry or cold, dry climates. They have become allergic to environmental moulds.

http://drmyhill.co.uk/wiki/Yeast_problems_and_candida

Tests that can be ordered from www.drmyhill.co.uk

Adrenal stress profile
Antioxidant status
Calcium studies
Carbonic anhydrase in red blood cells
Cardiolipin studies
Comprehensive digestive stool analysis
DNA adducts
Fat biopsy for toxins
Fructose investigations:
- Fructose-6-phosphate
- LDH iso-enzyme (indicative of liver damage)
- Short-chain fatty acids

Lactate dehydrogenase studies
Melatonin levels
Microrespirometry studies
Mitochondrial function profile combining the following tests:
- ATP profiles
- Coenzyme Q10
- Glutathione and glutathione peroxidase studies
- Plasma cell-free DNA
- Red cell NAD
- Serum L-carnitine
- Superoxide dismutase (SODase)

Salivary VEGF test
Short-chain polypeptides
Thyroid function profile – free T3, free T4, TSH
Translocator protein studies

Recommended products and suppliers

Biolab Medical Unit London England

A nutritional biochemistry medical laboratory measuring trace metals/ minerals, vitamins and toxins.

Website: www.biolab.co.uk

Bonematters

Heel bone density scan – which can be done using ultrasound – is very reliable, involves no radiation, and can be followed up within a few months to ensure progress.

Website: bonematters.org

Calibre – The Cassette Library

A registered charity providing tapes of books to the print disabled. The service is free, the voice on the end of the phone extremely friendly.

Tel: +44 (0)1296 432 339

Chloramine Information Center

For information about the effects of chloramine (a compound of chlorine and ammonia used in water purification) and how to protect against them.

Website: chloramineinfocenter.com

Detect & Protect

For the detection of electrosmog (invisible electromagnetic radiation).

Website: www.detect-protect.com/k/buzz/whatiselectrosmog.htm

Earthing

For products that connect to Earth's natural energy.

Website: www.earthing.com

Electric Forester Investigations

Electromagnetic surveys and investigations.

Website: www.electricforester.co.uk/electricforester/index.html

ElectroSensitivity UK

This is a registered charity (reg number 1103018).

Address: BM BOX ES-UK, London WC1N 3XX
Tel: +44 (0)845 643 9748 – freely available UK helpline staffed by volunteers
Website: www.es-uk.info

Friends of the Earth
Website: www.foe.co.uk

Garden Organic
Formerly known as Henry Doubleday Research Association, advice on how to garden organically whether your garden is large or small.
Website: www.gardenorganic.org.uk

Gluten-Free Society
For information about the effects of gluten on human health, tools to test for sensitivity and guidance on a gluten-free lifestyle.
Website: www.glutenfreesociety.org/gluten-and-the-autoimmune-disease-spectrum

Great Plains Laboratory, Inc.
A world leader in providing testing for metabolic, genetic, mitochondrial and environmental factors in chronic illness.
Website: www.greatplainslaboratory.com

The Healthy House
For an excellent range of products to help you detox your house including EMF detectors (just search for 'electrosmog detector' in their search box).
Tel: +44 (0)845 450 5950
Tel. from a mobile phone: +44 (0)1453 752216
Website: www.healthy-house.co.uk

MicroCell Essential Fatty Acids (on BioCare)
An omega-3 and omega-6 supplement for vegetarians, combining linseed and borage oils.
Website: www.biocare.co.uk/microcellr-essential-fatty-acids

Natural Health Worldwide
A website where any knowledgeable practitioner (experienced patient, health professional or doctor) can offer his/her opinion to any patient. This

opinion may be free, or for a fee, by telephone, email, or Skype. The practitioner needs no premises or support staff since bookings and payments are made online. Patients give feedback to that practitioner's Reputation page and star ratings evolve.
Website: www.naturalhealthworldwide.com

Powerwatch
A source of information about EMF issues.
Website: www.powerwatch.org.uk
Products website: www.emfields-solutions.com

SaferWave
Information on EMF for radiation emission.
Website: www.saferwave.com

Soil Association
For information about what the standards are to be classed as 'organic' in the UK.
Website: www.soilassociation.org

Tempur Mattresses and Pillows
Email: customerservice@tempur.co.uk
Tel: +44(0)800 0111 083
Website: uk.tempur.com

VegEpa (from Igennus)
Concentrated EPA supplement in a fish-gel capsule.
Email: sales@igennus.com
Tel: +44 (0) 845 13 00 424 or +44 (0) 845 13 00 424
Website: www.igennus.com

REFERENCES

Chapter 1: Why is CFS/ME the Worst-treated condition in Western Medicine?

1. White PD, Goldsmith KA, Johnson AL, et al. Comparison of adaptive pacing therapy, cognitive behaviour therapy, graded exercise therapy, and specialist medical care for chronic fatigue syndrome (PACE): a randomised trial. *The Lancet* 5 March 2011; 377(9768): 823-836. doi:10.1016/S0140-6736(11)60096-2
2. Courtney M. PACE Trial: Recovery rates and positive outcome rates. (Freedom of Information Request to Queen Mary, University of London, UK) What Do They Know. 26 October 2012. https://www.whatdotheyknow.com/request/pace_trial_recovery_rates_and_po (Accessed 28 September 2016)
3. ICO (Information Commissioner's Office). Freedom of Information Act 2000 (FOIA) Decision Notice Reference FS50565190. 27 October 2015. https://ico.org.uk/media/action-weve-taken/decision-notices/2015/1560081/fs_50565190.pdf (Accessed 28 September 2016)
4. First-Tier Tribunal, General Regulatory Chamber: Information Rights. Appeal Number EA/2015/0269. Queen Mary University of London v. The Information Commissioner. http://informationrights.decisions.tribunals.gov.uk/DBFiles/Decision/i1854/Queen%20Mary%20University%20of%20London%20EA-2015-0269%20(12-8-16).PDF (Accessed 13 October 2016)
5. McCrone P, Sharpe M, Chalder T, et al. Adaptive pacing, cognitive behaviour therapy, graded exercise and specialist medical care for chronic fatigue. *PLOS ONE* 1 August 2012; 7 (8): e40808. doi:10.1371/journal.pone.0040808
6. Tuller D. Trial by error: the troubling case of the PACE chronic fatigue syndrome study. *Virology Blog* 21 October 2015. http:// www.virology.ws/2015/10/21/trial-by-error-i (Accessed 28 September 2016)
7. Hooper M. *Magical Medicine: how to make an illness disappear*. February 2010. http://www.meactionuk.org.uk/magical-medicine.pdf (Accessed 28 September 2016)
8. Goldin R. PACE: the research that sparked a patient rebellion and challenged medicine. Sense about Science USA 21 March 2016. http://

senseaboutscienceusa.org/pace-research-sparked-patient-rebellion-challenged-medicine/ (Accessed 28 September 2016)

9. Matthees A, Kindlon T, Maryhew C, Stark P, Levin B. A preliminary analysis of 'recovery' from chronic fatigue syndrome in the PACE trial using individual participant data. *Virology Blog* 21 September 2016. http://www.virology.ws/wp-content/uploads/2016/09/preliminary-analysis.pdf (Accessed 13 October 2016)
10. Kindlon T. Reporting of harms associated with graded exercise therapy and cognitive behaviour therapy in myalgic encephalomyelitis/chronic fatigue syndrome. *Bulletin of the IACFS/ME* 2011; 19(2): 59–111. http://www.ncf-net.org/library/Reporting%20of%20Harms.pdf (Accessed 29 September 2016)
11. Grady D, Klimas NG. Readers ask: a virus linked to chronic fatigue syndrome. *New York Times* 15 October 2009. http://consults.blogs.nytimes.com/2009/10/15/readers-ask-a-virus-linked-to-chronic-fatigue-syndrome (Accessed 28 September 2016)

Chapter 3: The clinical picture of CFS/ME

12. Heckenlively K, Mikovits J. *Plague: one scientist's intrepid search for the truth about human retroviruses and chronic fatigue syndrome (ME/CFS), autism, and other diseases.* New York: Skyhorse Publishing, 2014.
13. Agence France-Presse. French court awards woman disability grant for 'allergy to gadgets'. *The Guardian* 27 August 2015. http://www.theguardian.com/world/2015/aug/27/french-court-awards-woman-disability-grant-for-allergy-to-gadgets
14. Hyde B. *Missed Diagnoses: myaglic encephalomyelitis & chronic fatigue syndrome, 2nd edition*. lulu.com 2011
15. Ravera S, Panfoli I, Calzia D, et al. Evidence for aerobic ATP synthesis in isolated myelin vesicles. *International Journal of Biochemistry & Cell Biology* January 2009; 41(7): 1581–91. doi:10.1016/j.biocel.2009.01.009
16. Fisher GC, Cheney P. *Chronic Fatigue Syndrome: a comprehensive guide to symptoms, treatments, and solving the practical problems of CFS.* New York: Warner Books, 1997.
17. Mansfield J. *Arthritis: allergy, nutrition and the environment*. London: Thorsons, 1990.

Chapter 4: The mechanisms of energy delivery in the body

18. Peckerman A, LacManca JJ, Dahl KA, et al. Abnormal impedance cardiography predicts symptom severity in chronic fatigue syndrome. *The American Journal of the Medical Sciences* August 2003; 326(2): 55–60.

19. Myhill S, Booth NE, McLaren-Howard J. Chronic fatigue syndrome and mitochondrial dysfunction. *International Journal of Clinical and Experimental Medicine* 2009; 2: 1–16. http://www.ijcem.com/files/IJCEM812001.pdf
20. Booth NE, Myhill S, McLaren-Howard J. Mitochondrial dysfunction and the pathophysiology of myalgic encephalomyelitis/chronic fatigue syndrome (ME/CFS). *International Journal of Clinical and Experimental Medicine* 2012; 5(3): 208–220. http://www.ijcem.com/files/IJCEM1204005.pdf
21. Myhill S, Booth NE, McLaren-Howard J. Targeting mitochondrial dysfunction in the treatment of myalgic encephalomyelitis/chronic fatigue syndrome (ME/CFS) – a clinical audit. *International Journal of Clinical and Experimental Medicine* 2013; 6(1): 1–15. http://www.ijcem.com/files/IJCEM1207003.pdf
22. Lengert N, Drossel B. In silico analysis of exercise intolerance in myalgic chronic fatigue syndrome. *Biophysical Chemistry Encephalomyelitis* July 2015; 202: 21–31. doi:10.1016/j.bpc.2015.03.009
23. Dykens JA. Drug-induced mitochondrial dysfunction: an emerging model for idiosyncratic drug toxicity. Pfizer Drug Safety Research & Development 2007. http://www.mitoaction.org/files/Dykens%20for%20Mitoaction.pdf (Accessed 28 September 2016); Dykens JA, Marroquin LD, Will Y. Strategies to reduce late-stage drug attrition due to mitochondrial toxicity. *Expert Review of Molecular Diagnostics* 2007; 7(2): 161-175.

Chapter 5: Energy delivery mechanisms

24. Toft AD. *Understanding Thyroid Disorders*. British Medical Association: Family Doctor Publications Ltd. First edition 1999; Revised edition 2000; Second edition 2008.
25. Koulouri O, Moran C, Halsall D, Chatterjee K, Gurnell M. Pitfalls in the measurement and interpretation of thyroid function tests. *Best Practices and Research: Clinical Endocrinology and Metabolism* December 2013; 27 (6): 745–62. doi:10.1016/j.beem.2013.10.003
26. Robinson P. *Recovering with T3: my journey from hypothyroidism to good health using the T3 thyroid hormone*. Elephant in the Room Books, 2013.

Chapter 7: The fermenting gut

27. Pond CM. *The Fats of Life*. New York: Cambridge University Press, 1998.
28. Nishihara K. Disclosure of the major causes of mental illness – mitochondrial deterioration in brain neurons via opportunistic infection. *Journal of Biological Physics and Chemistry* March 2012; 12: 11–18. doi:10.4024/38NI11A.jbpc.12.01

29. Meirleir K de, Roelant C, Fremont M, Metzger K, Butt HL. Research on extremely disabled ME patients reveals the true nature of the disorder.

Chapter 9: Inflammation: the general approach

30. Elia M. Organ and tissue contribution to metabolic rate. In: Kinney JM, Tucker HN, editors. *Energy Metabolism: tissue determinants and cellular corollaries*. New York: Raven Press; 1992. pp. 61–79.
31. Buttgereit FI, Burmester GR, Brand MD. Bioenergetics of immune functions: fundamental and therapeutic aspects. *Immunology Today* April 2000; 21(4): 192–99.
32. Berg RD. Bacterial translocation from the gastrointestinal tract. *Advances in Experimental Medicine and Biology* 1999; 473: 11–30.
33. Zimmer C. Our inner viruses: forty million years in the making. The Loom, National Geographic 1 Feb 2015. http://phenomena.nationalgeographic.com/2015/02/01/our-inner-viruses-forty-million-years-in-the-making (Accessed 28 September 2016)
34. Heckenlively K, Mikovits J. *Plague: one scientist's intrepid search for the truth about human retroviruses and chronic fatigue syndrome (ME/CFS), autism, and other diseases*. New York: Skyhorse Publishing, 2014.
35. Nathan CF. Macrophages, dendritic cells and pathogens. Weill Medical College of Cornell University. http://grantome.com/grant/NIH/P01-AI056293-04. Nathan CF. From transient infection to chronic illness'. Science 9 October 2015; 350(6257): 161. http://science.sciencemag.org/content/350/6257/161.figures-only (there is a paywall here)
36. Pall ML. Electromagnetic fields act via activation of voltage-gated calcium channels to produce benficial and adverse effects. *Journal of Cellular and Molecular Medicine* August 2013; 17(8): 958–65. doi:10.1111/jcmm.12088

Chapter 10: Inflammation: allergy and autoimmunity

37. WebMD. Asthma Health Centre: Asthma and sulfite allergies. http://www.webmd.com/asthma/asthma-and-sulfites-allergies (Accessed 27 September 2016)
38. Mansfield J. *The Six Secrets of Successful Weight Loss*. London: Hammersmith Health, 2012.
39. Ashford, N, Miller C. *Chemical Exposures: low levels and high stakes*. New York: John Wiley & Sons, 1998.
40. Agence France-Presse. French court awards woman disability grant for 'allergy to gadgets'. *The Guardian* 27 August 2015. http://www.theguardian

.com/world/2015/aug/27/french-court-awards-woman-disability-grant-for-allergy-to-gadgets

Chapter 11: Inflammation: chronic infections–Viral

41. Kingsley P. *The New Medicine: a modern approach to clinical illness*. Morley: SureScreen Life Sciences, 2013.
42. Abelin M. Treatment of herpes simplex with shock doses of vitamin B12 (Cycobemin) and Iloban. Svenska Lakartidningen 1961; 58: 1984–90. (Article in Swedish.)
43. Hawkes CH, Giovannoni G, Keir G, Cunnington M, Thompson EJ. Seroprevalence of herpes simplex virus type 2 in multiple sclerosis. *Acta Neurologica Scandinavica* December 2006; 114(6): 363–67. doi:10.1111/j.1600-0404.2006.00677.x
44. Alibek K, Baiken Y, Kakpenova A, et al. Implication of human herpesviruses in oncogenesis through immune evasion and suppression. *Infectious Agents and Cancer* 2014; 9: 3. doi:10.1186/1750-9378-9-3

Chapter 12: Inflammation: chronic infections–Bacterial

45. MacDonald AB. Alzheimer Borreliosis – My journal articles. http://alzheimerborreliosis.net/research (Accessed 28 September 2016)
46. ArminLabs – diagnosing tick-borne diseases. Our diagnostic tests. http://www.arminlabs.com/en/tests (Accessed 28 September 2016)
47. EliSpot. Applications in diagnosis and research & literature. http://www.elispot.com/ (Accessed 28 September 2016)
48. Theophilus PAS, Victoria MJ, Socarras KM, et al. Effectiveness of *Stevia redaudiana* whole leaf extract against the various morphological forms of *Borrelia burgdorferi* in vitro. *European Journal of Microbiology and Immunology* 2015 5(4): 268–80. doi:10.1556/1886.2015.00031

Chapter 13: Reprogramming the immune system

49. Anagnostou K, Islam S, King Y, et al. Assessing the efficacy of oral immunotherapy for the desensitisation of peanut allergy in children (STOP II): a phase 2 randomised controlled trial. *The Lancet* 12 April 2014; 383(9925): 1297–304. doi:10.1016/S0140-6736(13)62301-6
50. Tang MLK, Ponsonby A-L, Orsini F, et al. Administration of a probiotic with peanut oral immunotherapy: a randomized trial. *The Journal of Allergy and Clinical Immunology* March 2015; 135(3): 737–44. doi:10.1016/j.jaci.2014.11.034

Chapter 16: Sleep

51. Blanchard KR, Adams-Brill M. *What Your Doctor May Not Tell about Hypothryroidism: a simple plan for extraordinary results*. New York: Grand Central Publishing, 2004.
52. Richardson BA. Cot mattress biodeterioration and SIDS. *The Lancet* 17 March 1990; 335 (8690): 670 doi:10.1016/0140-6736(90)90463-F; Richardson BA. Sudden infant death syndrome: a possible primary cause. *Journal of the Forensic Science Society* July–September 1994; 34(3): 199–204.
53. Rechtschaffen A, Bergmann BM, Everson CA, Kushida CA, Gilliland MA. Sleep deprivation in the rat: X. integration and discussion of the findings. *Sleep* February 1989; 12(1):68–87; Rechtschaffen A, Bergmann BM. Sleep deprivation in the rat: an update of the 1989 paper. *Sleep* 1 February 2002; 25(1): 18–24.
54. Newsham GR, Aries MBC, Mancini S, Faye G. Individual control of electric lighting in a daylit space. *Lighting Research and Technology* 2008; 40(1): 25–41. doi:10.1177/1477153507081560
55. Shastri A, Bangar S, Holmes J. Obstructive sleep apnoea and dementia: is there a link? *International Journal of Geriatric Psychiatry* April 2016; 31(4): 400–05. doi:10.1002/gps.4345.

Chapter 17: The Paleo-ketogenic diet

56. Sharkey L. Revealed: Nike's 'Just Do It' slogan was inspired by a convicted killer's last words. *Independent* 18 March 2015. http://www.independent.co.uk/life-style/fashion/news/nike-s-just-do-it-slogan-was-inspired-by-a-convicted-killer-s-last-words-10117596.html

Chapter 20: Detoxing

57. Kane E, Kane P. Phosphatidylcholine: life's designer molecule. *BodyBio Bulletin* 2005 http://www.bodybio.com/BodyBio/docs/BodyBio Bulletin-Phosphatidylcholine.pdf (Accessed 28 September 2016)
58. Waring RH. Report on absorption of magnesium sulfate (Epsom salts) across the skin. http://www.epsomsaltcouncil.org/wp-content/uploads/2015/10/report_on_absorption_of_magnesium_sulfate.pdf (Accessed 28 September 2016)

Chapter 21: The emotional hole in the energy bucket

59. Colby J. False allegations of child abuse in cases of childhood myalgic encephalomyelitis (ME): Argument and Critique. July 2014. http://www

.doctormyhill.co.uk/drmyhill/images/6/65/False_Allegations_of_Child_Abuse_in_Childhood_ME_-_Jane_Colby.pdf (Accessed 28 September 2016)

60. Kindel MA. Three ways to help Karina Hansen – ME hostage in Denmark. ME Advocacy 19 October 2015. http://www.meadvocacy.org/3_ways_to_help_karina_hansen_me_hostage_in_denmark (Accessed 28 September 2016)
61. Gallagher P. Mother cleared of poisoning teenager daughter with hormones supplied by Belgian doctor says case should be landmark for patents' rights. *Independent* 30 October 2014. http://www.independent.co.uk/news/uk/crime/mother-cleared-of-poisoning-teenager-daughter-with-hormones-supplied-by-belgian-doctor-9829226.html (Accessed 28 September 2016)
62. Davies J. *Cracked: why psychiatry is doing more harm than good*. London: Icon Books, 2014.
63. American Psychiatry Association. *Diagnostic and Statistical Manual of Mental Disorders: DSM-5*. Londres: American Psychiatric Publishing, 2013.
64. Green B, Bruce M-A, Finn P, et al. Independent review of deaths of people with a learning disability or mental health problem in contact with Southern Health NHS Foundation Trust April 2011 to March 2015. Mazars, December 2015 https://www.england.nhs.uk/south/wp-content/uploads/sites/6/2015/12/mazars-rep.pdf (Accessed 28 September 2016)

Chapter 22: Reprogramming the brain

65. Kaiser JD. Combining the best of natural and standard therapies. www.jonkaiser.com (Accessed 28 September 2016); K-PAX Pharmaceuticals. The Synergy Trial: methylphenidate plus a CFS-specific nutrient formula as a treatment for chronic fatigue syndrome. Clinical Trials.gov September 2014. https://clinicaltrials.gov/ct2/show/study/NCT01966276 (Accessed 28 September 2016)

Chapter 23: Common associated problems

66. Michaëlsson K, Wolk A, Langenskiöld S, et al. Milk intake and risk of mortality and fractures in women and men: cohort studies. *BMJ* 2014; 349: g6015. doi:10.1136/bmj.g6015
67. Kennel KA, Drake MT. Adverse effects of bisphosphonates: implications for osteoporosis management. *Mayo Clinics Proceedings* July 2009; 84(7): 632–38. doi:10.1016/S0025-6196(11)60752-0

Appendix 1

68. Koulouri O, Moran C, Halsall D, Chatterjee K, Gurnell M. Pitfalls in the measurement and interpretation of thyroid function tests. *Best Practice and Research: Clinical Endocrinology and Metabolism* December 2013; 27(6): 745–62. doi:10.1016/j.beem.2013.10.003

Appendix 4

69. Lascaratos JG, Marketos SG. The carbon monoxide poisoning of two Byzantine emperors. *Journal of Toxicology: Clinical Toxicology* 1998; 36(1–2): 103–07.

Appendix 5

70. Baillie-Hamilton P. *The Detox Diet: eliminate chemical calories and restore your body's natural slimming system* London: Michael Joseph, 2002.
71. Food Standards Agency UK. The Natural Mineral Water, Spring Water and Bottled Drinking Water (England) Regulations 2007 (as ameneded). July 2010. http://www.food.gov.uk/sites/default/files/multimedia/pdfs/waterguideeng07updated.pdf (Accessed 28 September 2016)
72. Sarantis H, Naidenko OV, Gray S, Houlihan J, Malkan S. Not so sexy: the health risks of secret chemicals in fragrance. 12 May 2010. Breast Cancer Fund, Commonweal and Environmental Working Group. http://www.ewg.org/sites/default/files/report/SafeCosmetics_FragranceRpt.pdf (Accessed 28 September 2016)

Appendix 6

73. Lerner AM, Beqaj SH, Gill K, et al. An update on the management of glandular fever (infectious mononucleosis) and its sequelae caused by Epstein-Barr virus (HHV-4): new and emerging treatment strategies. *Virus Adaptation and Treatment* 23 September 2010; (2): 135–45.
74. Lerner AM, Beqaj SH, Deeter RG, et al. A six-month trial of valacyclovir in the Epstein-Barr virus subset of chronic fatigue syndrome: improvement in left ventricular function. *Drugs of Today* August 2002; 38(8): 549–61.
75. Lerner AM, Zervos M, Chang CH, et al. A small, randomized, placebo-controlled trial of the use of antiviral therapy for patients with chronic fatigue syndrome. *Clinical Infectious Diseases* 1 June 2001; 32(11): 1657–58. doi:10.1086/320530
76. Lerner AM, Beqaj SH, Deeter RG, Fitzgerald JT. Valacyclovir treatment in Epstein-Barr virus subset chronic fatigue syndrome: thirty-six months follow-up. *In Vivo* September/October 2007; 21(5): 707–13.

77. Lerner AM, Beqaj S, Fitzgerald JT, et al. Subset-directed antiviral treatment of 142 herpesvirus patients with chronic fatigue syndrome. *Virus Adaptation and Treatment* 24 May 2010; 2010(2): 47–52. doi:10.2147/VAAT.S10695.

INDEX

ABOUT THE AUTHOR AND EDITOR

Dr Sarah Myhill MB BS, the author, qualified in medicine (with Honours) from Middlesex Hospital Medical School in 1981 and has since focused tirelessly on identifying and treating the underlying causes of health problems, especially the 'diseases of civilisation' with which we are beset in the West. She has worked in the National Health Service and private practice and for 17 years was the Hon. Secretary of the British Society for Ecological Medicine, which focuses on the causes of disease and treating through diet, supplements and avoiding toxic stress. She helps to run, and lectures at, the Society's training courses and also lectures regularly on organophosphate poisoning, the problems of silicone, and chronic fatigue syndrome. Visit her website at www.drmyhill.co.uk

Craig Robinson MA, the editor, took a first in Mathematics at Oxford University in 1985. He then joined Price Waterhouse and qualified as a Chartered Accountant in 1988, after which he worked as a lecturer in the private sector, and also in the City of London, primarily in Financial Sector Regulation roles. Craig first met Sarah in 2001, as a patient for the treatment of his CFS, and since then they have developed a professional working relationship, where he helps with the maintenance of www.drmyhill.co.uk, the moderating of Dr Myhill's Facebook groups and other ad hoc projects, as well as with the editing and writing of her books.

the politics and practice of sustainable living

CHELSEA GREEN PUBLISHING

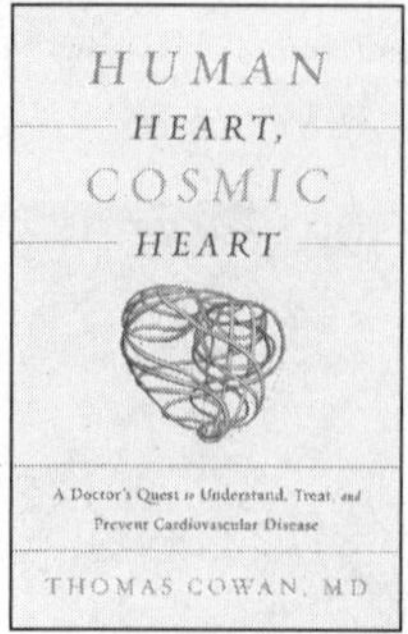

HUMAN HEART, COSMIC HEART
A Doctor's Quest to Understand, Treat, and Prevent Cardiovascular Disease
THOMAS COWAN, MD
9781603586191
Hardcover • $24.95

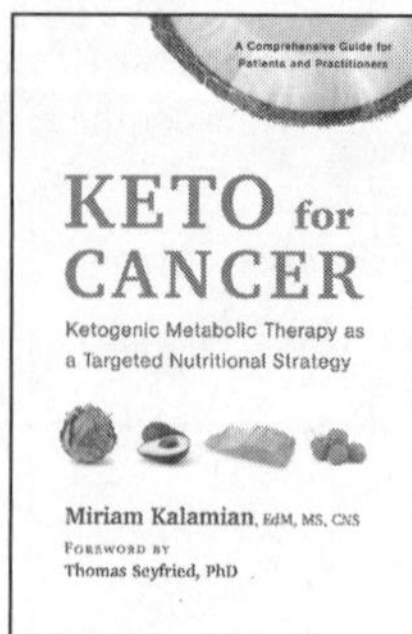

KETO FOR CANCER
Ketogenic Metabolic Therapy as a Targeted Nutritional Strategy
MIRIAM KALAMIAN, EdM, MS, CNS
9781603587013
Paperback • $29.95

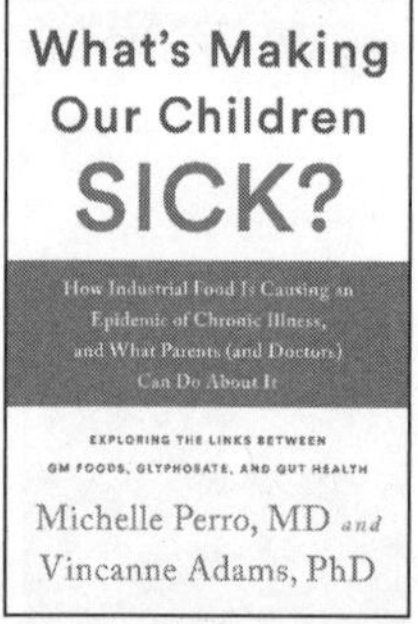

WHAT'S MAKING OUR CHILDREN SICK?
How Industrial Food Is Causing an Epidemic of Chronic Illness, and What Parents (and Doctors) Can Do About It
MICHELLE PERRO, MD
and VINCANNE ADAMS, PhD
9781603587570
Paperback • $24.95

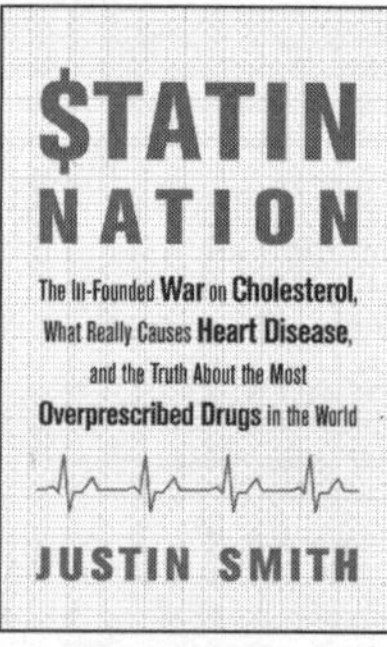

STATIN NATION
The Ill-Founded War on Cholesterol, What Really Causes Heart Disease, and the Truth About the Most Overprescribed Drugs in the World
JUSTIN SMITH
9781603587532
Paperback • $19.95

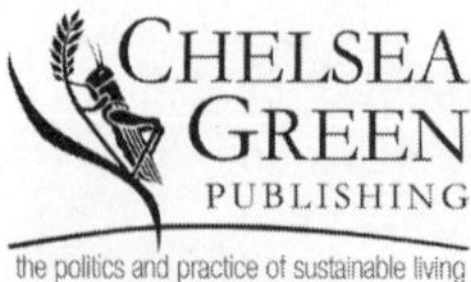

For more information or to request a catalog,
visit **www.chelseagreen.com** or
call toll-free **(800) 639-4099**.